HISTORY OF MEDICINE

A Scandalously Short Introduction

Jacalyn Duffin's *History of Medicine* provides a brief survey of the history of Western medicine with reference to recent scholarly literature and current issues in health care. Organized conceptually around the major fields of medical endeavour – anatomy, physiology, pathology, pharmacology, surgery, obstetrics, psychiatry, pediatrics, and family medicine – this book provides an accessible overview of medical history as a vibrant component of social, intellectual, and cultural history, and as a research discipline in its own right.

Each chapter begins in antiquity and ends in the twentieth century. Throughout, Duffin shows that alternative interpretations can be found for most elements of our past and that topics of interest can go well beyond 'great men' and 'great discoveries' to include ideas, diseases, patients, institutions, and great mistakes. This approach does not mean that the 'great men' and women are neglected; rather, they appear in context. Medical disasters, such as chloramphenicol and thalidomide, are covered along with the triumphs, and examples from Canada's past, largely ignored in other medical histories, are included. A chapter on methodology, suggestions for further reading with special attention to Canadian sources, and a careful index make it possible to research a specific event or historical debate, or to satisfy a more general curiosity.

By presenting the material in a structure that resonates with the broad outlines of medical training, and by focusing on the questions asked most often, this text is a relevant guide for students to the history of the profession they are about to embrace, and for those who would teach them, be they physicians or historians. Duffin's clear and entertaining prose and the many illustrations will help to demystify medicine for general readers and for students in other domains, such as history, philosophy, and sociology.

Jacalyn Duffin, MD, FRCP(C), PhD, is a historian and a practising hematologist. She is the author of two other books, *Langstaff: A Nineteenth-Century Medical Life* (1993) and *To See with a Better Eye: A Life of R.T.H. Laennec* (1998), and many journal articles on the history of medical practice, iconography, and disease. Since 1988 she has been the Jason A. Hannah Professor of the History of Medicine at Queen's University, where she teaches in medicine, philosophy, history, and law.

HISTORY OF MEDICINE

*A Scandalously
Short Introduction*

Jacalyn Duffin

UNIVERSITY OF TORONTO PRESS
Toronto Buffalo

Printed in Canada

Reprinted 2000

ISBN 0-8020-0949-2 (cloth)
ISBN 0-8020-7912-1 (paper)

∞

Printed on acid-free paper

Canadian Cataloguing in Publication Data

Duffin, Jacalyn
    History of medicine : a scandalously short introduction

    Includes bibliographical references and index.
    ISBN 0-8020-0949-2 (bound)   ISBN 0-8020-7912-1 (pbk.)

    1. Medicine – History.   I. Title.

    R131.D83 1999   610′.9   C99-930685-5

Excerpts of material written by L.M. Montgomery are published with the permission of David Macdonald and Ruth Macdonald, who are the heirs of L.M. Montgomery.

University of Toronto Press acknowledges the financial assistance to its publishing program of the Canada Council for the Arts and the Ontario Arts Council.

University of Toronto Press acknowledges the financial support for its publishing activities of the Government of Canada through the Book Publishing Industry Development Program (BPIDP).

Canadä

For my students,
past, present, and future,
with thanks

Doc, I have an earache.

2000 B.C.   Here, eat this root.

1000 B.C.   That root is heathen, say this prayer.

1850 A.D.   Prayer is superstition, drink this potion.

1930   That potion is snake oil, swallow this pill.

1970   That pill is ineffective, take this antibiotic.

2000   That antibiotic is artificial, here, eat this root.

Anon, 'History of Medicine,' circulating on the Internet 1997–8

Contents

Illustrations

Tables

Acknowledgments

Historical ideas, like disease ideas, can be both hereditary and communicable. In these pages my mentor, Mirko Grmek of Paris, will find many of his historical and medical concepts with my gratitude. The infectious enthusiasm and confidence of my editor, Gerald Hallowell, were essential catalysts for turning my thoughts into a book.

Many other people contributed to this work by reading chapters, answering questions, offering creative suggestions, and providing help with illustrations. Hannah Professors Paul Potter and Charles G. Roland, Professor Martin Friedland, Cherrilyn Yalin, and an anonymous reviewer for University of Toronto Press kindly commented on earlier drafts of the entire manuscript. I am also indebted to friends and colleagues, Ian Carr, Peter Cruse, Dale Dotten, Eleanor Enkin, Murray Enkin, Joel Howell, Bert Hansen, Anita Johnston, Olga Kits, Felicity Pope, Adrian Wilson, and Robert David Wolfe for their willing contributions. I gladly acknowledge the generosity of librarians, libraries, and colleagues at Queen's, in particular for advice on specific chapters, Alex Bryans, Prakash Burra, Neil Conacher, Gerald Evans, Pamela Frid, Charles Hayter, R. Neil Hobbs, Steve Iscoe, Gerald Marks, John Matthews, Terrie Romano, Joan Sherwood, Duncan G. Sinclair, Lucinda Walls, and James L. Wilson. They helped me to understand the lively debates and diversity of opinion in their fields.

My students are my newest teachers and toughest critics. Their persistent requests for an introductory text made me decide to do what I had long said I would never do. Several cheerfully read chapters in a test-drive exercise that shaped the final version. In particular, I thank former medical students Hershl Berman, Magdalena Biernacka, Ian Billingsley, Matthew Bowes, Ruttan Bhardwaj, Trevor Corneil, Darryl d'Costa, Leigh Eckler, Kymm Feldman, Diana Fort, Wael Haddara, Fiona Mattatall, and Matteus Zurowski, and former graduate students in history Elaine Berman, Jennifer Marotta, and Megan Nichols. Without their inspiring belief in its future utility, this book would not have been written.

HISTORY OF MEDICINE

A Scandalously Short Introduction

CHAPTER ONE

Introduction:
Heroes and Villains in
the History of Medicine*

My recommendation is that the doctor should be, plainly and unmistakably, a humanist.

Robertson Davies, 'Can a Doctor Be a Humanist?' 1984

The Heroes and Villains Game

In the early fall, incoming medical students at Queen's University play a game called Heroes and Villains. Acting like an icebreaker at a party, the game introduces them to three components of their education: the library, the information literacy course, and the history of medicine. The students are divided into teams to work with one or two partners of their choice. From a worksheet, they choose a name from medicine's past (see table 1.1). The task is to find something written by that historical figure (a primary source) and something written about the figure (a secondary source), and to decide whether the person is a hero, a villain, or both. The students then prepare to present their findings to the class and write a brief report with a bibliography. Prizes are promised.

The list of potential heroes and villains includes figures from antiquity, Nobel laureates, women, and local worthies. There is nothing special about our list; an endless number of alternatives could be

*Educational objectives for this book are found on p. 393.

Table 1.1
'Heroes' and 'villains' in medical history: Game worksheet

1 Divide the work among members of your team.
2 Use the electronic catalogue and the reference section of your library/libraries to find:
   (i) at least one item written by each person, and
   (ii) something about each person.
3 Decide whether the person is a hero, a villain, or both – and why.
4 Think about the objectives (below) and hand in brief written conclusions *with references*. Reports can be written by the whole team together or by groups within the team.

Team 1A
Herophilus
William Harvey
Maude Abbott
Gerhard Domagk
Robert Tait McKenzie
William Osler

Team 1B
Andreas Vesalius
Celsus
Elizabeth Smith-Shortt
Wilfred T. Grenfell
Alexis Carrel
William Osler

Team 2A
Avicenna
Ambroise Paré
Henry Morgentaler
James D. Watson
Helen MacMurchy
William Osler

Team 2B
Paracelsus
Rudolf Virchow
J. Lorimer 'Blimey' Austin
Robert Gallo
Marie Stopes
William Osler

Team 3A
Hippocrates
Norman Bethune
Emily Stowe
Linus Pauling
Thomas Sydenham
William Osler

Team 3B
Galen
Michel Sarrazin
Claude Bernard
Florence Nightingale
Frederick Banting
William Osler

Objectives
1 to distinguish the various types of monographs (single author, edited volume, posthumous collection, translation, facsimile, etc.)
2 to search the electronic catalogue for maximum effectiveness (author, subject, keyword)
3 to learn the basics of controlled vocabularies
4 to understand the meaning of primary sources (books by) and secondary source (books about)
5 to recognize that all history (even medical history) is a process of interpretation strongly influenced by the present

created to match the resources of other libraries and places. William Osler is in every list because of the eventual prize.

The whole-class session – nicknamed the 'debriefing' – usually takes place the following day. When the weather is fine, the class gathers outside.

'Who would like to speak first?' I ask. Rare volunteers are immediately given the floor; often, however, my question meets with dead silence.

'Who chose Hippocrates?' I try next. Groans and pointing fingers identify a reluctant but usually grinning pair, who tell their classmates what they have learned about the Greek physician of 2,500 years ago. As they wrap up, I ask, 'Is he a hero or a villain?'

'Definitely a hero.'

'Why?' A variety of answers justify the opinion.

I play devil's advocate: 'Hippocrates seemed to forbid abortion and use of the knife; he taught medicine only to men.' But the students' judgment proves unshakable, and we move on to the next example.

After one or two of these enforced mini-presentations, volunteers clamour to tell of the remarkable personage whose life and work they have just studied. Time will not permit all topics to be covered. Sometimes, I must interrupt a speaker to give others a chance. (Once, two students spontaneously adopted the personae of their subjects and treated their class to the spectacle of Avicenna and Paracelsus debating the symbolic need to burn books.)

As the hour flies by, I grow increasingly anxious that no one will win the prize, and the whole point of the game will be missed. Despite my best efforts at dredging up the shadier sides of these individual stories, the students keep resisting my attacks. Finally someone, perhaps an anonymous voice in the crowd, will answer the 'hero or villain' question with, 'It depends on how you look at it.'

'What did you say?' I ask. 'Louder.' Then I ask the whole class, 'What did she/he say?' The class repeats it. Then, amid laughter and clapping, the embarrassed student is conspicuously awarded the first prize, a book of Osler's writings, and I begin to relax.

Over the years, I have learned that medical students are intent on viewing their predecessors with unquestioning reverence, akin to religious awe. 'Yes, Hippocrates may have recommended never to use a knife, but he is a hero because he showed that disease had natural causes ...' 'Yes, Alexis Carrel may have been a Nazi sympathizer, but he is a hero because he made it possible to transplant organs ...' Even after the dramatic hints dished out in class, the majority of students will conclude their written assignments with the view that their subject is a hero. In a decade of playing this game, no student has yet proclaimed a subject to be a villain – though that judgment would not bring a prize either.

Few students question the premise of making value judgments about the past; but when one of them does, that person also wins a prize, just like the student who says, 'It depends.' Understandably, first-year students want to find heroes in the past. Relieved to have survived the stiff competition for admission, they anticipate forty years or more in their chosen profession with optimism and idealism. On graduation day, most will still remember the historical figure they researched in the first week of training. The game provides an historical role model, but it also draws attention to medicine's present and future too.

The premise of the game Heroes and Villains is the premise of this book. Medical history, like medical practice and medical science, is about questions and answers, evidence and interpretation. Some questions are better than others; some sources are more to be trusted than others; and some interpretations are stronger than others. Good historians are aware of the danger in projecting their own desires and values into historical scenarios and texts. History invites students to ponder why things came to be as they are and how they change. It reminds them of the future probability of having to relinquish the very ideas and 'facts' they are about to study. As a result, history is consistent with the medical education goals of lifelong learning.

How to Use This Book

Many essays and books have been written on the reasons why history should be taught to medical students, and at least as many publications offer advice on how to do it effectively. This book represents

> **What's Important**
>
> It is of small consequence for the student to know that an obscure book upon a recondite subject, by an author with an unpronounceable name, was published at a particular date. On the other hand it is of considerable importance for the students to be familiar with ... 'the climate of opinion' behind the intellectual deeds of a particular period.
>
> Cecilia Mettler, *History of Medicine*
> (Philadelphia and Toronto: Blakiston, 1947), xii

just one of numerous methods. At Queen's University, instead of being a separate course or seminar, history has infiltrated the entire curriculum and is taught as an integral component of the various medical disciplines under study.

The goals of our program are the goals of this book:

1 to raise awareness of history (and the humanities as a whole) as a research discipline that can enrich understanding of the present, and
2 to instill a sense of scepticism with regard to the 'dogma' of the rest of the curriculum.

These goals have been criticized for being insubstantial and unambitious. But we do not intend to turn future doctors into historians; rather we offer them an additional, conceptual tool for learning about medicine. Medical students are intelligent. Even if they last studied humanities in high school, they soon grasp the thrill and adventure of a debate over questions and context. In reaching for these modest goals, students learn something about the past; however, they can select the events that seem most relevant to their own personal lives and career goals. Names and dates are less important than ideas. Good history relies on accurate reference to such details, but it is, above all, a way of thinking.

This book does not pretend to be comprehensive, nor is its structure particularly original. Fifty years ago, Cecilia Mettler organized her textbook according to medical subjects and ideas. Several other weighty tomes provide far more information and many more pictures (see 'Suggestions for Further Readings,' below). This book attempts a brief survey of the history of Western medicine with reference to recent scholarly literature and current issues in health care, and with the recognition that practitioners can be of any sex, religion, race, or nationality. It is unapologetically aimed at Canadians.

The chapters do not follow an overriding chronology, and they can be read in any sequence. They are devoted to various disciplines of medical study, and the order in which they appear here roughly corresponds to the sequence followed in the medical curriculum at Queen's. Chronology will be found within each chapter, together with a sampling of themes or questions that govern historical research. Some events are developed with reference to recent literature, while others are ignored. Canadian examples are used often. The suggestions for further reading are not exhaustive, but they will orient the interested reader to background on most of the material covered; again, sources on Canadian subjects are included separately. In keeping with the message of the Heroes and Villains game, I have tried to show that alternative interpretations can be found for most elements of our past and that topics of interest can go well beyond 'great men' and 'great discoveries' to include ideas, diseases, patients, institutions, and great mistakes.

The final chapter offers advice on how to research a question in the history of medicine. Once again, it is neither infallible nor comprehensive. The appendices offer educational objectives and a few reference points for information on period, place, and ideas, including alternative health care and medicine in other times and places. Students often turn to the historian for information on other medical belief systems, which this book, being a history of our own dominant medicine, does not address; in appendix B4 some directions are given to compensate for this failing.

I wrote this book because my students asked me to do so. I hesitated for a long time because of the limitations of my expertise. After repeated requests, I finally embarked on the project, hoping that it would be a useful guide for students, for instructors wishing to incorporate history into their health-care teaching, and for interested practitioners. I also hoped that it might demystify medicine for students in other domains, such as history, philosophy, and sociology. But as soon as I began trying to turn those comfortably private, oral presentations into public print, I ran up against my own lack of erudition (as predicted) and was awed by the numerous places where I risked falling into the very traps described in chapter 15. Without the security of fudging footnotes and scholarly apparatus, I began to feel exposed on alien turf. Every sentence seemed like a minefield – each word, a bomb waiting to explode. I am indebted to many predecessors whose far more ambitious works resolved numerous problems, and I am grateful for the comments of the students and practitioners who were pestered to read portions of the work. Some readers will find errors that inevitably remain; others will no doubt complain that I have ignored their favourite topic. I hope that they will let me know and help to make the next edition better.

Suggestions for Further Reading
(See also appendices B3 and B4)

Ackerknecht, Erwin H. *A Short History of Medicine.* Baltimore: Johns Hopkins University Press, 1982

Castiglioni, Arturo. *A History of Medicine.* New York: Knopf, 1958

Garrison, Fielding H. *An Introduction to the History of Medicine.* 4th edn. Reprint, Philadelphia: Saunders, 1929

Hudson, Robert P. *Disease and Its Control: The Shaping of Modern Thought.* Westport, Conn.: Greenwood Press, 1983

King, Lester S. *Medical Thinking: A Historical Preface.* Princeton, N.J.: Princeton University Press, 1982

Kiple, Kenneth F. *The Cambridge World History of Human Disease.* Cambridge and New York: Cambridge University Press, 1993

Irvine Loudon, ed. *Western Medicine: An Illustrated History.* Oxford and New York: Oxford University Press, 1997

Lyons, Albert S., and R. Joseph Petrucelli. *Medicine: An Illustrated History.* New York: Abrams, 1978

Magner, Lois N. *A History of Medicine.* New York: Dekker, 1992

Mettler, Cecilia C. *History of Medicine: A Correlative Text, Arranged According to Subjects*, ed. Fred A. Mettler. Philadelphia and Toronto: Blakiston, 1947

Porter, Roy. *The Greatest Benefit to Mankind: A Medical History of Humanity from Antiquity to the Present.* London: HarperCollins, 1997

– ed. *The Cambridge Illustrated History of Medicine.* Cambridge: Cambridge University Press, 1996

Rullière, Roger. *Abrégé d'histoire de la médecine.* Paris: Masson, 1981

Singer, Charles Joseph, and E. Ashworth Underwood. *A Short History of Medicine.* Oxford: Clarendon Press, 1962

On Canada
(See also appendix B2 [ii])

Abbott, Maude Elizabeth Seymour. *History of Medicine in the Province of Quebec.* Toronto: Macmillan, 1931

Bernier, Jacques. *La médecine au Québec: Naissance et évolution d'une profession.* Québec: Presses de l'Université Laval, 1989

Canniff, William. *The Medical Profession in Upper Canada 1783–1850.* 1894. Reprint, published for the Hannah Institute for the History of Medicine. Toronto: Clarke, Irwin, 1980

Carr, Ian, and Robert Beamish. *Manitoba Medicine: A Brief History.* Winnipeg: University of Manitoba Press, 1999

Godfrey, Charles M. *Medicine for Ontario: A History.* Belleville, Ont.: Mika, 1979

Heagerty, John J. *Four Centuries of Medical History in Canada and a Sketch of the Medical History of Newfoundland.* Toronto: Macmillan, 1928

Jack, Donald Lamont. *Rogues, Rebels, and Geniuses: The Story of Canadian Medicine.* Toronto: Doubleday, 1981

Marble, Allan Everett. *Surgeons, Smallpox, and the Poor: A History of Medicine and Social Conditions in Nova Scotia, 1749–1799.* Montreal: McGill-Queen's University Press, 1993

CHAPTER TWO

The Fabricated Body:
History of Anatomy*

Anatomy is to physiology, as geography to history; it describes the theatre of events.

Jean Fernel, *On the Natural Part of Medicine*, 1542, preface (cited in Sherrington 1946, 64)

Anatomy is the study of the structure of the body. Today it seems integral to the study of medicine, but structural explanations of disease were long considered secondary to those of function (physiology). This chapter will explore the rise of anatomy from irrelevancy – even taboo – to its place as an institutional power in medical education.

The word 'anatomy' is derived from the Greek word ανατομη (dissection). It still implies cutting, but also structure (morphology) – the shape, size, and relationships of body parts. It is also a metaphor for the analysis of any problem.

Medicine is the study of disease and its treatments. To understand disease, doctors focus on abnormalities of structure and function, which are the objects of the complementary disciplines of anatomy and physiology. Traditionally, these two domains have competed for curriculum time, laboratory space, and pride of place in the minds of practitioners. Of course, considerable overlap takes place between structure and function: a broken leg does not work very well; neither

*Educational objectives for this chapter are found on pp. 393–4.

does a heart with a hole in its septum. But abnormal structure does not always imply disease; for example, congenital deformities, such as having six toes or a large birthmark, are not intrinsically associated with suffering or shortened life. Similarly, abnormal function can be compatible with healthy living; the heterozygous form of thalassemia, for example, conveys few consequences for affected individuals.

Medical cultures that emphasized the study of anatomy peaked centuries ago, in Alexandria, then declined, peaked again during the Renaissance, then declined, and peaked again in the last century. The present form of medical education still reflects this most recent heyday, but the perceived centrality of anatomy in modern medicine may be on the wane again.

Three themes recur throughout the history of anatomy:

1 Ambivalence, or 'approach-avoidance.' Should anatomical dissection be allowed or not? The desire to learn about illness often conflicted with religious or cultural aversions to the notion of cutting up dead bodies.
2 'The gift of art to medicine.' The expression of anatomical wisdom relied on visual forms of communication.
3 Anatomical study separate from medical wisdom. The pursuit of anatomy in art or science did not imply equal status in medicine.

Dissection and Anatomical Ideas in Antiquity

The elaborate burial practices of the ancient Egyptians provided frequent opportunities for the observation of body parts. Embalmers were adept at situating and extracting organs through tiny holes and slits in the body. Egyptian graphic art may have been stylized, but the statuary reveals a sensitive appreciation of surface and underlying structures. Unlike the embalmers and artists, however, the physicians do not appear to have used anatomy.

Our knowledge of ancient Egyptian medicine is based on a few surgical papyri (see chapter 10). Egyptian explanations of disease seem to have emphasized physiology, in which breath was the essence of life. Blood vessels were hypothesized rather than known, and only a

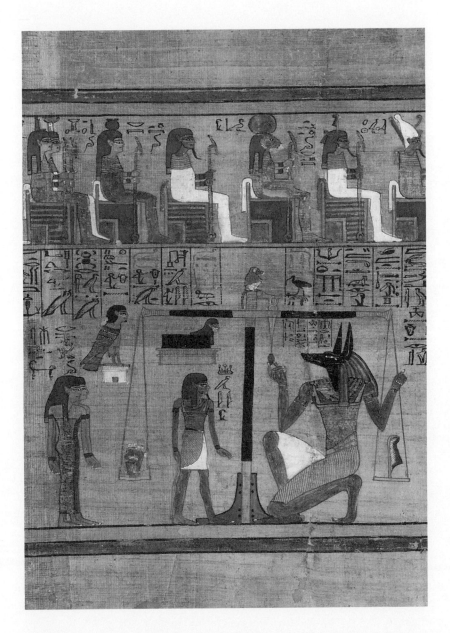

Weighing the heart. From the ancient Egyptian Book of the Dead, Papyrus of Ani, ca. 1420 B.C. British Museum, London

few organs were connected with specific functions. Some organs were associated with certain deities and used as hieroglyphics. For instance, a stylized uterus, or *sa*, represented the goddess of childbirth. Because this symbol was bicornuate (had two horns), scholars think that the model may have been animal rather than human. The heart symbolized the soul. In illustrations for the Book of the Dead, the heart of the deceased is weighed against the feather of truth; when the two balance, the soul may pass on to the next world.

Ancient Greek sculpture reflects a preoccupation with the accurate portrayal of surface anatomy, with attention to the underlying muscles and bones. Votive offerings left at temples by sick people hoping for cures were fashioned from clay or stone to resemble afflicted body parts – uterus, breasts, bladder, and limbs – sometimes with anatomical derangements such as varicose veins.

Despite these artistic influences and their skill in observation, Greek doctors were not especially interested in anatomy. Dissection of human bodies was forbidden, and funeral practices centred on cremation. Function was more important than structure. Explanation of illness relied on the four elements (earth, air, fire, and water) and their four cognate humours inside the body (see chapter 3). Given the laws and funeral customs, few opportunities arose for examination of internal structures of humans. Exceptions are found in Hippocratic treatises on fractures and dislocations, which reveal extensive knowledge of bones and joints.

Illustration is essential to the teaching of anatomy, and the ban on dissection did not extend to animals. The fourth-century B.C. philosopher and biologist, Aristotle, appears to have used large diagrams when he taught the comparative anatomy of animals. Unfortunately none of the original drawings have survived.

After about 300 B.C., the Greek city of Alexandria permitted dissection of the bodies of criminals, alive or dead. These public demonstrations were designed to horrify as much as instruct. That the practice was reserved for criminals indicates the social ambivalence regarding dissection, which could be seen as a desecration. Two Alexandrians, Herophilus and Erasistratus, described minute structures, including lymph lacteals, the meninges, and vascular structures such as the *torcular herophili* (named after Herophilus). None of their writings have survived. Our evidence for their work is based on other writers, including Galen, who lived some four hundred years later.

Galen on Herophilus

Herophilus 'attained the highest degree of accuracy in things which became known by dissection, and he obtained the greater part of his knowledge, not like the majority ... from irrational animals, but from human beings themselves.'

Galen, second century, A.D. (cited in von Staden 1989, 143)

Galen was born in 129 A.D. in Pergamum, on the Aegean coast of modern Turkey, but he lived much of his life in Rome. He deplored the laws that forbade human dissection; at least three of his many treatises were devoted to human anatomy, ostensibly as understood by the Alexandrians. Galen served as a physician to the gladiators, and he may have taken advantage of gaping wounds to observe internal structures. A great experimenter, he dissected animals, both living and dead, his preferred subjects being the pig and the rhesus monkey. He extrapolated from animals to humans and devised elaborate theories concerning anatomical structures, the motion of blood, and the origin and sustenance of life. Some observations were accurate for animals but missed their mark when applied to humans; for example, he ascribed five lobes to the liver and a vascular network in the brain called the *rete mirabile.*

Galen's writings are authoritative and bragging, and his teleological perspective allowed him to conceive of all structures as having been created for a purpose (see chapter 3). This confident philosophy corresponded well with the views of Christianity. As a result, his was the medical textbook of choice for more than a thousand years. His immediate successors may have carried out some human dissection, but anatomies became rare and ritualized exercises for endorsing Galen's authority, not for seeking truth.

The oldest known representation of what appears to be an anat-

Five figure drawings, from a twelfth-century Bavarian manuscript. They are typical of those found in a number of Persian and Latin manuscripts of the Middle Ages. Bayerische Staatsbibliothek, CLM 120002, fols. 2v–3r

omy lesson is a fourth-century A.D. wall painting from a Roman catacomb (Via Latina), which was discovered in 1957. The instructor sits a considerable distance from the cadaver. Neither he nor his students touch the body, which is prodded with a long pole as it lies on the ground as if to emphasize its base nature.

The oldest extant anatomical illustrations date from the early Middle Ages and are the work of Persian and Arab scholars, who preserved and transmitted the ancient Greek authors, illuminating the texts with stylized diagrams. The schematic figures squat in a froglike

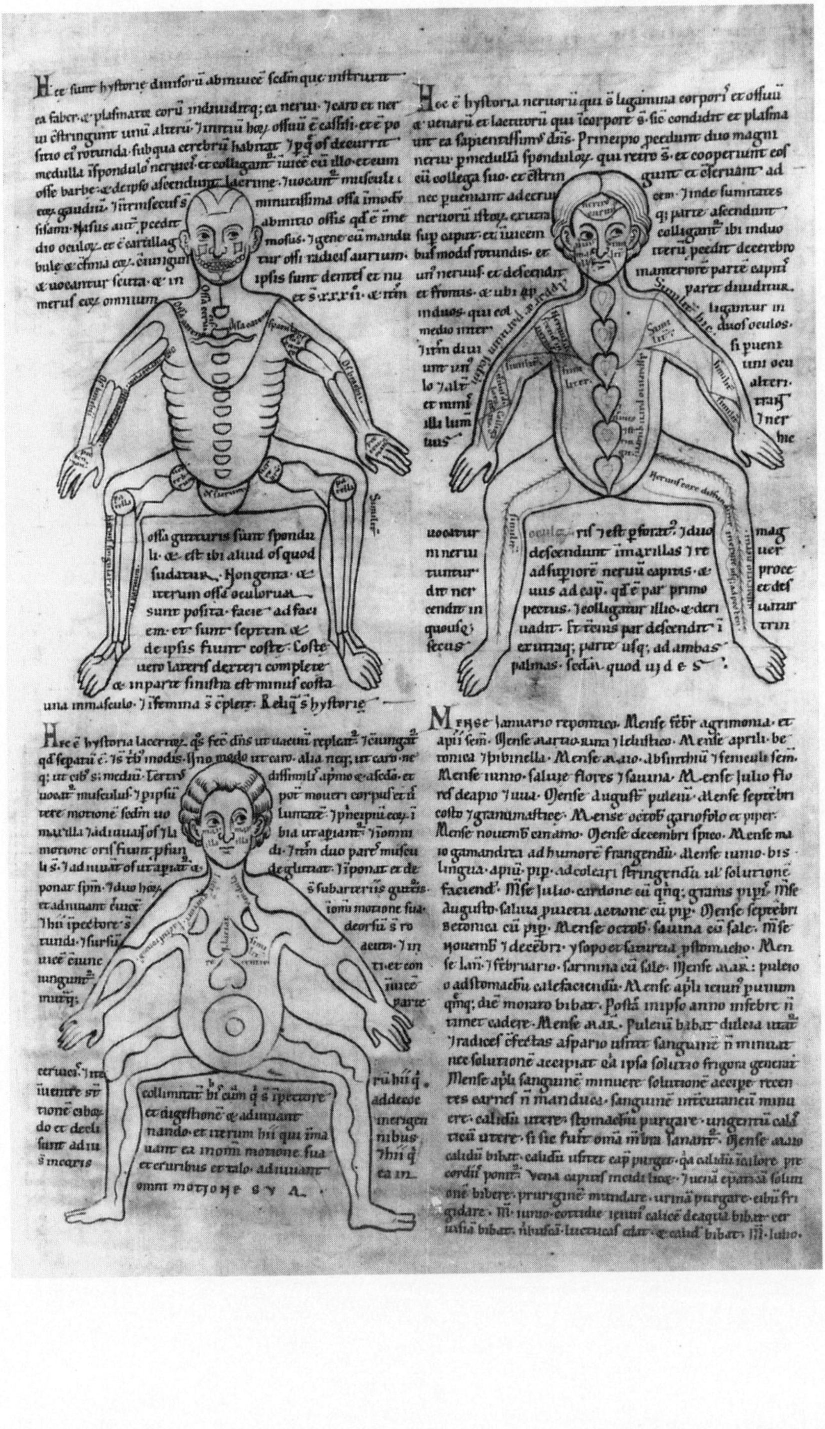

posture to expose the genitalia and the inner aspects of the limbs. Several drawings usually complete each series of five or six systems: vessels, muscles, nerves, organs, and bones. The practice extended into medieval Europe. The German medical historian Karl Sudhoff, who made a study of these drawings, concluded that their Greek precursors in Aristotle's work had probably come in similar series of five or six.

Medieval Treatises on the Body

In the thirteenth and fourteenth centuries, art and anatomy both experienced an awakening, fostered by legislative changes, the decline of religious teaching, and reactions to criminal violence or epidemic diseases. Municipalities, especially in Italy, were pressured to permit dissection in order to determine cause of death in cases of murder or other unusual situations (see table 2.1).

The rise of secular universities also contributed to the increase of dissection. In Christian tradition, the body was linked to sin and the temporal existence of the profane world. Learning about its inner workings was not only unnecessary but it could jeopardize salvation, because the literal interpretation of Scripture anticipated the resurrection of the soul within an intact body. As a result, the church did not condone dissection. Images of anatomies from the medieval period emphasize the barbarity of the act. Sometimes, the pope granted special dispensations for certain medical schools, such as Montpellier in southern France, but the subjects were executed criminals – or, on rare occasions, living criminals, who may have been sentenced to death by vivisection. Tension grew as schools yearned to practise dissection and the church refused; the resultant disorganization mirrored inconsistencies in the evolving power structure of society. Would-be anatomists were sometimes prosecuted.

Legal dissections were ritualized and infrequent – once or twice a year, for example; in some places, only once every five years. The professor sat high above the scene, reading from a Latin edition of Galen. The demonstrators were often illiterate barbers, who dissected in conjunction with the lesson. (On barber-surgeons, see

Table 2.1
Anatomy legislation in Europe, thirteenth to sixteenth centuries

Date	Place	Dissection permitted
1207	Normandy	Yes
1230	Saxony	No
1238	Sicily, Naples	Yes
	Salerno (Frederick II)	Yes – once every 5 years
1258	Bologna	Yes – victims of aggression
1300	Vatican (Boniface VIII)	No
1302	Bologna	Yes – autopsy for suspected poisoning
1308	Venice	Yes – once a year
1315	Padua	Yes – Mondino made public dissection
1319	Bologna	No – students arrested for dissecting
1366	Montpellier	Yes – occasional dissections
1374	Montpellier	Yes – once or twice a year
1391	Lerida, Spain	Yes – one criminal every three years
1404	Vienna	Yes – first public dissection
1540	England (Henry VIII)	Yes – four times a year
1565	England (Elizabeth I)	Yes – criminals after execution

chapter 10.) As a result, the words of Galen could persist unchallenged. Differences between the cadaver and a Galenic ideal were explained by the imperfection of the (usually criminal) mortal.

One anatomist who broke with tradition was the Italian, Mondino dei Luzzi. He emphasized the need for anatomists to do their own dissection, but his teachings differed little from Galen. His 1316 treatise, the *Anathomia Mondini*, became the standard reference for the next hundred and fifty years. Its manuscript editions were not illustrated, but later versions were: however, when his work was first printed in 1478, it was already being superseded by newer treatises.

The artistic awakening of the late Middle Ages was applied to portrayal of the body in several fourteenth-century anatomical treatises. In the *Chirurgia* (Surgery) of Henri de Mondeville, the image of the patient/cadaver is vertical and slightly more fluid than its rigid predecessors, as if captured in living action (see also chapter 10). The numerous images in the 1345 treatise of Guido de Vigevano (actually an illustrated edition of Mondino) display the anatomist himself conducting the dissection; however, the stylistic portrayal recalls the five-figure drawings from centuries before.

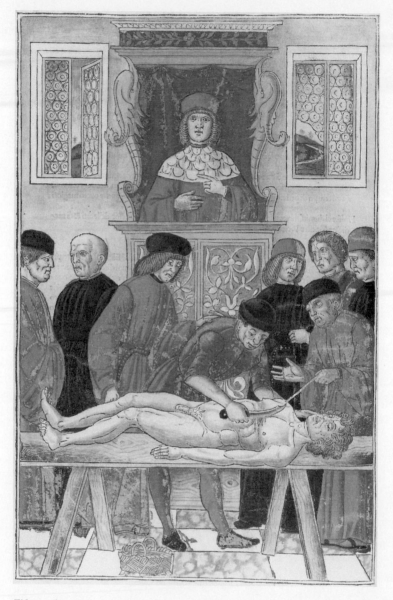

Fifteenth-century anatomy lesson. The professor reading from Galen sits high above the dissectors. From Johannes de Ketham, *Fasciculo di medicina,* 1493. Yale University Library

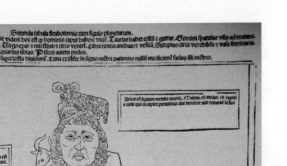
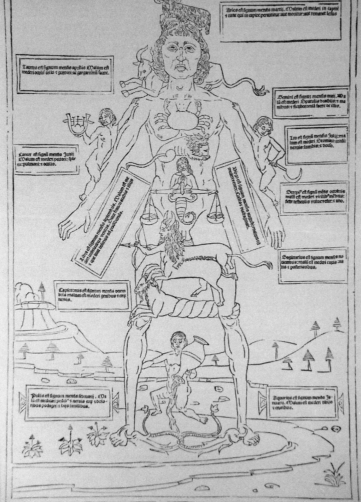

Zodiac man, Johannes de Ketham, *Fasciculus medicinae*, 1491[?], facsimile, Karl Sudhoff and Charles Singer, 1924

Sometimes the image of a 'zodiac man' was used to explain the relationship between the body and the external world and to indicate the auspicious times and sites to treat. These figures synthesized a large amount of information. Modifications were made to illustrate many potential injuries or diseases with the appropriate sites and methods of treatment: a 'wounds man,' a 'disease man,' and a 'bloodletting man.' Examples of these 'men' are found in the treatise *Fasciculus medicinae* (ca. 1491) by Johannes de Ketham. Despite its apparent artistic and intellectual conservatism, the *Fasciculus* relied on one important innovation: printing. It could be said to mark a symbolic beginning of the anatomical Renaissance.

Art and Renaissance Anatomy

The Renaissance is a period in Western European history – roughly from 1400 to 1600 – when an artistic and intellectual awakening coincided with a reappreciation of the ancients. Many causes – economic, social, and demographic – can be cited for the Renaissance. From the perspective of medical history, one of the most intriguing and debated 'causes' is the fourteenth-century plague, which depopulated Europe and radically altered its economic structure (see chapter 7). Plague endorsed a certain scepticism toward Galen, who had not described it, and toward the church, because the 'good' seemed to die as readily as the 'sinful.' It also affected art. People became inured to the spectacle of corpses in the street, and the horror of human remains tended to fade. Prominent citizens took to having themselves portrayed on their future tombs as rotting corpses – *memento mori* – gruesome anatomical reminders of death, which not even the church could challenge. With this revival, or rebirth (*renaissance*), came a reappreciation of classical authors, art, and language, and a rediscovery of the beauty of the human body and the various modes of portraying it. If the exterior of the body could be glorified, it was a simple matter to extrapolate attention to its interior.

Renaissance art contributed to anatomy, and artists were anatomists. For example, Leonardo da Vinci – architect, painter, engineer, scientist, and philosopher – claimed to have practised thirty dissections himself, although scholars now think it was fewer than ten. He

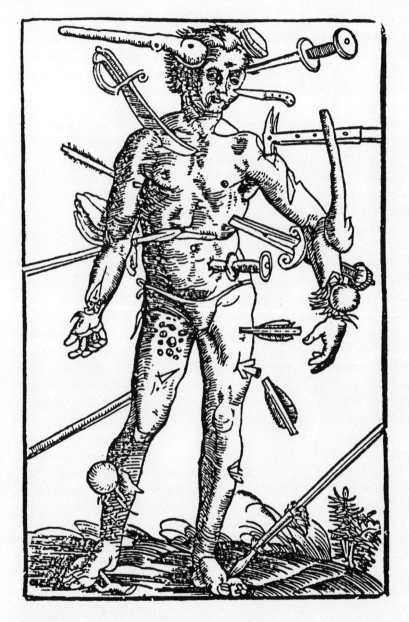

Wounds man, from Hans Gersdorff, *Feldbuch der Wundartznei*, 1517, facsimile, Wissenschaftliche Buchgesellschaft, 1967, xviii verso

planned a treatise of anatomy, maintaining that to elucidate the structure of the human body, several 'anatomies' must be conducted – one devoted to each structural system: bones, muscles, vessels, nerves, and organs. Two hundred pages of Leonardo's anatomical sketches and writings are kept in the Royal Library at Windsor Castle, England. His famous 'Vitruvian man' was drawn in the same year as the printing of Ketham's more static figures; the contrast between them demonstrates that artists were more preoccupied with anatomical detail than physicians were.

Leonardo was interested in the finer points of structure for scientific and artistic reasons, but contemporary medicine remained ignorant or uninterested, and doctors continued to recite Galen as told by Mondino. Thirty years after Leonardo's drawings, yet another commentary on Mondino was published, by Giacomo Berengario da Carpi, who provided pleasing but stylistically simple woodcut images of cadavers, sometimes in the lifelike act of helping out with the dissection.

Why were medical practitioners less interested in anatomical wisdom than they are now? Doctors treated the sick for subjective illness, suffering, and dysfunction, but except for fractures and dislocations, alterations in structure were impossible to fix. Consequently, trying to correlate disease with dead internal organs, which could be neither visualized nor altered during life, seemed to be a waste of time (see chapter 4). Clinicians did not reject dissection as an intellectual pursuit, so much as they thought it lacked practical application.

Vesalius and the *Fabrica* (The Structure of the Human Body)

The magnificent *De humani corporis fabrica* of Andreas Vesalius was published in 1543, fifty years after Leonardo's drawings. Born in Brussels in 1514, Vesalius studied medicine at Louvain, in his native Belgium, before travelling to France. In Paris he was taught by a professor who read Renaissance-style from Galen while prosectors dissected below. Vesalius later claimed to have dissected, boiled, and reassembled his first skeleton from the corpse of an executed criminal stolen from a gibbet. He moved on to Padua near Venice, where anatomy was more an integral part of medical studies than it was in Paris. Shortly after his arrival, he was awarded a doctorate in medicine. The following day, according to an oft-repeated legend, he was appointed 'professor' of surgery at the age of twenty-three. Vesalius then began anatomical teaching in earnest.

Not only did Vesalius conduct his own dissections, but he befriended artists of the nearby city states in Venice and Florence. Scholars have suggested that the contact was fostered by apothecary shops, where doctors went for their medicines and artists bought their pigments. As a result of this contact, Vesalius obtained the best possible artistic advice for his work, and therein lay his success.

In 1538 Vesalius published his first book, a sort of *hors d'oeuvre* that preceded his *chef d'oeuvre* by five years. Called the *Tabulae sex* (Six tables), this short book was astonishingly popular because it was illustrated with high-quality images. In keeping with long-standing tradition, it contained only six illustrations with narrative; reflecting Renaissance ideals, three ancient languages were used: Latin, Greek, and Hebrew. Despite the evident care taken in artistic preparation, some morphologic features and body proportions seem not quite right; the spine is a little too straight, the ribs shortened. More surprising are the residual Galenic features: a five-lobed liver and the *rete mirabile!* Surely, after all his personal experience, the young Vesalius knew that these structures did not exist. Why did he leave them there? Some historians think that it was a deliberate attempt to soften the reaction to his future work and spare himself the hostility of his older colleagues. The *Tabulae sex* sold out rapidly and was 'read to bits' as students hung the large images above their dissecting tables. Copies of the *Tabulae* are more scarce than original editions of the much bigger and more famous *Fabrica*.

On the title page of the 1543 *Fabrica*, Vesalius shows himself surrounded by a huge crowd at the Padua faculty; he is looking boldly at the reader while he dissects the corpse of a woman. The cadaver, he tells us, was the mistress of a monk; he and his students had acted quickly to remove identifying features before the body could be taken by the grieving cleric. The title page is full of symbolism. Below are the barbers, displaced from the table and squabbling. Cast off to the side are animals – dogs and monkeys, Galen's subjects and the source of his errors. Above, in the traditional place reserved for the recitation of Galen, is a skeleton. In the crowd are Vesalius's students and colleagues, including ancient savants, the bearded Realdo Colombo, who described the pulmonary circulation, and a youth writing or drawing, who, some think, may be the artist. Despite the emphasis on innovation, historian Andrew Cunningham has drawn attention to Vesalius's connections with the anatomists of antiquity; he found impressive clues, not only on the title page, that the anatomist was actually 'emulating' Galen.

Who was the artist? Similarities in the Mannerist style with the landscape background and architectural elements lead some to claim that it was the great Titian. The most likely candidate, according to a letter by Vesalius, is his fellow Belgian, Jan Stefan van Kalkar, who worked in Titian's studios. Another meticulous craftsman was probably engaged to sculpt the wood blocks from the original drawings. The blocks were then carried across the Alps for printing by the leading house of Johannes Oporinus in Basel, Switzerland.

The *Fabrica* contained not six drawings but seven books of many drawings each. The first book was devoted to the skeleton. The second featured the muscle men, the most famous series in the treatise, beginning with eight poses in the front view, including the *écorché*, a body with only the skin removed. Commentary explained what had been done to create each successive image by cutting the muscles at their origins to leave them dangling by their insertions. Ironic humour pervades the artwork: as the layers of muscle are removed, the poor cadaver became the worse for wear, moving from athletic exuberance to needing ropes and walls for support. The anatomical decay is reflected in the landscape background, which becomes increasingly barren as summer turns to winter. After the eighth pose, the whole process is repeated for the back view of the body.

The third book was devoted to the veins and arteries – gone was the *rete mirabile* of 1538. The fourth book described the nerves. The fifth explored the abdominal organs, with the liver's lobes reduced to two. It also included dissections of the genitalia, which have become the object of scholarly curiosity. The vulva, vagina, and uterus of the monk's defunct mistress are shown without adnexal attachments; the image resembles a penis, inviting speculation about

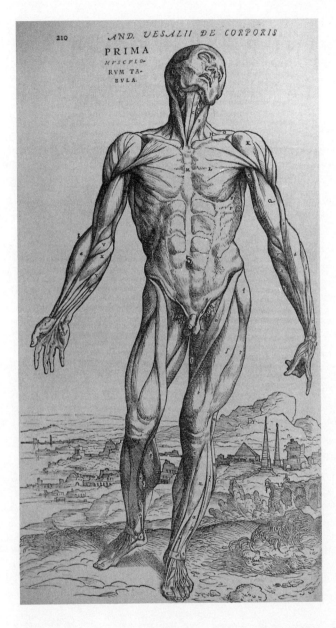

The *écorché*, one of the muscle men from Vesalius's *Fabrica* [1543], 2nd edn, 1555

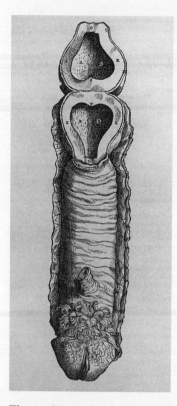

The vagina and vulva from Vesalius's *Fabrica* [1543], 2nd edn, 1555. The resemblence to the male organ is no accident. Vesalius was interested in homology, and the fallopian tubes had yet to be described.

a message of homology. The sixth book focused on the thoracic organs, and the seventh, on the brain.

Andrew Cunningham has argued convincingly that Vesalius – by his method, with its emphasis on personal exploration and vivisection, and despite his refutation of some Galenic anatomy – 'was simply Galen restored to life,' a true Renaissance man (Cunningham 1997, 114).

Some anatomical inaccuracies can be identified in these images; for example, the rectus abdominus muscle extends too far up the rib cage. In contrast to its predecessors and many of its successors, however, Vesalius's achievement was unequalled. The *Fabrica* has become an object of veneration; first editions have been tracked down, and new translations made. Terence Cavanagh has shown that placing the reversed muscle figures in a series creates a continuous landscape. Some scholars locate the scenery in the Eugenean Hills near Padua, where scores of doctors have travelled in search of the exact site.

Vesalius soon gave up academic life, and he successively went into the private service of various crowned heads: the Holy Roman Emperor Charles V, Philip II of Spain, and Henri II of France. He then seems to have left royal service to travel, only to die while on a pilgrimage to the Holy Land. His unmarked grave is thought to be on the small Mediterranean island of Zante, but circumstances surrounding his demise are obscure. The carved woodblocks for the illustrations of the *Fabrica* survived into the twentieth century and were used for a facsimile edition in 1934. But during the Second World War, they were destroyed in the bombing of Munich.

After the *Fabrica*, scientists began to pay more attention to structure. Several similar works followed, each an artistic achievement in itself. A series of brilliant dissections resulted in the discovery of hitherto forgotten or unknown body parts. In 1545, Charles E[s]tienne published an atlas that gave special attention to nerves and vessels. In 1561 Gabriele Fallopio (or Fallopius) described the inner ear, the cranial nerves, and the fallopian tubes that had been missing in the *Fabrica*. Bartolomeo Eustachio (or Eustachius) demonstrated the adrenals, the vena cavae, the sympathetic ganglions, and the inner ear, including the tube that bears his name. Girolamo Fabrizio da Aquapendente (or Hieronymous Fabricius) described the valves of the veins in 1603, and twenty years later Gaspare Aselli found the lymph lacteals while dissecting a living animal that was in the process of digestion. In 1747 Bernard Siegfried Weiss (or Albinus) published his celebrated atlas, which featured engravings of muscled and unmuscled human skeletons in a lush forest with other exotic marvels, including a rhinoceros.

Despite these accomplishments, anatomy still had little to do with bedside medicine. The sixteenth- and seventeenth-century anatomists concentrated mostly on the discovery and artistic portrayal of the normal, or healthy, human form. They did not relate structure to disease. But early in the seventeenth century, scientists did begin to apply the new knowledge about structure to the study of function. Physiology, rather than medicine, was the first to find applications for the new anatomical research. For example, William Harvey discovered the circulation of blood by relying heavily (but not exclusively) on his teacher Fabrizio's demonstration of the valves in the veins (see chapter 3).

With the exceptions of Antonio Benivieni in the fifteenth century and Jean Fernel in the sixteenth, few writers were interested in abnormal anatomy until nearly a century and a half after the *Fabrica*. Théophile Bonet and Giovanni Battista Morgagni wrote massive compendia of anatomical pathology as a basis for disease; but their works were not illustrated (see chapter 4).

By the eighteenth century, dissection had become more respectable. A new philosophy of knowledge, called sensualism, was predicated on the view that all wisdom came from observation through the senses; observation was venerated, while theorizing was supposedly set aside. Anatomical studies could be seen to fit this new tradition. Artists painted distinguished anatomists at work surrounded by their students, a prime example being Rembrandt's famous painting of the lesson of Dr Tulp. Others created wax models, which became an important tool of medical education. Museums were founded to preserve elegant dissections and waxes for future reference. Spectacular remainders are the eighteenth-century collections of John Hunter in London, England, of Honoré Fragonard in Maisons Alfort, near Paris, and of the Mutter Museum in Philadelphia.

But anatomy's relevance to medicine continued to be ill-defined. Why? First, aversion to human remains persisted. Eighteenth-century caricaturists such as William Hogarth derided dissection as a vile act, an appropriate 'reward for cruelty.' Second, even doctors who practised anatomy had difficulty imagining how to apply it; the same sensualism that celebrated anatomy made it an object of suspicion when it came to medicine. Doctors could not diagnose internal changes until the patient was dead; nor could they correct them. Diseases and diagnosis were based on symptoms (see chapter 4).

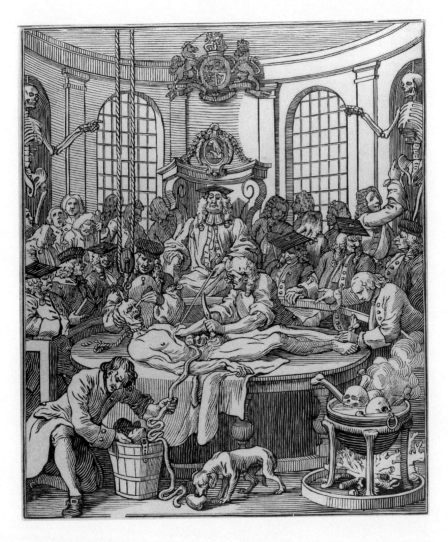

The Reward of Cruelty. Engraving by John Bell [prior to 1750], after William Hogarth. Yale University Library

---

Medical Mistrust of Anatomy

Others ... have pompously and speciously prosecuted the promoting of this art by searching into the bowels of dead and living creatures, as well sound as diseased ... but with how little
success such endeavors have been or are likely to be attended I
shall here in some measure make appear ...

Thomas Sydenham, ca. 1668 (cited in Dewhurst 1958, 3)

All that anatomy can doe is only to shew us the gross and sensi-
ble parts of the body, or the vapid and dead juices all which,
after the most diligent search, will be not much able to direct a
physician how to cure a disease than how to make a man ... If
anatomy shew us neither the causes nor cures of most diseases
I think it is not very likely to bring any great advantages for
removeing the pains and maladys of mankind.

John Locke, ca. 1668 (cited in Dewhurst 1958, 3–4)

And over a century later ...

Anatomy, though so carefully cultivated, has yet not supplied
medicine with any truly important observations. One may
scrupulously examine a corpse, yet the necessities on which
life depends escape one ... Anatomy may cure a sword wound,
but will prove powerless when the invisible dart of a particular
miasma has penetrated beneath our skin.

Louis Sebastien Mercier, *The Picture of Paris before and after the Revolution*, 1788.
Trans. Wilfrid and Emilie Jackson (London: Routledge, 1929), 97

Anatomy Goes Medical

At the beginning of the nineteenth century, technology and a recon-
figuration of disease concepts changed medical attitudes to anatomy.
The diagnostic techniques of percussion and auscultation made it

possible to detect structural changes inside the chest. Names and concepts of diseases changed from being subjective symptoms, such as hemoptysis and shortness of breath, to associated anatomical lesions, such as pulmonary effusion, pulmonary consolidation, and emphysema (see chapters 4 and 9).

As diseases became increasingly anatomical, medicine had to move in the same direction. Anatomy and dissection suddenly became not only interesting but essential for medical training. Chairs of anatomy, which had once been independent, became a feature of every well-dressed medical school. Pathological anatomy soon followed: the first British chair of pathological anatomy was awarded to Robert Carswell in 1828; the first French professorship went to Jean Cruveilhier in 1835. By 1848, twenty-five of the approximately forty medical schools in the United States offered instruction in dissection.

New problems soon arose because of the limited supply of bodies. Dissection may have become acceptable to academics, but the general public was not eager to see the corpses of its loved ones displayed and opened for instruction. Few places enjoyed legal mechanisms for obtaining anatomic material. In cities with large poorhouses and public hospitals, such as postrevolutionary Paris and New Orleans, unclaimed bodies were automatically given to medical educators. Elsewhere, cadavers were retrieved from cemeteries or were purchased on the sly.

The new occupation of 'resurrection man' emerged. Fabled in song and story, it satisfied the growing market for fresh bodies with the newly buried corpses of private citizens. The public was offended by the outrageous practice, and turned on the grave robbers' clients too. In the United States, physicians' homes and medical schools were mobbed and burned on several occasions. Cemeteries were guarded; following a burial, wealthy citizens posted sentries to protect family plots from violation. The Canadian medical teacher John Rolph, temporarily in exile at Rochester, New York, for his part in the 1837 Rebellion, had a former student in Toronto ship anatomical subjects across Lake Ontario in whisky barrels. To avoid middleman costs, medical students became adept at grave-robbing; those in Kingston, Ontario were notorious despoilers of patrician plots.

Where medical schools operated in proximity to graveyards, the trade in human bodies could be brisk and ruthlessly competitive.

The inevitable happened: murder for the sale of corpses. Unknown numbers of disadvantaged people may have been killed to this end. Students and professors might have guessed the provenance of especially fresh or healthy looking cadavers; however, in their eagerness both to dissect and to maintain supplies, they asked no questions. In the famous case of 1823, the Scotsmen William Burke and William Hare murdered at least sixteen people and sold the corpses to Robert Knox, anatomist at the leading medical school in Edinburgh. Knox took pains to remove the heads and other identifying features from the bodies as soon as he received them. First, the pair preyed on the poverty-stricken elderly tenants in Burke's home. Then they murdered a local prostitute, well known to the students; but the lads merrily dissected her corpse without comment. Only when Burke and Hare kidnapped a well-known boy with mental retardation, James Wilson ('Daft Jamie'), was suspicion aroused. A few days later, the body of Margery Docherty, a healthy woman who had been reported missing, was found in the anatomist's laboratory. Burke and Hare were charged with her murder. Hare was excused by testifying against his accomplice. Burke was hanged, his body dissected in public, and the remains displayed for hundreds of onlookers. His fate indicated that dissection was still a ghastly 'reward for cruelty': his name is a synonym for murder. Neither Knox nor his students were charged, but the professor's career was in ruins.

Soon after, legislation restricted the sale of bodies and provided medical schools with access to unclaimed corpses in hospitals, prisons, and poorhouses (see table 2.2). In Britain, the Anatomy Act was passed into law nine years after the Burke and Hare affair. Massachusetts also moved early in this regard, but most American states revealed their chronic ambivalence to the issue by failing to pass legislation until after the Civil War. Canada's anatomy legislation was the special project of the colourful physician pioneer, William 'Tiger' Dunlop.

Dissection slowly became acceptable to the public. Scenes of anatomy lessons relinquished their ghoulishness for an aura of solemnity,

Table 2.2
Nineteenth-century anatomy legislation

1798	France
1831	Massachusetts
1832	England, Warburton's Anatomy Act
1843	Canada (revised 1859 and 1864)
1844	Prussia
1865 +	Most states of USA
1883	Pennsylvania

which symbolized the seriousness of medicine itself. Improved techniques of preservation and injection of blood vessels have enhanced the longevity and utility of each corpse. Gender became an issue as women entered medicine in the late nineteenth century. Many schools believed that ladies were too delicate to confront corpses or to look on naked male bodies, especially in the presence of living men, and some schools exempted women from dissection or stipulated that they take their classes separately. Problems with the supply of cadaveric material remained, partly because medical students were fond of joking about cadavers and skeletons, and regularly had themselves photographed with the specimens in disrespectful poses. But gradually the stigma was removed, and people became willing to leave their bodies to science. Most schools mark the donation with an annual service of thanksgiving and respect.

Anatomy Today: Basic Science or Hazing Ritual?

When health-care practitioners look back on the past that has just been described, it is difficult for them to see it as anything other than a logical series of progressive steps leading to openness and tolerance about the body that is the essence of medical wisdom and practice. For them, the body is a neutral and obvious assemblage of structural 'facts.' Recently, cultural historians have shown that the story is not quite so straightforward. In a new trend called 'body history,' they challenge the idea of the body as an immutable entity that is simply waiting to be discovered and explored. They have shown how its 'construction' was influenced by social and cultural pressures

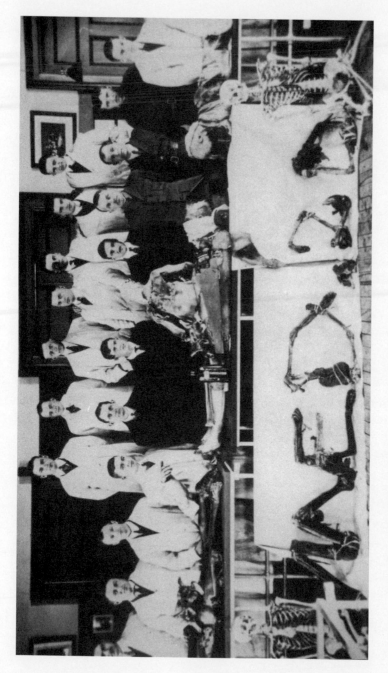

Queen's medical class of 1920 posing with anatomical parts. The words 'Med 20' are spelled in cadaver limbs. Friend-Vandewater Gallery, Botterell Hall, Queen's University. Photo by Queen's Medical Art and Photography Services

of time and place. Instead of tracing a story about the 'fabric' of the body, historians are interested in how it may have been 'fabricated.'

For example, Londa Schiebinger pointed out that the shapes imputed by eighteenth-century anatomists to the female pelvis exaggerated natural proportions in a manner that emphasized women's role in childbearing. Similarly, Thomas Laqueur examined structural representations of femaleness as vehicles for the expression of political and cultural attitudes toward women. Sander Gilman and John Efron showed how anti-Semitism contributed to the 'normal' but deviant anatomies of Jews. Concepts of normalcy are culturally contingent; for example, excess weight can be a manifestation of health in one culture and a sign of illness in another. Other ideals of size and proportion, including height, skull capacity, and brain size, also have been influenced by notions of racial, cultural, and gender superiority. David Armstrong has shown that the constructing influences now include anatomy itself, which has become so pervasive in medical thought that many immaterial problems, such as illnesses, are reified as if they were material entities (see chapter 4).

If the history of anatomy is no longer quite as obvious as it once was, its future seems equally in doubt. Where exactly is anatomy going? Is it a pillar in the institutions of learning or has its time passed? Are we witnessing a new rise in the relative significance of function over structure? The evidence is mounting to suggest that anatomy as an investigative discipline may be in decline once again.

After the hard-won legacy of Mondino and Vesalius, it is surprising that students rarely do their own dissecting. Demonstrators prepare specimens in advance. Some demonstrators are surgical residents who need refresher courses because their anatomy has been forgotten in the subsequent training. Why? Because detailed anatomy is not reinforced by the general practice of medicine. In acknowledgment of this reality, the innovative medical school at McMaster University in Hamilton, Ontario (founded in the late 1960s), has never taught anatomy through formal dissections.

Anatomy continues to hold departmental status in many health science faculties; however, it has difficulty claiming to be a discrete research discipline. The publications of anatomy professors rarely address the elucidation of gross or even microscopic structure.

At best, they investigate ultrastructure, growth, and function of embryos, cells, genes, and molecules. Often their research bears little connection to anatomy at all. Department names are being changed to include the words 'cell biology,' while the seemingly old-fashioned museums are dubbed 'learning centres.'

These observations are not meant to imply that study of body structure is irrelevant to medical practice or that it does not deserve a prominent place early in medical training. On the contrary. Illness is felt and diagnosed within the body. But we can ask why anatomy continues as a form of academic organization if it is no longer a field of active research. The once-excluded discipline is now the establishment – the product of a two-hundred-year-old tradition, consolidated wisdom, reduced into Galenic compendia available on CD-Rom. Even as the hours devoted to its study are shrinking, the long-contested privilege to dissect will not be relinquished easily.

Our teachers dissected, we dissect, and our students must dissect too. Moreover – and in striking contrast to the past – society now expects future doctors to cut up dead bodies. While continuing to condone the practice, awe-struck relatives and friends betray traces of retained revulsion when they ask medical students for the gory details: 'Ooooo! What's it like?' Anatomy distinguishes doctors from others; it demarcates modern medicine, both intellectually and socially. Aside from its many other intrinsic merits, the study of anatomy is now a symbolic rite of initiation that socializes members into a professional tradition.

Suggestions for Further Reading

Armstrong, David. *Political Anatomy of the Body: Medical Knowledge in Britain in the Twentieth Century*. Cambridge and New York: Cambridge University Press, 1983

Barzun, Jacques, ed. *Burke and Hare: The Resurrection Men*. Metuchen, N.J.: Scarecrow Press and New York Academy of Medicine, 1974

Cavanagh, G.S. Terence. *The Panorama of Vesalius: A 'Lost' Design from Titian's Studio*. Athens, Ga: Sacrum Press, 1996; also *Medical History* 27 (1983), 77–9

Cazort, Mimi. *The Ingenious Machine of Nature: Four Centuries of Art and Anatomy*. Ottawa: National Gallery of Canada, 1996

Choulant, Ludwig. *History and Bibliography of Anatomic Illustration*. 1852. Trans. Mortimer Frank. New York: Hafner, 1962

Cunningham, Andrew. *The Anatomical Renaissance: The Resurrection of the Anatomical Projects of the Ancients*. Aldershot, England: Scolar Press; Brookfield, Vt: Ashgate, 1997

Dewhurst, Kenneth. 'Locke and Sydenham on the Teaching of Anatomy.' *Medical History* 2 (1958), 1–12

Efron, John M. 'Images of the Jewish Body: Three Medical Views from the Jewish Enlightenment.' *Bulletin of the History of Medicine* 69 (1995), 349–66

Gilman, Sander L. *Difference and Pathology: Stereotypes of Sexuality, Race, and Madness*. Ithaca, N.Y.: Cornell University Press, 1985

Herrlinger, Robert. *History of Medical Illustration from Antiquity to 1600*. Trans. Graham Fulton-Smith. Munich: Editions Medicina Rara and Heinz Moos Verlagsgesellschaft, 1970

Laqueur, Thomas. *Making Sex: Body and Gender from the Greeks to Freud*. Cambridge, Mass.: Harvard University Press, 1990

O'Malley, C.D., and J.B. de C.M. Saunders. *Leonardo da Vinci on the Human Body*. New York: Schuman, 1952

Persaud, T.V.N. *Early History of Human Anatomy: From Antiquity to the Beginning of the Modern Era*. Springfield, Ill.: Charles C. Thomas, 1984

– *A History of Anatomy in the Post-Vesalian Era*. Springfield, Ill.: Charles C. Thomas, 1997

Richardson W.F., and J.B. Carman. 'On Translating Vesalius.' *Medical History* 38 (1994), 281–302

Roberts, K.B., and J.D.W. Tomlinson. *The Fabric of the Body: European Traditions of Anatomical Illustration*. Oxford: Clarendon Press, 1992

Schiebinger, Londa. 'Skeletons in the Closet: The First Illustrations of the Female Skeleton in Eighteenth-Century Anatomy.' In *The Making of the Modern Body: Sexuality and Society in the Nineteenth Century*, ed. Catherine Gallagher and Thomas Laqueur, 42–82. Berkeley: University of California Press, 1987

– *Nature's Body: Gender in the Making of Modern Science*. Boston: Beacon Press, 1993

Schultz, Bernard. *Art and Anatomy in Renaissance Italy*. Ann Arbor, Mich.: UMI Research Press, 1985

Sherrington, Charles. *The Endeavour of John Fernel*. Cambridge: Cambridge University Press, 1946.

Singer, Charles Joseph. *A Short History of Anatomy from the Greeks to Harvey*. 2nd edn. New York: Dover Publications, 1957

Stafford, Barbara Maria. *Body Criticism: Imaging the Unseen in Enlightenment Art and Medicine*. Cambridge, Mass., and London: MIT Press, 1991

Von Staden, Heinrich. *Herophilus: The Art of Medicine in Early Alexandria: Edition, Translation, Essays.* Cambridge: Cambridge University Press, 1989

Wolfe, D.E. 'Sydenham and Locke on the Limits of Anatomy.' *Bulletin of the History of Medicine* 35 (1961), 193–220

On Canada

Leblond, Sylvio. 'Anatomistes et résurrectionistes au Canada, et plus particulièrement dans la province de Québec.' *Canadian Medical Association Journal* 95 (1966), 1193–7, 1247–51

MacGillivray, Royce. 'Body Snatching in Ontario.' *Canadian Bulletin of Medical History* 5 (1988), 51–60

Robinson, Clayton L.N. *J.C. Boileau Grant: Anatomist Extraordinary.* Canadian Medical Lives Series, no. 14. Toronto: Hannah Institute and Dundurn Press, 1993

Shepherd, Francis J. *Reminiscences of Student Days and Dissecting Room.* Montreal: The Author, 1919

CHAPTER THREE

Interrogating Life: History of Physiology*

We must never make experiments to confirm our ideas, but simply to control them.

Claude Bernard, *An Introduction to the Study of Experimental Medicine*, 1865, 38

Definition

Physiology is the study of the function of living beings. From a medical perspective, it stands both in relation and in opposition to anatomy, the study of structure. The word 'physiology,' derived from Greek, means the study of nature. It was used infrequently in antiquity by Galen and others; however, in modern times, it has come to represent a separate discipline with well-defined methods.

Four Recurrent Themes

Throughout history, physiology has attempted to identify and classify the fundamental properties of life. Functions of living beings are divided into smaller tasks, each a physiological process in itself. For example, nutrition can be divided into alimentation, mastication, swallowing, digestion, absorption, transportation, growth, repair, and excretion. Similarly, other functions – such as locomotion and

*Educational objectives for this chapter are found on p. 394.

reproduction – can be treated as ensembles of smaller tasks. In various permutations and combinations, these properties have always been the focus of physiology. Sometimes they were given different names or were grouped in different patterns, but in virtually every period the functions have been 'reified' until they became concrete objects or beings in themselves.

Three of the four themes in this chapter are dualistic. The first is conceptual: the relationship between mechanism and vitalism. Mechanism is the reduction of life to physical and chemical forces; it is sometimes related to materialism, which defines all existence in terms of tangible matter. Vitalism is the view that life is governed by forces peculiar only to living beings – forces which cannot be reduced to physical laws. The life force of vitalism has often been associated with theological notions of spirit or soul, and its proponents have sometimes been devoutly religious. But the vital force of physiologists should not be equated with divine spirits. Neither mechanism nor vitalism satisfies all explanatory problems. When one mode of thinking dominates, a reactive swing back toward the other usually follows.

The second dualistic theme is about method of inquiry: the relationship between teleology and empiricism. The word 'teleology,' often defined as 'the doctrine of first [or final] causes,' refers to knowledge of purpose. 'Empiricism' refers to knowledge obtained through 'pure' observation without theoretical bias. Both methods deal with cause and effect. But teleology implies a confident belief in the possibility of uncovering the ultimate reason for a certain function. Empirical methods, on the other hand, are supposedly confined only to observed events and their immediate (and equally observable) causes. Teleology was more influential in ancient physiology than it is today; a few centuries ago, it was devalued by scientists who preferred empirical methods and explanations as they established principles for experimentation on life. Virtually every problem in physiology could be reformulated with the question 'Why?' But the search for purpose is no longer the overtly stated aim of scientific experiments. Rather, the scientific method now purports to explore 'how' and confines experiments to observation of events in natural or manipulated environments.

The dualistic tensions between mechanism and vitalism and

between teleology and empiricism are directly connected to a third – the relationship between speculation and experimentation. 'Armchair physiology,' as the speculative type has been called, refers to the physiology practised until modern times. But the dominance of speculation in the past did not exclude experimentation. The experimental *method* is relatively modern, but physiological experiments have been conducted for at least two thousand years. Nor should we think that speculation has no role in scientific investigation today.

The final theme is sociological: the rise of physiology as a separate discipline or profession. A desire to explain life phenomena has always been part of human character; in antiquity, however, a physiologist was most likely to be a philosopher. After the sixteenth century, a physiologist was an anatomist, or perhaps a doctor. In the nineteenth century, separate chairs or departments of physiology were founded. Now, physiology is its own unique discipline with institutes, societies, journals, chairs, departments, and conferences. But we may be witnessing a decline in the generic all-purpose physiologist as subspecialties emerge, such as respirology, endocrinology, and neurophysiology. Psychology has invaded physiology, and it is through this window that I will bring the chapter back to the first theme of vitalism and mechanism.

An Overview of the History of Physiology

Throughout most of human history, a knowledge of physiology was far more important to medicine than a knowledge of anatomy. Structure had little to do with concepts of disease, nor was it essential for explaining how bodies work (see chapter 2). To explain life function, the Greeks embraced the notion of balance in four humours: black bile, yellow bile, phlegm, and blood. The four humours were cognates of, and combined the characteristics of, the four elements in the Greek 'periodic table': earth, air, fire, and water. The power of this theory can be found in the works of many ancient writers, including Hippocrates and Galen. Its roots may extend to an even older tradition, for the Ayurvedic writings of ancient India refer to three similar humours: *vayu* (air), *pitta* (bile), and *kapha* (phlegm). These three combined with other nutrients to

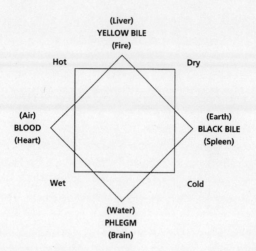

Schematic arrangement illustrating the properties and relationship of the four humours and four elements in Greek science. Mark Howes, Queen's University

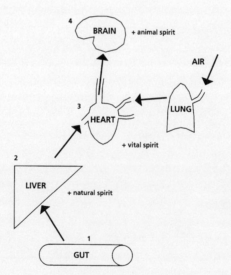

Schematic illustration of Galen's physiology. Mark Howes, Queen's University

form seven basic tissues, one of which was blood (*rakta*). The ancient Greeks also conceived of a life force (*enhormonta*, or *pneuma*) that permeated and sustained living beings.

Much simplified, Galenic understanding of nutrition and circulation proceeded as follows: Food is consumed, absorbed, and transformed in the liver into blood with natural spirit. It passes to the lung, where it is imbued with air or vital spirit (*pneuma zoticon*). It then flows outward, in both arteries and veins, to all the organs including the brain, which employs it to make additional animal spirit (*pneuma psychicon*), the source of motion. The health of an individual depends on the balance of humours and the strength of the life forces.

Galen imagined that blood constantly flowed outward from the heart, like water in an irrigation ditch. To make the concept 'work,' he postulated the existence of pores in the heart. Incredulous observers wonder how Galen could have mistaken the anatomy of the heart and the direction of blood flow, but human dissections were largely forbidden during his time.

A Thought Experiment

Limit yourself to what Galen knew and the methods of investigation available to him. Then try to refute his theory.

Galen was not an 'armchair physiologist'; he performed many experiments on animals to determine the relative importance of the brain, heart, lungs, and liver. A teleological framework is evident in his writing – each body part had certain specific faculties: attractive, retentive, alterative, repulsive, or eliminative. The following passage from his treatise *On the Natural Faculties* is derived from an experiment in which he tied the ureters and the urethra. It displays both teleology and vitalism:

In fact, those who are enslaved to their sects are not merely devoid of all knowledge, but they will not even stop to learn! Instead of listening as they ought, to the reasons why liquid can enter the bladder through the ureters, but is unable to go back the same way ... they refuse to learn; they even go so far as to scoff and maintain that the kidneys as well as many other things have been made by nature *for no purpose!* ...

If we are not going to grant the kidneys a faculty for attracting this particular quality ... we shall discover no other reason. For surely as everyone sees that either the kidneys must attract the urine or the veins propel it. (Bk. 1:13, 15)

Galen's physiology appealed to the Christian church. His references to the life force were conflated with the 'soul,' and his dogmatic formulations took on the aura of biblical edict. As a result, Galenic notions were repeated, commented on, and copied for generations. If doubts arose, they were not expressed until the fifteenth and sixteenth centuries (see chapter 2).

The overthrow of Galenic theory was gradual. For example, in 1553, a decade after Vesalius's great *Fabrica*, the Spanish physician and cleric Michael Servetus was denounced as a heretic by the religious reformer John Calvin. Servetus had refuted Galen by announcing that blood did not pass through the cardiac septum but went from the right heart to the left through the lungs – an early description of the pulmonary circulation. For this and other 'heresies,' he was jailed and then burned alive.

The Advent of Mechanism

Despite draconian measures to preserve Galenic authority, attacks eventually arose on all sides. Galen's critics claimed that he had ignored effective therapies and that he had failed to describe two important scourges of more recent times: plague and syphilis (see chapter 7). Then, in 1628, the English physician William Harvey published his famous book *On the Motion of the Heart*, explaining how blood circulated through the lungs and the body.

Harvey's discovery was no accident. Several preconditions, both anatomical and conceptual, had set the stage. First, at Padua he had learned of the valves in the veins from anatomy teachers who had known of Vesalius. Anatomically, then, he knew that blood in the veins flowed toward the heart. Second, using mathematical calculations based on the pulse and the stroke volume, he reasoned that if blood did not circulate, the liver would have to manufacture four hundred gallons (1,800 litres) of blood a day – vastly more, it seemed, than could be fabricated from average daily food intake. Third, Harvey was influenced by philosophical notions of cycles in nature and by the new mechanical pumps and fire engines in the world around him.

Harvey's experiments on animals merely confirmed this prior reasoning; yet he appears to have hesitated for more than a decade before publishing what would be seen as a radical revision. His argument relied on anatomical observations and calculations, and was removed from ancient theorizing or speculation. As a result, many cite his book as the beginning of modern physiology.

Following Harvey, others were inspired to seek mechanistic explanations for life functions. A numerical passion flowed into medicine from other disciplines preoccupied with finding simpler ways of describing events. Typifying the agenda of his era, Harvey's contemporary Galileo Galilei said, 'Measure all that is measurable and make those things measurable which have hitherto not been measured' (Rothschuh 1973, 76). In this new tradition, the Italian physician Santorio Santorio of Venice and Padua invented a pendulum machine to count the pulse. To measure body heat, he devised a large, unwieldy thermometer, an elaborate precursor of the smaller instruments that were used in clinical practice two centuries later. But the best known of Santorio's inventions was a metabolic balance chair, in which he spent much of his life, often eating and sleeping there. By carefully weighing his ingesta and excreta, Santorio calculated a daily average loss of 1.25 kg in the form of 'insensible perspiration.'

René Descartes, the seventeenth-century French philosopher and mathematician, expressed the philosophic mood by explaining bodily functions according to mechanical laws and without denying the existence of God. To explain sensation and reaction, Descartes invoked small, rapidly moving particles – 'animal spirits' – which travelled in hollow nerves. Muscles contracted on hydraulic principles, swollen by the in-rush of animal spirits. Descartes knew of

> **Descartes Compares a Sick Man to a Poorly Made Clock**
> (in contrast to a healthy man and a well-made clock)
>
> A sick man is in truth no less the creation of God than is man
> in full health ... A clock, composed of wheels and counter-
> weights, is no less exactly obeying all the laws of nature when it
> is badly made and does not mark the time correctly than when
> it completely fulfills the intention of its maker; so also the
> human body may be considered as a machine, so built and
> composed of bones, nerves, muscles, veins, blood, and skin
> that even if there were no mind in it, it would not cease to
> move in all the ways it does at present when it is not moved
> under the direction of the will.
>
> Descartes, *Meditations*, 1641. Trans. Lawrence J. Lafleur
> (Indianapolis and New York: Bobbs Merrill, 1960), 138–9

Harvey's treatise; in his theory, however, blood circulated, not
because it was pumped by the heart but because it was heated in the
heart to projectile expansion.

For Descartes, heat, not life force, was the major characteristic of
life. He recognized the existence of a divinely created soul, which he
equated with the mind and located in the pineal gland. But this soul
was separate from bodily operations. Animals were alive, but they did
not have souls. This separation of soul from body, expressed by Descartes (although he had predecessors), is often referred to as Carte-
sian 'mind-body dualism.' Ignoring the mind to focus on the body
resulted in a number of scientific treatises that represented the body
in mechanistic terms. Mind-body dualism also provoked debate over
the relationship between experience, structure, and illness. Critics
soon challenged the inadequacies of dualism. In many ways, the controversy has yet to be resolved, although it is largely ignored in biomedical research. The medicine subtended by such a philosophy was
called 'iatromechanism.'

Iatromechanists defined and described disease through physical

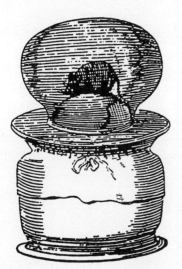

Mouse in a jar. From John Mayow, *Tracta-
tus duo quorum*, 1668. The consumed air
is measured by displacement of the mem-
brane.

analogies involving pumps, levers, springs, and pulleys. These physiologists also noticed that chemistry could mimic the living phenomena of fermentation, combustion, and decomposition. Because
bodily processes could be described in similar terms, iatrochemistry
became a specialized subset of early modern physiology. By the
seventeenth century, sulphur, mercury, and salt had expanded the
traditional four elements of the periodic table. All elements, old and
new, participated in explanations of life and disease.

The English iatrochemist John Mayow, taking his lead from Descartes's equation of heat and life, studied living beings as units of
combustion – a candle needs air to burn, just as animals need air to
live. Placing a lit candle under a jar inverted in water, he used the
rising level of water to measure the air consumed. He observed that
the candle went out when about one-fifth of the air was gone and
concluded that only some, not all, air could sustain burning. He
repeated the experiment using a mouse instead of a candle and
noticed that the mouse died when the same proportion of air had
been consumed. Again he concluded that only some air was able to
support life. But was the 'breathable air' the same as the 'burnable
air'? To answer the question, he placed a mouse and a candle
together in the jar. Both were extinguished faster than they had

been when alone, and still only one-fifth of the air had been consumed. Mayow thereby brought life closer to combustion.

During the late-seventeenth and early-eighteenth centuries, several physiologists reacted to what they considered the exaggerated mechanism of the times. Among them were the German Georg Stahl and the French physician Julien Offray de La Mettrie. Stahl, who began as a mechanist, provided the label 'phlogiston' for the combustible portion of air. It had been interesting, even useful, he said, to separate the soul from the body. But he soon found that the separation hindered investigation of problems such as voluntary motion. Stahl thought that in emphasizing the physical sciences, the iatro-mechanists had fostered a trend away from life itself. How, he asked, could attractive but simplistic analogies – describing the heart as a pump, or heat as a driving force – refute the existence of an underlying life force that moves the heart or generates heat? Mechanistic physiologists simply ignored these questions.

Stahl reintroduced the ancient concept of a life force in terms of a gaslike *anima* that acted like the newly discovered but invisible gravity of Isaac Newton. For Stahl, a lifeless body was a chemical soup that would simply decompose. The *anima* was the force that kept it alive, in good repair, and moving. Eighteenth-century Europe divided into two camps, physiologically speaking: the mechanistic and the vitalistic.

The Swiss physician-naturalist Albrecht von Haller was perhaps the most prolific physiologist of the eighteenth century. In his *Physiological Elements of the Human Body* (1757–66), he redefined two previously known properties of life: sensibility (perception) and irritability (response). All living beings – plants and animals – were said to possess both. Study of these properties, which we would now call neurophysiology, was the central focus of life research for at least a century. Von Haller based his conclusions on anatomical observations, and he conducted animal experiments. Using similar methods, his Italian contemporary, Lazzaro Spallanzani, studied reproduction, concluding that all living beings were descended from others and that spontaneous generation did not occur. But the debate over spontaneous generation raged on for another century before it was put to rest by Louis Pasteur.

Oxygen was discovered in the eighteenth century by Joseph B. Priestley and Antoine-Laurent Lavoisier (see chapter 8). Soon it was generally accepted that all animal life required oxygen. Life, like a flame, could be seen as combustion of carbon in the presence of oxygen. This idea corresponded well with the parallel notion of heat as life.

In 1780, the Italian Aloisius Galvani made the startling observation that passage of an electric current through the leg of a frog could produce reflex movement. Electricity thus joined gravity and the life force as an invisible but powerful entity that produced movement.

Positivism and the Rise of Experimental Physiology

In the eighteenth century, physiologists had been preoccupied with the causes of life functions, but in the nineteenth century they turned to the more elemental definition of 'facts.' This trend was a product of the rise of positivism, a rigid extrapolation of the older sensualism, a philosophy of knowledge preoccupied with observation (see chapter 2).

Positive philosophy was named and described by Auguste Comte of France, who is often called 'the founder of sociology.' Its tenets were already unarticulated ideals for many of his scientific contemporaries. Postmodern philosophy has criticized positivism, especially its confidence in the existence of immutable 'facts,' which are now seen as constructs susceptible to the biases of the observer (see, for example, Fleck 1979). Nevertheless, physiology and medicine are still strongly positivistic.

Physiological research in the early nineteenth century continued to focus on anatomical structure to locate the site of biological processes and elucidate their nature. By the time anatomy became essential to medical education, physiologists were well placed to profit; however, virtually all medical anatomy was done on cadavers. Because a dead body was unsuitable for the study of life, physiologists conducted their experiments on living animals, and usually not at medical schools. Sometimes, like Santorio, they used themselves as subjects.

Tenets of Positivism

- All knowledge evolves through three increasingly sophisticated stages:

  theological: explanations based on gods or supernatural powers

  metaphysical: explanations based on immaterial forces

  positive: explanations based only on direct observations.

  The most positive systems of knowledge are mathematics and astronomy; the least are biology and the social sciences.
- A search for cause(s) of events is futile, because causes are unknowable.
- Instead, positive knowledge stems from observed events or 'facts.'
- Numbers should be used to describe observations to avoid subjective verbal metaphors that drag science back into metaphysics or theology.
- Positivism seeks to establish laws through correlation of facts.

Based on Auguste Comte, *Cours de philosophie positive*, 1830–42.
Trans. Frederick Ferré (Indianapolis: Hackett, 1988)

In a few years of vigorous research following the French Revolution, François Xavier Bichat, a young genius from Lyons working in Paris, attempted to define the properties of life by exploring aspects of existence that disappeared with death. His methods were both anatomical (he adopted the notion of tissues as anatomical structures and used surgical methods) and philosophical (he classified life functions into two types: animal and organic). After a winter of frenzied investigation – during which he dissected six hundred corpses, taught at least two courses, and worked on several books – Bichat died of a sudden febrile illness at the age of thirty.

Inspired by Bichat, the French physician François Magendie vivisected unanesthetized animals to explore the properties of life.

Table 3.1
First national periodicals in physiology

Date	Country	Editor	Title
1795	Germany	Reil	*Archiv für Physiologie*
1821	France	Magendie	*Journal de physiologie*
1896	England	Foster	*Journal of Physiology*
1898	United States	Porter	*American Journal of Physiology*
1929	Canada	Collip	*Canadian Journal of Research*
1950	Worldwide		250 titles
1990	Worldwide		Thousands (or very few?)

In some famously cruel experiments, he showed that sensory and motor nerve fibres travelled together in the whole nerve, except near the spinal cord, where sensory fibres occupied the dorsal root and motor fibres, the ventral. Priority for this discovery resulted in a dispute with Charles Bell of England, who also had experimented on motor function. Bell went on to make other observations, especially on cranial nerves and the facial palsy that bears his name. Magendie extended his investigations to circulation, digestion, and the effects of drugs and 'poisons,' including rabies virus in saliva (see chapter 5). He hesitated to draw sweeping conclusions from his work, but he dismissed the vital forces of his predecessors as arbitrary assumptions. Yet he too was unable to avoid certain vitalistic concepts in his interpretations.

Magendie founded one of the first periodicals of physiology (see table 3.1). Essays on life function had been published since scholarly journalism began, but the creation of periodicals devoted to physiology was a nineteenth-century development.

A materialistic view of life appealed to many of Magendie's contemporaries. In 1828 Friedrich Wöhler, working in Berlin, synthesized urea, a substance previously thought to be a product of living processes only. It was said that vitalism was dead: no special forces were needed to explain life, because all vital functions, like urea, would eventually be reproduced in the laboratory. The research of the German chemist Justus von Liebig and his colleagues at Giessen was devoted to similar chemical interpretations of life processes. Liebig synthesized chloroform (1830), studied fermentation, discovered the amino acid tyrosine (1846), and wrote an influential textbook on what he called 'animal chemistry.'

Features of *Naturphilosophie*

Nature is a hierarchy, ranging from:
plants, characterized by a vegetative preoccupation with
  reproduction; to
insects and animals, characterized by their irritability; to
humans, characterized by their sensibility.

Not everyone agreed with the empirical spirit that had informed the investigations of Liebig and Magendie. A counter-movement, *Naturphilosophie*, emphasized intuition over empiricism and scorned experimentation. Its advocate, Friedrich von Schelling, described *Naturphilosophie* as speculation about life in terms of hierarchies and orders; it was based on the principle that nature was visible spirit, and spirit was invisible nature. Influenced by the ideas of the writer, J.W. von Goethe, who had studied the morphology of plants, Schelling urged a search for similarities in life functions in order to uncover the general cosmic patterns governing nature. *Naturphilosophie* appealed to many prominent German physicians, including J.C. Reil, F. Blumenbach, and Johannes Müller. Müller's influential handbook of physiology blended these ideas with evidence from experimental science.

Many histories recount how Schelling's *Nature Philosophy* 'retarded' the growth of 'real' science. But we might ask, Why did it develop when it did? Like many before him, Schelling was concerned with the mind-body problem. Even his critics seem to have regarded body organization as the product of an immaterial force – vital, spiritual, or creative. Both structure and function had to have some antecedent cause, yet the new positivistic experimentation rejected the search for causes as unwelcome teleological thinking. A debate over these modes of reasoning about life began in earnest. At the time, few could predict which perspective would emerge victorious; however, overt teleology would soon be hounded from the scientific method.

The most famous physiologists of the mid-nineteenth century were Claude Bernard of France and Karl Friedrich Wilhelm Ludwig of Germany. Their work formed the methodological basis of today's experimental physiology. A student of Magendie, Bernard was educated as a doctor but spent his life in animal research, making many discoveries on the formation of glycogen and other life processes. His main contribution, however, was the elaboration of an approach to experimentation, now known as the scientific method. Bernard would observe a phenomenon, localize it to an anatomical structure, and then surgically alter that structure in order to study its effects. His *Introduction to Experimental Physiology* (1865) laid out the philosophical and methodological principles of investigation. Bernard advocated isolating the event under study by controlling all conditions of the experiment. He endorsed the empirical view that everything needed to understand an event can be derived from rigorous observation of that event. Without denying a vital force, he claimed that only its consequences could be observed.

Bernard recognized that the living organism reacts to change in its environment to maintain a constant, or homeostatic, *milieu intérieur*. His work on both glycogen and diabetes was permeated with this ideal. At the end of his life, experimental physiology was greatly admired, especially in drug testing, but it was still peripheral to medical studies, which continued to be preoccupied with cadaveric research. Bernard never became a professor in a medical school; he worked at the Collège de France in Paris.

A Vignette

Bernard's home life was said to be unhappy because both his wife and daughter were antivivisectionists. My friend François Gallouin, also a physiologist, suggests that domestic discord may be beneficial to scientific work, since it favours long hours in the lab.

Germany poured uniquely large sums into education and purpose-built laboratories for scientific research, and soon became the leader in the establishment of physiological journals, chairs, and laboratories. Müller taught several scientists who went on to establish distinguished careers, including the Swiss histologist R.A. von Kolliker, the German neurologist Emil Du Bois-Reymond, and the German pathologist Rudolf Virchow. But Karl Ludwig's institute at Leipzig was the mecca for physiology.

Ludwig was firmly convinced that physics and chemistry could explain all life functions. Politically he was a liberal, and spiritually he was an atheist. His social and philosophic views were associated with his reductionist science, providing yet more fodder for the debate over the nature of life. He analysed renal and cardiovascular physiology, inventing mechanical devices to measure the previously unmeasurable – the kymograph (1846), and a *Stromuhr*, or 'stream clock' (1867), which monitored blood flow. Genealogies of Ludwig's disciples illustrate his powerful influence on physiology in Russia, Italy, England, Scandinavia, and the United States.

The surgeon William Beaumont was the first American to attract international fame for physiological investigation of an unusual case. In 1822 he treated the abdominal gunshot wound of a French Canadian, Alexis St Martin. Because the wound healed with an external fistula to the stomach, Beaumont could experiment on St Martin's digestion by tying string around pieces of meat and other foods, inserting them through the fistula, and retrieving them after varied periods of time. So eager was he to maintain the investigations that he often had St Martin live with him for up to two years at a time during the next decade. But the patient grew tired of the arrangement and returned to his home at St Thomas, in Joliette County, Quebec. At the age of seventy-eight, he was reported to be healthy with his fistula still open, but he was apprehensive of scientific designs upon him. When he died in 1880, William Osler received a telegram from St Martin's family, warning him to stay away and describing a deliberate delay before the exceptionally deep burial of the body. They hoped that decomposition and depth would dissuade doctors from attempts to dissect it.

Physiology in the Twentieth Century

Osler saw the integration of physiology in medicine as the 'growth of truth.' The rise of the discipline has been charted through the

On Accident in Discovery

Chance favours the prepared mind

> Saying attributed to Louis Pasteur, ca. 1854 (cited in
> Vallery-Radot 1927, 76–9)

Many inventors and discoverers ascribe their findings to 'accident,' 'serendipity,' or 'chance.' First-hand accounts notwithstanding, historians and philosophers of science regard chance as a bit-player rather than the *magister ludi*. Only when an observer knows that something is missing or needed is it likely to be found. An unexpected coincidence can bring a juxtaposition of circumstances to the attention of an observer who may be looking for something else. But a discovery will be made only if that observer has some insight or special knowledge – a 'lucky ticket' – that allows for correlation. The chance occurrence may have taken place many times in the past without a 'discovery.' For example, 'accidents' such as St Martin's may have occurred before, but it was Beaumont's prior knowledge of research elsewhere that enabled him to take full advantage of that particular fistulous stomach. Patterns of scientific communication, the conscious development of a method, and the existence of laboratories – and even, to a certain extent, relative amounts of research funding – tend to diminish the role left to chance.

increased attendance at international conferences – from 124 delegates representing eighteen countries at the first meeting in 1889, to 4,300 delegates from fifty-one countries by 1968. Once physiology became an experimental discipline, its relevance to medicine increased. First awarded in 1901, the Nobel prizes in medicine were also prizes in physiology; in general, they have been given for the reduction of life processes to physicochemical terms (see appendix A). Cardiac contraction and circulation were now electrical as well as muscular. Respiration was no longer a phenomenon of the lungs alone, but a physical and chemical event also operating at the level of cells, subcellular organelles, and molecules (see chapter 8). In the early twentieth century, hormones and vitamins were isolated and identified as the enzymes of living processes – the former being an intrinsic product of the organism; the latter, extrinsic and synthesized by other organisms (see chapter 13). In 1944, DNA was recognized as the stuff of heredity by Nova Scotia–born Oswald T. Avery.

Hormones, in particular, offer an interesting bridge between vitalistic and mechanistic views. The word 'hormone,' derived from the Greek ὁρμῶντα (hormonta), meaning 'I arouse' or 'I excite,' was used by Hippocrates and two millennia of other medical writers to describe the life force. 'Hormone,' as a modern scientific word, was coined in 1902 by the British physiologists W.M. Bayliss and E.H. Starling when they announced their discovery of secretin. In other words, when modern hormones were first conceived, they were recognized as the chemical translation of the life force. Among the most recent of hormone finds are the endorphins (found in the mid-1970s). Secreted in response to pleasurable events, they bind to internal receptors, which can also bind various narcotic drugs. More than any other product, the endorphins seem to fit into a mechanical conception of the mind-body link. The intellectual fervour over each endocrine or vitamin discovery was reflected in the Nobel Prizes. (On insulin, see chapter 5; on sex hormones, chapter 11; on endocrinology and stress, chapter 12; and on vitamins, chapter 13.)

Since the 1950s, psychology and psychiatry have both become increasingly physiological as perception and movement have been described in mechanical terms that can be measured and manipulated. The advent of major tranquillizers (neuroleptics) that help schizophrenics to manage their symptoms seemed to endorse a chemical theory of mind, as did the advent of lithium for bipolar disorders (see chapter 12). Oncology is now struggling to find methods to study the role of mind, thought, emotion, personality, spirituality, and behaviour in cancer outcomes.

The continued dominance of positivism means that our methods demand numbers. For example, the Quality of Life Index (1981), the McMaster Health Index Questionnaire (1982), and similar tools were invented to express qualitative information as a quantity. Here is the same mind-body problem that disturbed Stahl, Schelling, and others who are now known (and sometimes scorned) as vitalists. Our society, which derives quantitative indices to express quality, may do well to remember Claude Bernard's idea that most of life is qualitative: we use numbers simply to facilitate our understanding of it, not to define it.

Western society celebrates explanations of motion, will, and thought in terms of chemistry and physics as the most important accomplishments in medicine and physiology. One well might ask why physicochemical discoveries attract fame and reward while other less reductionist observations are not celebrated. For example, why is it that the efforts of scientist Linus Pauling and the founders of International Physicians for the Prevention of Nuclear War (see chapter 6) were rewarded with Nobel prizes for peace, not medicine, although their actions may have prevented millions of deaths if not global annihilation? Does medicine's close identification with experimental physiology (and its attendant positivism) explain its difficulty with the less measurable social, cultural, environmental, and economic determinants of health? Is medicine's focus on cure rather than prevention a product of its link to experimental physiology? Does this link explain medical preference for biological therapies over others?

Historians have tried to connect philosophical attitudes in biological science to the political and religious views of individual scientists. Some correlations have been found, but no pervasive consensus can be reached. Indeed, the most convincing arguments suggest that all science partakes of both vitalism and mechanism – what differs is the extent to which scientists are willing to admit it. Recognizing that 'vitalism' had taken on pejorative connotations in scientific circles, one historian characterized the debate between vitalists and mechanists as a fight between the 'modest' and the 'arrogant' (Canguilhem 1965, 86, 95, 99). Those who try to address aspects of life that cannot yet be expressed in 'scientific' terms are called vitalists, usually by others and not by themselves. Vitalists offend reductionists by being perceived as too humble – possessed of a fatal modesty, *sophrosyne*, the opposite of *hubris* (see Ingelfinger 1980). In return, reductionists offend vitalists not only for arrogance (although that is

Another Vignette: What Does the Author Think of Vitalism? of Religion?

Both [Francis] Crick and [James] Watson [Nobel laureates 1962] had been influenced by Erwin Schrödinger's *What Is Life?*, a popularization of genetics seen from a physicist's perspective. Crick's approach to biology was quite different from Schrödinger's because Crick was an atheist and Schrödinger's perception of life was vitalistic. What Crick found of value, however, was Schrödinger's recognition that many of the uniquely biological properties, such as heredity, were amenable to an analysis that physicists had successfully used for the structure of inanimate matter.

Elof Axel Carlson, 'Francis Crick,' in Daniel Fox et al.,
Nobel Laureates in Physiology or Medicine (New York: Garland,
1990), 111–12

part of it) but also for the necessary limitations that they are forced to impose on their investigations, because certain conditions, such as attitude, personality, pleasure, and value, cannot be controlled or measured. Nobel laureate Peter Medawar wrote that biologists no longer need to invoke vital forces, and vitalistic ideas fall into the 'limbo of that which is disregarded' (Medawar and Medawar 1983, 277). But so-called vitalists refuse to disregard or discount the as yet unmeasurable phenomena.

Teleology may be unacceptable as a framework for the scientific exploration of life, but 'Why?' is the most seductive question we can ask of science (and of history!). Speculation will continue to thrive in the minds of creative scientists, and consequently thinking that gets labelled as 'vitalistic' cannot be suppressed. The concept of irreducible complex processes still proves to be useful – even for those who pretend to repudiate vitalism – if only for providing a language to address the unexplained: What makes a DNA molecule unzip? Why are some of us sane and others insane? Why do we not decompose during life? Why are some physicochemical mixtures alive and some dead? It is fascinating to notice how often scientists who win the Nobel Prize eventually write philosophic works, in which they acknowledge questions that are not (yet) amenable to laboratory investigation as a stimulus to further research. (On reading this chapter my physiologist colleague Steven Iscoe observed how rarely award-winning humanists ever do the reverse!)

Suggestions for Further Reading

Bernard, Claude. *An Introduction to the Study of Experimental Medicine.* 1865. Trans. Henry Copley Green, 1927. Reprint, New York: Dover, 1957

Canguilhem, Georges. *La connaissance de la vie.* 1965. 2nd edn. Paris: Vrin, 1980

– *Ideology and Rationality in the History of the Life Sciences.* Trans. Arthur Goldhammer. Cambridge, Mass., and London: MIT Press, 1988

Coleman, William. *Biology in the Nineteenth Century.* London and New York: Cambridge University Press, 1977

Coleman, William, and Frederic L. Holmes, eds. *The Investigative Enterprise: Experimental Physiology in Nineteenth-Century Medicine.* Berkeley; Los Angeles; London: University of California Press, 1988

Cranefield, Paul F. *The Way In and the Way Out.* Mt Kisco, N.Y.: Futura, 1974 [on the Bell-Magendie controversy]

Duchesneau, F. *La physiologie des lumières: Empirisme, modèles, et théories.* The Hague, Boston, London: Martinus Nijhoff, 1982

Farley, John. *The Spontaneous Generation Controversy from Descartes to Oparin.* Baltimore: Johns Hopkins University Press, 1977

Fleck, Ludwik. *Genesis and Development of a Scientific Fact.* Chicago: University of Chicago Press, 1979

Fox, Daniel M., Marcia Meldrum, and Ira Rezak, eds. *Nobel Laureates in Physiology or Medicine: A Biographical Dictionary.* New York: Garland, 1990

Frank, Robert Gregg. *Harvey and the Oxford Physiologists: A Study of Scientific Ideas and Social Interaction.* Berkeley: University of California Press, 1980

French, R.K. *William Harvey's Natural Philosophy.* Cambridge and New York: Cambridge University Press, 1994

French, Richard D. *Antivivisection and Medical Science in Victorian Society.* Princeton, N.J.: Princeton University Press, 1975

Fye, Bruce. *The Development of American Physiology: Scientific Medicine in the Nineteenth Century.* Baltimore and London: Johns Hopkins University Press, 1987

Geison, Gerald L. *Michael Foster and the Cambridge School of Physiology: The Scientific Enterprise in Late Victorian Society.* Princeton: Princeton University Press, 1978
– ed. *Physiology in the American Context, 1850–1940.* Bethesda, American Physiological Society, 1987
Goodfield, G.J. *The Growth of Scientific Physiology.* London: Hutchinson, 1960
Grmek, Mirko D. 'Le rôle du hasard dans le genèse des découvertes scientifiques.' *Medicina nei secolo* 13 (1976), 277–305
– *Première revolution biologigue: Reflexions sur la physiologie et la médecine du XVIIe siècle.* Paris: Payot, 1990
– *Claude Bernard et la méthode expérimentale.* Paris: Payot, 1991
Haigh, Elizabeth. *Xavier Bichat and the Medical Theory of the Eighteenth Century.* London: Wellcome Institute for the History of Medicine, 1984
Hall, Diana Long. *Why Do Animals Breathe?* New York: Arno Press, 1981
Hall, Thomas S. *Ideas of Life and Matter: Studies in the History of General Physiology, 600 BC–1900 AD.* 2 vols. Chicago: University of Chicago Press, 1969
Holmes, Frederic L. *Claude Bernard and Animal Chemistry: The Emergence of a Scientist.* Cambridge: Harvard University Press, 1974
– *Hans Krebs.* 2 vols. New York: Oxford University Press, 1991–3
– *Between Biology and Medicine: The Formation of Intermediary Metabolism.* Berkeley: University of California at Berkeley, 1992
Ingelfinger, F.J. 'Arrogance.' *New England J. Medicine* 303 (1980), 1507–11
Judson, Horace Freeland. *The Eighth Day of Creation: Makers of the Revolution in Biology.* New York: Simon and Schuster, 1979
Kawakita, Yosio, Shizu Sakai, and Yasuo Otsuka. *The Comparison between Concepts of Life Breath in East and West. Proceedings of the 15th International Symposium on the Comparative History of Medicine – East and West.* Tokyo: Ishiyaku EuroAmerica, 1995
Lesch, John E. *Science and Medicine in France: The Emergence of Experimental Physiology, 1790–1855.* Cambridge, Mass. and London: Harvard University Press, 1984
Medawar, Peter B., and J.S. Medawar. *Aristotle to Zoos: A Philosophical Dictionary of Biology.* Cambridge, Mass.: Harvard University Press, 1983
Olby, Robert. *The Path to the Double Helix.* Seattle: University of Washington, 1974
Osler, William. *The Growth of Truth.* London: H. Frowde, 1906
Paton, William D.M. *Man and Mouse: Animals in Medical Research.* Oxford and New York: Oxford University Press, 1984
Rothschuh, Karl E. *History of Physiology.* Trans. Guenter B. Risse. New York: Robert E. Krieger, 1973
Taton, René. *Reason and Chance in Scientific Discovery.* London: Hutchinson Scientific and Technical, 1957

Tuchman, Arleen Marcia. *Science, Medicine, and the State in Germany: The Case of Baden, 1815–1871.* New York and Oxford: Oxford University Press, 1993
Vallery-Radot, René. *Life of Pasteur.* Trans. R.I. Devonshire. Garden City, N.Y.: Garden City Publishing, 1927
Williams, Elizabeth A. *The Physical and the Moral: Anthropology, Physiology, and Philosophical Medicine in France, 1750–1850.* Cambridge and New York: Cambridge University Press, 1994

On Canada

Bensley, Edward H. 'Alexis St Martin.' *Canadian Medical Association Journal* 80 (1959), 907–9
Connor, J.T.H. 'Cruel Knives? Vivisection and Biomedical Research in Victorian English Canada.' *Canadian Bulletin of Medical History* 14 (1997), 37–64
Fournier, Marcel, Yves Gingras, and Othmar Keel, eds. *Sciences et médecine au Québec: Perspectives sociohistoriques.* Québec: Institut québécois de recherche sur la culture, 1987
Fox, Michael Allen. *The Case for Animal Experimentation: An Evolutionary and Ethical Perspective.* Berkeley: University of California Press, 1986
Moore, Terence. *Joe Doupe: Bedside Physiologist.* Toronto: Hannah Institute for the History of Medicine and Dundurn Press, 1989
Pitcock, C.H. 'William Beaumont, M.D. and Malpractice: The Mary Dugan Case, 1844.' *Journal of the History of Medicine and Allied Sciences* 47 (1992), 153–62
Potter, Paul, and Hubert Soltan. 'Murray Llewellyn Barr, O.C.: 20 June 1908– 4 May 1995.' *Bibliographical Memoirs of the Royal Society of London* 43 (1997), 31–46
Segall, Harold N. 'William Stairs Morrow: Canada's First Physiologist-Cardiologist.' *Canadian Medical Association Journal* 114 (1976), 543–5

CHAPTER FOUR

Science of Suffering: History of Pathology*

Life is short, the Art long, opportunity fleeting, experience treacherous, judgment difficult.

Hippocrates, *Aphorisms*, I, 1

Pathology as a System of Medical Knowledge

Medicine is not a science; rather, it is an applied technology or an art that makes extensive use of science. Medicine's claims to being scientific are anchored in pathology as the study of disease. Pathology, from the Greek words for 'suffering' and 'theory about,' is literally the study of suffering. But its meaning has narrowed to represent material knowledge about disease.

Humans have always tried to understand illness, injury, and death. In other words, pathology has always been practised, even if it was not explicitly named. Pathology is a system of knowledge used to draw conclusions about illness. It changed through the centuries, but in every time and place it was validated by current science and philosophy. Past pathologies may not resemble our own, but they have always acknowledged the contemporary view of 'science.'

Functions of Pathology

Despite differences in content, the functions of pathology are uni-

*Educational objectives for this chapter are found on p. 394.

versal. First, pathology is used to explain suffering, to account for why and how humans are subject to pain and death. 'Why me?' ask sick people. Illness demands a 'logical' explanation, rooted either in the cultural and spiritual ideas of sin and blame or in the more material and 'scientific' ideas of structure, function, heredity, contagion, and risk.

Second, pathology is used to identify or *define* the ailment from which a person suffers: the process of diagnosis. Doctors use signs that point – just like signs on the highway – to the diagnosis or prognosis. Good clinical skills convert subjective symptoms into objective signs. A physical examination yields more signs. Signs are not simply the product of observation; they also contain knowledge. For example, the symptom of squeezing chest pain becomes a sign of heart disease with the addition of medical knowledge.

This diagnostic function of pathology has an important corollary: in identifying that which is 'abnormal' or sick, pathology also tends to identify that which is 'normal.' The line between normal and abnormal is conditioned by culture, religion, economics, race, class, gender, and other social and biological factors. Phenomena once thought to be 'abnormal,' or 'diseased,' are now considered variants of normal. Examples include visceroptosis (the drooping gut syndrome) and homosexuality (see chapters 10 and 12). Conversely, other phenomena now thought to be diseases were inconceivable only a short time ago. Examples include psychiatric problems, hypertension, carcinoma *in situ*, and AIDS.

Third, pathology is used to predict outcomes. In some cultures, especially in antiquity, accurate prognosis was at least as important as an ability to cure. Medical prediction based on a few reliable signs relating to an individual resembles priestly divination: 'You will die on the seventh day.' Prognosis is still an important function of pathology, but it is now couched in statistics, derived from the experience of a cohort, and defined by age, sex, diagnosis, and extent of lesion. For example, we speak of five-year survival, the 50 per cent mortality index, and risk.

Fourth, pathology is used to justify treatments. As we will see in chapter 5, most treatments were discovered through observation rather than reasoning (i.e., empirically). Therapeutic rationales were often applied post hoc; in some cases, they still are. They relate an apparently effective treatment to the scientific formulation of a problem. Sometimes, a remedy of choice persists while the explanation of how it works alters considerably.

Finally, pathology has been used to prove the reasonableness of an explanation, a diagnosis, or a course of action. Postmortem examination is the most obvious form of this function. In Europe, occasional records of autopsies for retrospective diagnosis can be traced to the late thirteenth century. For both legal and medical reasons, autopsy is still the ultimate challenge of our knowledge system. Was the diagnosis correct? Could anything else have been done? Anatomical proof became more important after 1800, when diseases were linked to organic changes and when the number of lawsuits for malpractice began to rise.

Disease versus Illness   *(F.   P. / 93 FF.*

Humans still suffer from the illnesses that plagued our prehistoric and simian ancestors. The subjective aspects of being sick do not change – pain, fever, swelling, vomiting, diarrhea, deformity, injury, loss of weight, loss of blood, loss of function, loss of life – but medical *ideas* about illness change. They are what we call disease.

We tend to think of illness and disease as identical and use the words interchangeably. For this discussion, however, and following philosophers, the word 'illness' is used to designate individual suffering; the word 'disease,' pertains to ideas about the illness. 'Illness' exists as the real suffering felt by a person; 'disease' exists only as a theory constructed to explain the illness, its presumed cause, and its target. More than semantic, the distinction is useful in the philosophy of medical knowledge, or medical epistemology, the study of how we know what we think we know.

Medical knowledge is the ability to recognize and respond to disease. Therefore, constructing, recognizing, and treating disease is its central enterprise. Disease concepts are 'built' from observations of many individual sufferings of a similar nature. They take into account the patient, the illness, and the presumed cause, but they are also influenced by the observer/doctor. Diseases are given characteristics (symptoms), names (diagnoses), life expectancies (course), antici-

---

The Hippocratic Triangle

The art has three factors, the disease, the patient, the physician. The physician is the servant of the art. The patient must cooperate with the physician in combatting the disease.

Hippocrates, *Epidemics I*, 11

---

pated outcomes (prognoses), and recommended treatments. A cause is implied in the concept constructed for a disease even when the cause is unknown.

If diseases are intangible thoughts about various illnesses, then what single theory or definition can be found to explain all diseases? In other words, what do all diseases have in common? So far, no single explanation has been found that successfully applies to every account of disease. However, one theory dominates medical practice – the *organismic, or individual, theory* of disease.

The organismic theory holds that diseases are bad, discontinuous, and affect individuals. From the perspective of an organism (individual), this theory is difficult to refute. By its very name, medicine subscribes to this ideal: diseases must be bad, because individuals seek help to be rid of them. Medical education is aimed at how to recognize and cure disease. Most medical accounts of disease have conformed to this view even if the authors had never heard of the theory.

Now the basis of the medical model, the organismic theory comfortably addresses the issue of the disease target, but offers little to explain what causes it. Throughout history, two additional perspectives about cause have vied for dominance. The first is the *ontological theory*, which holds that the causes come from outside the patient, that diseases vary one from another, and that they exist separate from the patient. The word 'ontology' stems from nouns derived from the Greek verb 'to be'; it emphasizes the idea of disease as a separate 'be-ing,' or entity.

A Thought Experiment about 'Illness' and 'Disease'

'Does smallpox exist?'

'No,' says the student aware of WHO's eradication of small-pox in 1979.

'Yes,' says the clever student, who read that the planned destruction of the remaining vials of smallpox virus has been deferred once again.

'But,' comes the philosophic reply, 'do the vials contain "smallpox" or do they contain the virus, which, when introduced into a human being, produces the illness that we label "smallpox" disease?'

Does smallpox exist? Is it a disease? An entity? An illness? An idea?

The second theory about the cause of disease is the *physiological theory*, which holds that causes emerge from inside the patient, that patients vary, and that diseases do not exist separate from patients.

These theories of disease can be used to analyse any account of illness and disease. A medical practitioner who approaches disease through the ontological theory will be concerned with what the patient *has*; conversely, a physiological perspective would emphasize who or what the patient *is*. Both cause-based theories have currency in modern medicine, and some disease descriptions seem to correspond to a combination of the two. At the end of this chapter, we will explore some criticisms of medical reasoning and another theory of disease that challenges the medical model.

Historical Overview of Pathology

Construction of disease concepts moved from spiritualistic accounts of nature, to careful bedside descriptions of illness, and then to the laboratory enterprise that is familiar to us today. The following pages briefly summarize the shift.

Supernatural Causes of Disease

At the beginning of Homer's epic poem, *The Iliad* (which originated sometime before 700 B.C.), the Greeks suffer a deadly pestilence, but they do not understand its cause. Few details about the illness are provided. They consult an oracle, who proclaims that their king has refused to return the daughter of a priest of Apollo for ransom and that the priest had appealed to his god who has punished all Greeks with the disease. The crowd confronts the king, the daughter is released, and the pestilence goes away.

The Book of Job from the Old Testament of the Bible (which also dates from the eighth century B.C.), describes another illness with a supernatural cause. The devout Job has a fine family, good health, and great wealth, but Satan tells God that Job is devout because he has everything. To prove that Job is constant, God wagers with Satan, who then destroys Job's family, his wealth, and his health. The bereaved Job suffers festering boils over his whole body, but he does not curse God, and after forty chapters of agony, God rewards him by restoring all his losses.

Both these accounts of illness conform to organismic and onto-logical views. The disease is bad and it comes from powers beyond the individual in order either to punish or to test the sufferers. The associated terror and misery are apparent, but the features of the illnesses seem unimportant, since few details are given. The pro-fessional healer or priest does not concentrate on the symptoms but looks widely for signs to determine why the deity has sent the afflic-tion. In this context, the patient's subjective opinion about the causes of the illness are given serious consideration, including the possibility that the disease may have moral, spiritual, or pedagogic functions. Treatment is the maintenance or restoration of integrity – righting wrongs, keeping faith.

Supernatural accounts of illness may have little currency in the modern science of pathology, but they continue to influence patients and policymakers. Diseases viewed as punishments include AIDS, eating disorders, and conditions related to smoking and alco-hol. On this view, some people are thought to deserve their illness and others feel outraged at being sick without having committed a 'sinful' act. The healthy can accept their good fortune as a token of their superiority. Similarly, chronic ailments such as arthritis and multiple sclerosis are called 'trials' – tests of character – and people who suffer uncomplainingly are said to have 'the patience of Job.'

Pathology at the Bedside

Greco-Roman Antiquity: Disease = Natural Imbalance

In the West, medical writings began in approximately the fifth century B.C. with a self-conscious refutation of the supernatural origins of disease. The Greco-Roman world had a pantheon of gods and an extensive mythology, but it also recognized a natural world of four elements and a healthy balance in the human body of four humours (see chapter 3).

The seventy treatises that make up the Hippocratic Corpus contain writings on medical philosophy and duties, for example, the *Oath*. Some disease descriptions from this period are classic examples of clinical observation, because they are recognizable as conditions diagnosed today. But pathology also looms large in the case histories, the descriptions of diseases and wounds, and the aphorisms. These last are sentences that summarize knowledge, usually for the elaboration of signs – for example, 'In athletes a perfect condition that is at its highest pitch is treacherous' (*Aphorisms*, I, 3); 'Old men endure fasting most easily, then men of middle age, youths very badly, and worst of all children, especially those of a liveliness greater than the ordinary' (*Aphorisms*, I, 13); and '[In] acute pain of the ear with ... high fever ... younger patients die ... on the seventh day or even earlier; old men die much later' (*Prognostic*, XXII).

Hippocratic pathology predicted, interpreted, and justified diseases and their treatments in concert with the best science of the day – clinical observation and reasoning. A good example is the famous text *The Sacred Disease*, a masterful description of what we now call epilepsy. The name was derived from the even older view that the sufferer was possessed by demons or touched by gods. But the author began with a clear statement: 'It is not, in my opinion, any more divine or more sacred than other diseases, but has a natural cause, and its supposed divine origin is due to men's inexperience and to their wonder at its peculiar character' (*Sacred Disease*, I). The clinical symptoms were described in detail: falling, shaking, loss of consciousness, incontinence. Affected children sensing the onset of an attack ('aura') would run to their mothers for comfort. This essay was based on the observation of many illness patterns. In explaining the cause, the author appealed to current science and attributed the disease to an obstruction of phlegm in the brain.

Many other diseases were associated with imbalance in the humours – too much or too little blood, too much or too little phlegm. Some were located to specific body parts. Treatments of bleeding, baths, fumigations, and diets were intended to restore the disrupted balance. External causes, such as trauma, noxious air, and unhealthy places, worked their harmful influence through the physical structures of the body. Like most other medical writings, these accounts are organismic (disease affects individuals, is bad and discontinuous). In contrast to earlier texts, however, their reliance on the theory of imbalance in the humours tends to make them physiological. Concepts similar to this imbalance, such as disharmony or conflict in the natural components of the body, can be found in the medical systems of ancient India and China.

Another writer famed for his classic descriptions was Aretaeus of Cappadocia, who lived around 100 A.D. His vivid accounts of the symptoms of diabetes and disorders of liver, kidney, and gut sometimes ornament modern texts. The extensive works of Galen in the second century A.D. also contain case histories, as well as essays on diseases, diagnosis, and therapeutics, and commentaries on earlier authors. Galen's pathology was eclectic, but its five functions are easily found. Frequently his pathology was used to justify his success as a practitioner; few examples of unanticipated therapeutic failure are described. Galen anchored some explanations in anatomy, although he did not dissect human subjects (see chapter 2). But he also made reference to the four humours and the life force. Except in cases of trauma or harmful airs, his disease concepts, like those of Hippocrates, tended to be organismic and physiological.

Galen's ideas dominated pathology in Europe, just as they dominated physiology, until early modern times (see chapter 3). Medieval philosophy advocated complete submission to the will of God. Galenical remedies could be attempted for sickness, but cure was the product of divine will. Attempts to refine diagnosis by distinguishing between diseases or by improving on Galen were considered arrogant. Some historians accused Galenism of 'preventing the advancement of medical science' because of its vitalistic reasoning, theory of blood flow, and therapeutics (Garrison 1929, 106). But it is unfair to blame Galen for his successors' lack of imagination. The longevity of his influence was neither his idea nor his fault; rather it was a manifestation of prevailing attitudes and practices.

Disease = Patterns of Suffering (Nosology)

Gradually medical authors began to distinguish between diseases on the basis of their symptoms in a practice called nosology (derived from the Greek words for 'disease' and 'theory about'). Hippocrates, Galen, and other ancient writers had described fevers with and without skin rash, and fevers with diurnal variations. In the ninth century A.D. a specific clinical distinction was made between the two febrile diseases with rashes, measles and smallpox, by the Persian physician-encyclopedist Rhazes (Abu-Bakr Mohammed Ibn Zakaria Al-Razi). Rhazes' twenty-volume compendium, *Continents*, was translated from Arabic into Latin in 1280. In the fourteenth century, after Europe was ravaged by the bubonic plague – a disease that could not be found in Galen – scholars looked for new ways of identifying disease. By 1476 Rhazes' *Continents* had been summarized in Padua. Twelve years later, his treatise on plague was translated into Latin.

In the Renaissance, spiritualistic and vitalistic explanations of the natural world lost credibility. Hippocratic observation was glorified, while rigid Galenism waned, together with the interdictions on human dissection. Physiological experimentation was revived with iatromechanism and iatrochemistry (see chapter 3). Doctors developed techniques to integrate the new sciences of chemistry. For example, uroscopy (the examination of urine) became a new diagnostic tool added to examination of the pulse. Charts were constructed to allow physicians to associate the colour, odour, turbidity, sweetness, and other chemical properties of urine with a specific diagnosis.

But medical practitioners were caught up in the realities of the bedside. People suffered from symptoms, such as pain and shortness of breath, not from acid urine; making a link between acid urine and the illness rarely led to benefits. These new scientific endeavours could not yet be mapped onto the analysis of a sick person, and their effects on pathology were modest. Nevertheless, with the decline in Galen and the rise of sensualist observation, doctors hesitated to invoke unknown causes for disease. Instead, they built a new system of diagnosis eventually known as nosology, which was self-consciously based on the careful observation of symptoms.

The English physician Thomas Sydenham, writing in Latin, published his clinical observations about diseases, especially fevers, and their treatment. In the tradition of Rhazes, he separated scarlet fever from measles (1676), and he described chorea (1686), the movement disorder that follows scarlet fever and now bears his name. With his friend, the physician-philosopher John Locke, he emphasized the importance of observation and the dangers of theory. Sydenham's treatise on podagra, or gout (1683), has become a classic for its rich description of the manifestations of the disease, from which he himself suffered.

Sydenham made reference to humours, but in his writings, diseases had well-developed characteristics, which were the basis of diagnosis. His diseases existed independent of the patient, as 'tyrants' or 'friends.'

In the century after Sydenham, nosology became an established enterprise, which effectively comprised a new kind of pathology. Medical writers, who actually called themselves nosologists, classified diseases into conceptual trees with branches for classes, orders, genera, and species. Symptoms and their sequence categorized diseases as if they were entities, or 'beings.' Authors devised their own systems, each hoping to find the perfect reflection of natural order. Some classifications recognized several thousand species of disease. Among the nosologists were François Boissier de Sauvages and Philippe Pinel of France, William Cullen of Scotland, and Carolus Linnaeus of Sweden – the same man who classified animals and plants.

Diseases with Personality

If [bleeding] be continued ... gout will take up its quarters even in a young subject, and its empire will be no government, but a tyranny.

> Thomas Sydenham on Gout, 1683, in *The Works of Thomas Sydenham*, trans. R.G. Latham (London: New Sydenham Society, 1848), 2:131

Osler on Pneumonia

Pneumonia may well be called the friend of the aged. Taken off by it in an acute, short, not often painful illness, the old man escapes those 'cold gradations of decay' so distressing to himself and to his friends.

> William Osler, *Principles and Practice of Medicine* (1892; 3rd edn, Edinburgh: Young J. Pentland, 1898), 109

Working mostly from books and only rarely at the bedside, medical students were obliged to memorize the 'correct' classification and the characteristics of each disease, depending on their place of study. The disease theories that apply best to Rhazes's measles, Sydenham's gout, and the nosological classifications include the organismic theory – as usual – and the ontological theory.

Nosological classifications are still used today in pathology and clinical medicine. In a manner reminiscent of the Hippocratic epigraph of this chapter, they simplify the mass of information gleaned from an accumulation of rare opportunities in clinical experience by giving it order and structure, to serve judgment in diagnosis and prognosis. Most nosological systems make reference to anatomical or chemical changes in radical contrast with eighteenth-century nosology. Only in psychiatry, where physical lesions are usually absent, do we continue to find a similar ordering of knowledge, based on observation of symptoms and behaviour (see chapter 12).

Pathology Moves into the Morgue

Disease = Altered Anatomy

Our present concepts of pathology are almost inseparable from anatomical change. Two centuries ago, however, the relevance of anatomy to bedside medicine was obscure, for three reasons: (1) changes inside the body were hidden until the patient was dead; (2) alterations visible at autopsy might have been due to death not to disease; and (3) internal changes could not be repaired. Nevertheless, anatomists continued to dissect, establishing the boundaries of normal and abnormal structure (see chapter 2).

While clinicians organized disease by its symptoms, some anatomists began to codify abnormalities found in cadavers. Four treatises, in particular, are worthy of note. The treatise of the Italian physician Antonio Benivieni, was published posthumously in 1507, nearly forty years before Vesalius's *Fabrica*. The Latin title, *De abditis nonnulis ac mirandis morborum et sanationum causis*, referred to the 'hidden' and 'wondrous' causes of disease that were revealed by autopsies in the 111 case histories. Benivieni was among the first to relate diseases to organic change.

In 1679 the Swiss physician Théophile Bonet published another collection of abnormal anatomy, which contained more than three thousand observations from his own practice and those of other writers since antiquity. He divided the work into four sections: head, thorax, abdomen, and systemic conditions such as fevers and wounds. Emphasizing the somewhat *para*medical nature of his endeavour, he called his treatise *Sepulchretum anatomicum* (Anatomical Graveyard). Bonet's book may have been longer and more developed than that of Benivieni, but his title reflected the marginal status of anatomy in medicine.

Nearly a century later, Giovanni Battista Morgagni of Padua published a prolix three-volume treatise, amplifying the work of his predecessor with his own experience. Unlike Bonet's title, Morgagni's *The Seats and Causes of Diseases Investigated by Anatomy* (1761) emphasized the importance of pathological anatomy to medical practice. He tried to make it more accessible to clinicians by including an

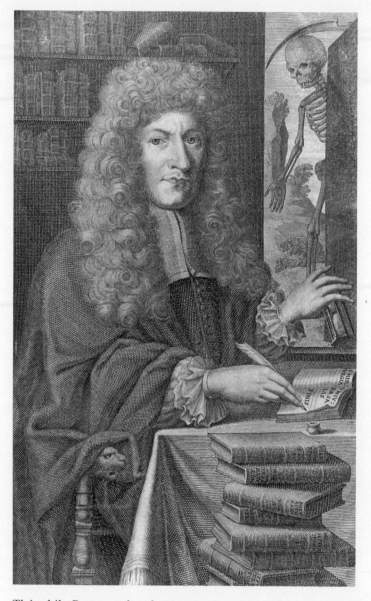

Théophile Bonet, as he chose to portray himself. Notice the grim reaper peeking through the door. *Sepulchretum anatomicum*, 1700, frontispiece

index for diseases and another for lesions; knowledge of one might lead a reader to knowledge of the other. A shorter and more accessible work was published in 1793 by Matthew Baillie, called *The Morbid Anatomy of Some of the Most Important Parts of the Human Body*. Many doctors were interested in pathological anatomy, but they were baffled by its relevance to diagnosis and therapeutics, since both were predicated on symptoms. Methods of examination before death revealed little about the internal organs. To have a 'disease' in the eighteenth century, a person had to feel sick.

A synthesis between anatomy and clinical medicine took place in the early nineteenth century with the advent of physical diagnosis – an approach that incorporated the inventions of thoracic percussion by Leopold Auenbrugger of Vienna and auscultation by R.T.H. Laennec of Paris. Symptoms of living patients could now be linked to anatomical changes. In 1830 Jean Cruveilhier published the first volume of his lavishly illustrated treatise on pathological anatomy. New trends in disease concepts had fostered this technology; once established, however, the techniques stimulated a further shift in disease concepts – from an emphasis on how the patient felt to an emphasis on what lesion could be discovered (see chapter 9). Reflecting the rise of anatomy in pathology, disease names changed, for example, from phthisis (or consumption) to tuberculosis.

In the early nineteenth century, doctors realized that not all patients would display all the 'classic' symptoms of any given disease: some might have a few symptoms; others might have all. In 1825 P.C.A. Louis of Paris analysed two thousand cases of tuberculosis by correlating mortality with the frequency of various symptoms and the age and sex of sufferers. Well before the mathematical tools of probability and statistics had been fully elaborated, he founded 'numerical medicine,' which was further systematized by his student L.D.J. Gavarret. Numerical medicine was pathology's response to the positivism that had permeated experimental physiology (see chapter 3). Its many successors include the 'evidence-based' medicine of the late twentieth century. The word 'natural,' meaning health, was gradually replaced by the mathematically loaded word 'normal' (see Warner 1986, 89–91).

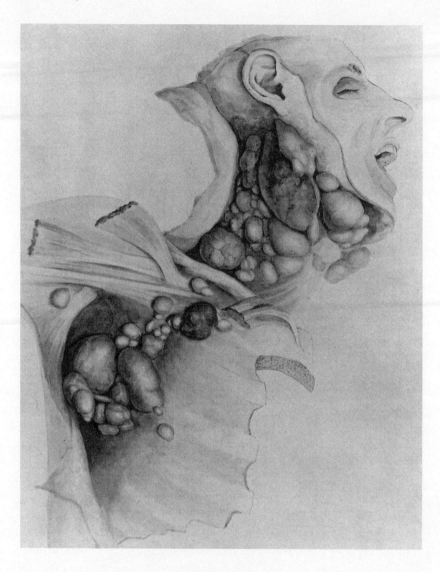

Hodgkin's disease. Watercolour by Robert Carswell, used to illustrate the reading of Thomas Hodgkin's original paper, 1832. The enlarged lymph glands were the anatomical definition of this disease. Medical School Library, University College, London

In this period, several more 'classic' descriptions of disease appeared, each reflecting the new scientific preoccupation with anatomy. Named for their discoverers, they were connected to the specific organic change that constituted their diagnosis; for example, Bright's disease of kidney (1827), Hodgkin's disease (1832), Graves' disease (1835), and Addison's disease (1855). The anchoring of diseases to three-dimensional anatomical forms, which could be illustrated, may have triggered the current passion for images in medical communication.

By the 1830s, microscopy had entered the realm of diagnosis. Diseases could be identified and classified by their changes at the level of tissues, in a process that had originated three decades earlier in the macroscopic observations of J.C. Smyth, P. Pinel, and Xavier Bichat. For example, the ancient concept of 'inflammation,' characterized by redness, swelling, heat, pain, and loss of function, took on new characteristics derived from microscopy. Czech-born Karl Rokitansky of Vienna wrote a German-language text of pathological anatomy and is said to have performed more than thirty thousand autopsies in his career. Rudolf Virchow, described leukemia (1846), founded a journal of pathological anatomy (1847) and wrote a treatise on cellular pathology (1858), which is often called a 'cornerstone' of the discipline (see also chapter 8). Based on his study of tumors, Virchow concluded that the anatomy and physiology of a single cell was passed on to all its 'daughter' cells – the idea now called cell theory. He was also a much-loved liberal politician (see chapter 7).

Elegant technological innovations linked microscopic and submicroscopic changes in structure to illness. This method prevails in our present system of medical knowledge. To determine what disease a patient has, doctors seek lesions, be they anatomical, chemical (such as high blood sugar), or physical (such as an elevated blood pressure). The clue to diagnosis is not so much how the patient feels but what the doctor finds. A person no longer needs to feel sick to have a disease (see chapter 9).

Anatomical methods of describing and identifying disease correspond to the organismic theory, and they can be both external (ontological) and internal (physiological) with respect to causes.

Disease = Damaged Organs

Symptoms, then, are in reality nothing but the cry from suffering organs.

> J.M. Charcot, *Clinical Lectures on the Senile and Chronic Diseases* (1868; English edn, London: Sydenham Society, 1881), 4

Surgery does the ideal thing – it separates the patient from his disease. It puts the patient back to bed and the disease in a bottle.

> Logan Clendening, *Modern Methods of Treatment* (St Louis: Mosby, 1925), 17

Favouring the ontological view is the fact that the physical lesion – a three-dimensional entity – is equated with the disease. Conversely, and favouring the physiological view, lesions seemed to emerge from within the patient – and may somehow depend on who she is. In the late nineteenth century, germ theory challenged that idea.

Disease = Invasion by Living Organisms

An ontological view of disease was consolidated in the 1880s with the triumph of germ theory, as a result of the work of a French chemist, a British surgeon, and a German physician, who approached the problem simultaneously, each from a different angle. Despite their numerous predecessors, medicine had long hesitated to accept the idea that diseases were caused by germs (see chapter 7).

Chemist Louis Pasteur studied fermentation to explore (and refute) the notion of spontaneous generation of living organisms. He demonstrated the link between bacteria and diseases, and in some impressive public demonstrations he proved that inoculation could convey immunity to domestic animals. Doctors were sceptical of his work for a variety of reasons: germs could be found everywhere, even in the healthy; furthermore, Pasteur was not a physician.

The surgeon Joseph Lister applied Pasteur's germ theory to the practice of wound dressing, using carbolic acid to deliberately 'kill germs' and seal wounds. His 1865 success with an open fracture of a young boy's leg was published in the *Lancet* in 1867. Acceptance of antiseptic technique varied, but the news spread quickly, publicizing the practical consequences of germ theory (see also chapter 10).

In 1882 Robert Koch identified *mycobacterium tuberculosis* as the cause of pulmonary tuberculosis, relying on the development of staining and culture techniques. He laid down rules to establish how a bacterium can be proved to be the cause of a disease. Finding the organism in every case was a necessary prerequisite, he said, but it was not sufficient evidence for believing that the organism was the cause of the disease. This observation became the first of four criteria. To be the proven cause of a disease, the organism must (1) be found in every case; (2) be isolated and grown in pure culture; (3) produce the same disease when injected into animals; (4) be recovered in all experimental cases. Satisfaction of these logical criteria, known as 'Koch's postulates,' is still a standard part of etiological investigation.

The triumph of germ theory immediately ratified the search for effective vaccines to convey immunity and for chemical therapies to kill the invading organisms. Initial research concentrated on vaccines, and Pasteur's most famous experiment concerned his efforts to find a vaccine for rabies.

Since antiquity, rabies had been known to be a lethal disease communicated by the bite of an infected creature. Pasteur was working with dogs to develop an attenuated vaccine; he made repeated injections of increasingly virulent material taken from rabies-infected rabbit nerve tissue, which was weakened by incubation in air. At his door on the evening of 4 July 1885 appeared three people: nine-year-old Joseph Meister, who had been viciously attacked by a rabid dog, the boy's unharmed mother, and the dog's owner, who had himself been bitten in rescuing the child and killing his animal. Sticks, stones, and straw in the dog's stomach were the diagnostic sign of rabies. The owner was thought to be out of danger (his skin had not been broken), but the physicians whom Pasteur consulted concluded that the boy would die. The vaccine should be given, they thought, even if it offered only a slight chance of recovery. In a series of injections reminiscent of Jenner's experiment (see chapter 7), Pasteur gave the child a series of solutions prepared from rabies-infected rabbit tissue that had been incubated for less and less time; the last injection contained fresh material. The child lived and grew to be a man, ending his days as the gatekeeper at the Pasteur Institute in Paris. Using Pasteur's notebooks, historian Gerald Geison has shown that at least two other 'private' patients had been injected with rabies vaccine before young Meister, and one had died.

Germ theory shifted the cause of disease away from internal organs to external invaders. Social purity movements could now marshal science to the aid of pre-existing efforts to clean up the world in a joint campaign against a living 'enemy' (see chapter 5). By 1906, germ theory had become so popular that it was mocked by George Bernard Shaw.

The Overworked Germ of Overwork

Ridgeon. It's nothing. I was a little giddy just now. Overwork I suppose ...

B.B. [Sir Ralph Bloomfield Bonington]. Overwork! There's no such thing. I do the work of ten men. Am I giddy? No. NO. If you're not well, you have a disease. It may be a slight one, but it's a disease. And what is a disease? The lodgment in the system of a pathogenic germ, and the multiplication of that germ. What is the remedy? A very simple one. Find the germ and kill it.

Sir Patrick. Suppose there's no germ.

B.B. Impossible ... there must be a germ: else how could the patient be ill? ... [*severely*] There is nothing that cannot be explained by science.

> G.B. Shaw, *The Doctor's Dilemma* (1906; reprint, Harmondsworth: Penguin, 1957), 102, 112

Opponents to germ theory worked to soften this increasingly ontological view of disease. They observed that heredity and vaccines could create or alter natural susceptibility to infection, and they concluded that infection with germs had something to do with the host as well as the invader.

Similarly, work on genetics early in the twentieth century demonstrated that some diseases long thought of as 'running in families' could be given a scientific rather than a biblical basis. A priority dispute in 1900 led to the rediscovery of the laws of heredity that had been published more than thirty years earlier by the Austrian botanist and cleric Gregor Mendel. Two years later, Archibald Edward Garrod of England announced that alcaptonuria was the first human disorder shown to follow Mendelian laws. Multiple-symptom constellations can now be reduced to a chromosomal abnormality or even to a single molecular substitution in DNA. For example, in 1959 Jérôme Lejeune linked a complex form of mental retardation to an extra chromosome. Lejeune also pointed out the racist implications in the term 'mongolism' chosen by his predecessor, J. Langdon Down. Alterations that result in many inherited disorders have now been defined at the phenotypic, chromosomal, and nucleic acid levels – for example, Tay-Sachs disease (assay of hexosaminidase A, 1970), sickle-cell anemia (locus on small arm of chromosome 11 of ß-globin chain synthesis, 1980); muscular dystrophy (gene mapping, 1987), and cystic fibrosis (gene mapping, 1989).

Over the course of a century, microscopic anatomy, bacteriology, immunology, and genetics, carried pathology into the laboratory, where it remains. Genetic diseases, immune dysfunction, and HLA phenotypes still provide a vehicle for physiological views of disease. Medical statistics continue to have great explanatory power, especially in discussions of incidence, prognosis, and survival, and in clinical trials. These trends were reflected in Canada.

The Canadian-born William Osler was fascinated by the potential of laboratory science in diagnosis. He was appointed pathologist at McGill University in 1874. Two decades later, as a founding professor at the influential Johns Hopkins medical school in Baltimore, he used his insights from pathology to advocate the widely copied system of educating young doctors: two years of basic science followed by two years of clinical training. Osler's *Principles and Practice of Medicine* (1892) exemplified the blend of scientific pathology with lucid

clinical descriptions, making it the most durable and influential textbook in the early twentieth century. His protégé Maude Abbott
founded McGill's superb museum of pathological specimens, and
her classification of congenital abnormalities of the heart was an
essential prerequisite for open-heart surgery. In the same tradition,
the Scottish-Canadian pathologist William Boyd published the first
of his many pathology texts in 1925. Admired for its use of science,
his writing was also hailed for its riveting prose. In bacteriology, Félix
d'Hérelle of Montreal studied bacteriophage, the viruses whose
nucleic acid became the prototype for molecular genetics.

William Boyd's Textbook of 1925

On bronchiectasis
'Stinking pools of pus' accumulate to cause 'exceedingly foul
breath which makes a social outcast of the unfortunate victim
so that he tends to live a life alone, apart, helpless and hope-
less.'

On villous papilloma of the bladder viewed with the cystoscope
The 'delicate many fingered growth ... unfolds its fragile processes when the bladder is filled with water until it looks like a
piece of seaweed floating in a marine pool.'

William Boyd, *A Textbook of Pathology* (1925; 8th edn,
Philadelphia: Lea and Febiger, 1970), 698, 945

The Medical Model of Today and Its Problems

Elements of both external (ontological) and internal (physiological)
causes can now be found in the current medical model. The former
are seen in diseases caused by viruses or bacteria, modified physiologically by the accompanying immune status of the host; the latter
are seen in genetic or autoimmune disorders, modified ontologically
by concepts such as oncogenes or post-viral autoimmunity for condi-

tions such as diabetes and multiple sclerosis. Nevertheless, disease descriptions in medical textbooks conform to an overriding organismic view of disease – something undesirable and hopefully discontinuous that affects individuals.

In embracing science, pathology was also vulnerable to the distortions, abuses, and errors of science. For example, the ontological view of disease as the product of demonized external invaders has led society to recoil from people who appear to be at risk. In nineteenth-century Canada, immigrants thought to be at risk of typhus or cholera were forcibly confined in unhygienic sheds, where those who had not previously been infected soon sickened and died. Similarly, in more recent times, homosexuals and Haitians have been equated with AIDS. Controls are proposed against these groups as if their members were equivalent to the disease or its cause (see chapter 7).

Physiological views of disease tend to allow observers to blame the patients for their illnesses. For example, some disease descriptions have incorporated prejudicial notions of race, gender, and class; 'Jewish' diseases, women's diseases, and diseases of poverty. Diseases are built of words and metaphors. Sometimes deliberately, sometimes unintentionally, metaphors convey social attitudes as they try to express dispassionate science. Consequently, disease can be 'socially constructed' (see also chapter 7). As literary critic Susan Sontag has shown, attitudes might be triggered by the status of the illness itself.

Science can also turn out to be 'wrong.' For example, phrenology is the study of character, intelligence, and other traits by reading the shape of the head. All too easily discredited now, phrenology was indeed scientific when the doctors were intent on finding external clues to hidden changes of the internal organs. Many distinguished physicians were students of phrenology.

Are there any heresies in our current pathology? Such a question is impossible to answer 'from within.' The heresies of the past persisted because they seemed to fit the observed data, held promise for its explanation, and corresponded to contemporary science. Medical authorities have been mistaken in views that they once expressed with great confidence. Popular critics of modern medicine point to these errors, complaining that the study of suffering takes a back seat to the study of objective lesions. Their complaints have philo-

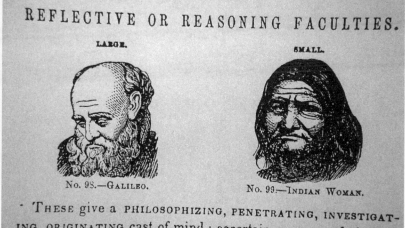

Phrenological comparison illustrating the relative reasoning power (and head shape) of Galileo and an Indian woman. From O.S. and L.N. Fowler, *Self-Instructor in Phrenology and Physiology*, 1859, 159

sophical implications. For example, people with 'chronic fatigue syndrome' have many symptoms, but the credibility of their disorder is low compared with that of symptomless but lesion-based conditions such as carcinoma *in situ* or hypertension. Those who turn to alternative or complementary medicines yearn for a holistic integration of body and mind. But holism is increasingly out of reach for a medicine predicated on the demonstration of material change. The popular neurologist-writer Oliver Sacks calls for a re-evaluation of medical knowledge. Citing the inadequacies of disease definitions that are confined to mechanical or chemical terms, he describes the metaphysical components of illness and human adaptation in organization and design. 'Nearly all my patients,' he says, 'whatever their problems, reach out to life – and not only despite their conditions, but often because of them, and even with their aid' (Sacks 1995, xviii). In other words, the subjective should be part of a disease, just as it is part of being ill. If we find a way to include the subjective in our concepts of disease, maybe we will also discover purpose and meaning.

Finally, the unquestioned acceptance of an organismic view of disease may be at odds with the political values of our world. If, for the purpose of argument, we contemplate the opposite, a population-based view of disease, we find a world in which disease is constant and cannot be eradicated – indeed, probably should not be eradicated – a world in which some disease might actually be beneficial. This 'nonorganismic,' or population-based, theory has also been called the ecological theory of disease. Traces of it have surfaced in the past, but rarely in medical texts. Medieval accounts of illness by writers such as Hildegard of Bingen emphasized the moral strength derived from a period of suffering. Closer to our own time, Social Darwinism or Malthusian concepts of the survival of the fittest might correspond to those ideals. For example, reference is often made to the supposed malaria-protection provided by sickle hemoglobin, which favours persistence of the sickle allele in various populations.

But we do not need to examine the past for examples of a nonorganismic view. Current issues of health-care funding juxtapose hard fiscal realities against medical ideals and the rights of individuals to the pursuit of a cure. Governments may decide that persons over a certain age are not entitled to expensive procedures such as dialysis and coronary bypass, or that infants under a certain gestational age do not warrant intensive care. They may also decide where and how physicians are to practise, or what groups are to be served by hospitals. This population view would hold, together with Oliver Sacks, that disease may not actually be 'good' but that in creating the greatest good for the greatest number, some disease, at least, is 'tolerable' (see chapter 6).

Pathology is a sophisticated science that defines material change in reliable ways. It has been reduced, however, from a holistic study of suffering to a laboratory-based study of what can be proved to be wrong. The answer – the diagnosis – almost always lies in the least material change.

Suggestions for Further Reading

Bates, Don, ed. *Knowledge and the Scholarly Medical Traditions.* Cambridge: Cambridge University Press, 1995

Canguilhem, Georges. *The Normal and the Pathological.* Trans. Carolyn R. Fawcett and Robert S. Cohen. New York: Zone Books, 1989

Cooter, Roger. *Cultural Meanings of Popular Science: Phrenology and the Organization of Consent in Nineteenth-Century Britain.* Cambridge and New York: Cambridge University Press, 1984

Garrison, Fielding H. *An Introduction to the History of Medicine.* 4th edn. Philadelphia: Saunders, 1929

Geison, Gerald L. *The Private Science of Louis Pasteur.* Princeton, N.J.: Princeton University Press, 1995.

Gundert, Beate. 'Parts and their Roles in Hippocratic Medicine.' *Isis* 83 (1992), 453–65

Hudson, Robert. *Disease and Its Control: The Shaping of Modern Thought.* Westport: Praeger/Greenwood, 1983

King, Lester S. *Medical Thinking: A Historical Preface.* Princeton, N.J.: Princeton University Press, 1982

– *Transformations in American Medicine: From Benjamin Rush to William Osler.* Baltimore: Johns Hopkins University Press, 1991

Long, Esmond R. *A History of Pathology.* Baltimore: Williams & Wilkins, 1928

Major, Ralph H. *Classic Descriptions of Disease.* Springfield: Charles C. Thomas, 1945, 1978

Maulitz, Russell C. *Morbid Appearances: The Anatomy of Pathology in the Early Nineteenth Century.* Cambridge: Cambridge University Press, 1987

Risse, Guenter B. 'History of the Concepts of Health and Disease.' In *Encyclopedia of Bioethics,* ed. Warren T. Reich, 2:578–91. 4 vols. New York: Free Press, 1978

Rose, Jeffrey. 'Sick Individuals and Sick Populations.' *International Journal of Epidemiology* 14 (1985), 32–8

Rosenberg, Charles E., and Janet Golden, eds. *Framing Disease: Studies in Cultural History.* New Brunswick, N.J.: Rutgers University Press, 1992

Sacks, Oliver. *An Anthropologist on Mars: Seven Paradoxical Tales.* Toronto: Alfred A. Knopf, 1995

Shorter, Edward. *From Paralysis to Fatigue: A History of Psychosomatic Illness in the Modern Era.* New York and Toronto: Free Press, 1992

Singer, Charles Joseph. *From Magic to Science: Essays on the Scientific Twilight.* 1928. Reprint, New York: Dover Publications, 1958 [on Hildegard of Bingen]

Sontag, Susan. *Illness as Metaphor.* New York: Farrar, Strauss, and Giroux, 1977

Warner, John Harley. *The Therapeutic Perspective: Medical Practice, Knowledge, and Identity in America, 1820–1885.* Cambridge, Mass. and London: Harvard University Press, 1986

Ziporyn, Terra. *Nameless Diseases.* New Brunswick, N.J.: Rutgers University Press, 1992

On Canada

Bliss, Michael. *William Osler: A Life in Medicine.* Toronto: University of Toronto Press, 1999

Carr, Ian. *William Boyd: Silver Tongue and Golden Pen.* Canadian Medical Lives Series, no. 15. Markham, Ont.: Hannah Institute and Fitzhenry & Whiteside, 1993

Cushing, Harvey. *The Life of Sir William Osler.* London and Toronto: Oxford University Press, 1940

Letts, Harry, and John Jacques. *A History of the Canadian Association of Pathologists / Histoire de l'Association canadienne des pathologistes.* 2nd edn. Kingston, Ont.: Allan Graphics, 1994

Rheault, M.J. 'Pierre Masson: His Influence on the Teaching of Pathology in Canada,' *Canadian Journal of Surgery* 28 (1985), 456–7

Rodin, Alvin E. *Oslerian Pathology: An Assessment and Annotated Atlas of Museum Specimens.* Lawrence, Kans.: Coronado Press, 1981

Summers, William C. 'On the Origins of the Science in *Arrowsmith*: Paul de Kruif, Felix d'Herelle, and Phage.' *Journal of the History of Medicine and Allied Sciences* 46 (1991), 315–32

Waugh, Douglas. *Maudie of McGill: Dr Maude Abbott and the Foundations of Heart Surgery.* Canadian Medical Lives Series, no. 13. Toronto: Hannah Institute and Dundurn Press

CHAPTER FIVE

First Do No Harm:
History of Pharmacology*

If the whole materia medica as used, could be sunk in the bottom of the sea, it would be all the better for mankind and all the worse for the fishes.

Oliver Wendell Holmes, 1883

In June 1991 the body of American President Zachary Taylor was exhumed for a medico-legal examination. He had been dead since 1850 – officially of diarrhea – but a question of poisoning had been raised. The president may not have been murdered, the papers claimed, but he had been killed by his physicians.

Stories like this one irritate me. The writers presume that the patient was not seriously ill until after he sought medical drugs or bleedings and that the illness did not contribute to his demise. Without denying the dangers of past therapy, I find these tales disturbing, because they hit close to hematologic home. Chemotherapy makes people vomit and lose their hair and reduces their immunity – and, by the way, it also shrinks tumors. One of my teachers used to call it 'poison with anti-cancer side effects.' We hope that safer and more effective treatments will be found in the future. In the meantime however, we give these potentially lethal drugs – not to kill our patients but to help them live longer and better. Are we deluding ourselves?

*Educational objectives for this chapter are found on pp. 394–5.

The Latest Frontier

The history of therapeutics is the latest frontier of medical history because it is so embarrassing. Until recently, ridicule was an aim of the few who wrote about past medicines. Current practices are assumed to be rational and scientific, while those of predecessors are not; what we do now is flawless, and what they did back then could not possibly have worked. History conducted through such a prejudicial lens (called 'presentism' by historians, see chapter 15) will be limited and insensitive even if it is lively and well written. Only recently have some historians begun to study why certain drugs were once endorsed by orthodox medicine. Others have begun to examine the parallel folk medicines of self-help – a much more difficult task, lacking sources that can easily be identified.

Most therapies were discovered by empirical means – observation, accident, and trial and error. But this method does not prevent 'reasoning' from participating in the transformation of observation into medical lore. The so-called empirical discovery of therapies relies on at least two prior conditions: agreement on what constitutes the disease (i.e., the need), and an opportunity to observe. For pharmacology, these conditions comprise the Pastorian 'preparation of the mind' (see chapter 3). Therapeutic rationale may be subject to historical vogue; however, a rationale for why the treatment was presumed to work will always have been applied – in many cases, *after* the drug's benefits were noticed.

Change in a disease concept can alter the rationale without necessarily altering the treatment. By the same token, a drug's mechanism of action can shift without refuting its benefits. For example, in the 1970s hydrochlorothiazide was thought to lower blood pressure through its diuretic and saliuretic effect; now it is thought to have an additional effect on the smooth muscle of blood vessels. A similar revision can be applied to digitalis, as we will see below.

Undesirable side effects can also lead to new applications. For example, minoxidil was introduced in the mid-1970s as a powerful antihypertensive, with the depressing side effect of hirsutism; now it is prescribed for external use as a treatment for baldness. Similarly, the adrenergic drug methylphenidate (Ritalin) was originally used as a stimulant, but its paradoxically calming side effect on children with hyperactivity (now called 'attention deficit disorder') became its principal application.

In their heyday, now defunct medical practices were neither irrational nor unscientific; the rationale was reconciled with prevailing science and concepts of disease. For example, when medicine looked for acids or bases in urine, remedies were selected to alter urinary acidity toward health. When syphilis first appeared as an import from the New World, the wood product guaiacum was thought to 'work' for two reasons: first, like the ailment, it came from America; second, the naturally occurring, spontaneous remissions could be attributed to whatever intervention had preceded them. Similarly, the colour red was a therapy for smallpox since at least the tenth century in Japan and Europe: red clothes, red rooms, red food, and red light. This idea persisted into the twentieth century with the work of the 1903 Nobel laureate Niels R. Finsen.

Reasoning is involved in all medical systems, including the past of orthodox medicine and the present of 'unorthodox,' or 'alternative,' medicine. In homeopathy, invented in the late eighteenth century by Samuel Hahnemann, the dominant assumption is that 'like cures like' – often expressed in Latin as *similia similibus curantur*. The best remedy will be the one which, when taken in large doses, produces symptoms similar to the disease to be cured; treatment then consists of giving that remedy in small 'homeopathic doses.'

Therapeutic rationale changes with perceptions of disease. For example, when peptic ulcer was thought to be associated with stress, hyperacidity, and disordered motility, the correct treatments dealt with those problems. But in the late 1970s, histamine-2 antagonists dramatically altered prescribing practices for ulcer; and in the early 1990s, a microbial explanation came to the fore, and management of the condition changed accordingly.

Perceptions of patients can also alter through time. In the medical journals of the 1950s and 1960s, tranquillizers promised to help women cope with the stress of housework. The idea that increased opportunities for outside employment might offer a better solution did not seem to have been a therapeutic consideration. Since then, tranquillizer remedies have not been discarded, but their target population has altered in conjunction with normative definitions of health and behaviour.

Some medically sanctioned treatments once hailed as miracle cures turned out to be useless or harmful. In the last century, increasing awareness of this possibility led to legislation designed to protect professionals and their patients from unjustified claims and unforeseen side effects. Pharmaceutical literature changed accordingly, and the 'small print' increased with time. Advertisements from a century ago contain few warnings about contents, side effects, drug interactions, and contraindications. The less than noble therapeutic past has itself become a mover in the history of pharmacology.

Mysticism, Religion, and Magic. Do They Work?

Since prehistoric times, doctors have been making recommendations for therapeutic intervention. Ancient remedies 'worked,' and some still work, including magic, prayer, and divine supplication. Ailing people are among the pilgrims who flock to shrines such as Lourdes in France, Fatima in Portugal, Santiago de Compostella in Spain, and the Oratoire St-Joseph, Cap-de-la-Madeleine, and Ste-Anne-de-Beaupré in Quebec. Sites of divine healing enjoy a charisma akin to that of medical meccas such as the Mayo Clinic. In our time, however, physicians leave the prescription of pilgrimages to other professionals.

The spiritualistic or vitalistic aspect of treatment has been reified in the concept of 'placebo' (from Latin 'to please'). The term 'placebo' long signified the administration of harmless but inert compounds; however, in the mid-twentieth century, placebo was found to be effective in virtually every form of intervention and disease.

Greco-Roman Treatments and Medical Botany

Since Greco-Roman diseases arose from an imbalance in the humours (see chapter 3), treatment consisted of trying to re-establish the balance. Modification of diet and life style were intended to alter the relative proportions of the elemental substances. After spiritual therapies, they are probably the oldest forms of medicine.

The Hippocratic treatises of the fifth century B.C. refer to many

---

An Experiment: Shifting Therapeutic Claims

Go to the library and examine drug advertisements in the medical journals of the past. You will find:

- drugs that are no longer used because they have since been recognized as dangerous;
- drugs that have been replaced by others with completely different actions, because our idea of the disease has changed (e.g., anxiolytics and antispasmodics for ulcers);
- treatments for conditions no longer considered to be diseases (e.g., agents to promote weight gain);
- tranquillizers to help women cope with housework and school meetings;
- advertisements that are tasteless, humourless, or corny because esthetic standards have changed too.

The older the journal, the more curiosities will be encountered. But recent publications also contain advertisements for products that are now considered inefficacious or harmful.

Finally, imagine how advertisements for present practice might appear to observers in fifty or one hundred years from now.

---

non-drug remedies, such as bloodletting, special diets, baths, exercise or rest, and applications of heat or cold. In addition, more than three hundred medications are cited, most of plant origin; they could be administered either externally or internally by mouth, rectum, vagina, and other orifices. Hippocratic doctors tended to be conservative in their treatment philosophy. They believed in the healing power of nature (*vis medicatrix naturae*), which governed the body's response to illness. Medicine was to help the body heal itself; it was not supposed to hurt, but the Hippocratics readily acknowledged that, sometimes, it could: 'to help, or at least to do no harm'

(*Epidemics* I, 11), a saying often written in Latin as *primum non nocere* (first, do no harm).

'Expectant' treatment – patiently waiting for nature's cure – has wandered in and out of fashion since the fifth century B.C. In their eagerness to glorify Hippocrates, some historians may have projected more caution onto their Greek predecessors than the texts would justify. At the time of writing, expectant medicine is no longer in vogue despite an energetic public lobby for its rediscovery. Folk medicines, herbal remedies, and natural products now compete for market share with the purveyors of gleaming capsules. Because medical practice tends to follow demand, orthodoxy may eventually bend toward *la médecine douce* (gentle medicine).

The Greek word for drug, *pharmakon*, from which pharmacology is derived, means a drug, a remedy, and a poison. In the earliest classifications, drugs were either toxins or antidotes, the antidotes were medicinal. In the first century B.C., King Mithridates VI of Pontus in Asia Minor feared being murdered by the Romans, with whom he was often at war. He is thought to have experimentally immunized himself against poisons by drinking the blood of ducks fed on toxic substances. A universal antidote bore his name. Ironically, the king was later unable to commit suicide with poison and had to ask a servant to polish him off with a sword.

Another ancient antidote was theriac, which was developed to counteract animal poisons. The word 'theriac,' is derived from the Greek word *therion* (wild beast) and reflects the composition as well as the purpose. Depending on which of the many recipes was used, theriac contained up to seventy ingredients, including the flesh of vipers. Both theriac and mithridates were used to treat infectious diseases, conceived of as 'pests,' or poisons. These remedies enjoyed almost mystical stature into the nineteenth century, and medical museums display magnificent faience jars for their keeping. The nineteenth-century physiologist Claude Bernard, who worked in a pharmacy in his youth, recalled that theriac was made by mixing the dregs of all the other preparations in a vat.

Galen, of the second century A.D., was a successful therapist. Among his many medications were vegetable derivatives, which came to be known as galenicals, or simples. His treatments could be aggressive, but he knew that his patients' confidence in his reputation could help him to effect cures. He was ready to take credit for the healing accomplished by nature or by stealth.

A Galenic Therapeutic Strategy: Winning Confidence

I completely won the admiration of the philosopher Glaucon by the diagnosis which I made in the case of one of his friends ... Observing on the window sill a vessel containing a mixture of hyssop and honey, I made up my mind that the patient, who was himself a physician, believed that the malady from which he was suffering was a pleurisy ... Placing my hand on the patient's right side ... I remarked: 'This is the spot where the disease is located.' He ... replied with a look which plainly expressed admiration mingled with astonishment.

Galen, *De locis affectis* (cited in Clendening [1942] 1960, 45–7)

Galen's pharmacopoeia embraced the therapies of his predecessor, Dioscorides, a first-century Greek surgeon who served the army of the Roman Emperor Nero. Dioscorides' medical botany described more than six hundred plants, animals, and their derivatives. He classified his remedies by their physical qualities: oils, animals, cereals, herbs, roots, and wines. Wine made with *mandragora* (mandrake root) was a love potion and anesthetic. Mandrake's anthropoid appearance may have had something to do with its legendary powers. Humans daring to pull it from the ground would be killed by its screams; a dog should be tied to the root and tempted to 'harvest' it by a nearby dish of meat.

Dioscorides' botany remained the most influential book on *materia medica* (medical substances) for fourteen hundred years. Most other medical botanies were simply commentaries on his work. The first medical book printed by the German inventor Johannes Gutenberg was the 1457 *Laxierkalender,* a collection of laxative remedies. Some herbals were written first in Greek, translated into Arabic,

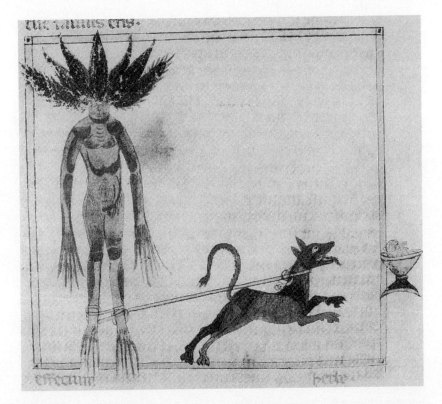

Mandragora (mandrake root) from a mid-thirteenth-century manuscript copy of a herbal by Apuleius. Wellcome Institute Library, London, WMS 573

then Latin, and finally a modern language. Often the texts are garbled with missing passages. None of the original Greek illustrations have survived. Illustrations in later manuscripts or books are highly stylized or are mismatched, or they describe plants that are difficult to identify or no longer exist, as in the illustrated commentary of Pietro Andrea Matthioli of 1554. Research on the ancient writings of Dioscorides and other botanists continues; its success relies on accurate translation and knowledge of manuscript sources.

Botany was a standard subject in medical education until about 1900. Medical schools and hospitals maintained botanical gardens,

not only for academic reasons but also for a reliable supply of remedies. Reflecting the intimate relationship between medicines and
growing plants, the first Europeans to cultivate land in Canada are
said to have been the family of the apothecary-settler, Louis Hébert,
who arrived in 1617. Similarly, it is no accident that, some eighty
years later, the first herbarium of North American plants was collected by a physician and surgeon, Michel Sarrazin of Quebec, who
first described the pitcher plant (*Sarracenia purpurea*).

Many drugs in use today were originally derived from plants,
although most are now synthesized in laboratories for commercial
distribution. Some have been around for a long time. Senna has
been known as a laxative since at least 1550 B.C.; castor oil comes
from the garden plant ricinus, which also was known to the Egyptians; foxglove has provided digitalis since at least the eighteenth
century; and an aspirinlike substance is found in the bark of willow
trees and yellow birch. The benefits of some vegetable remedies are
rediscovered with much fanfare, as was the case with the gastrointestinal effects of bran, promoted by Denis P. Burkitt in 1973.
Similarly, the cholesterol-lowering value of oat bran was widely publicized in the 1980s. Modern treatments originally derived from
plants include the anti-leukemia drug vincristine, found in the
Madagascar periwinkle; the podophyllotoxins (VP-16 and etopi-
side), derived from the root of the may-apple; and the breast cancer agent taxol, found in the ancient yew trees of Japan and the
Pacific Northwest.

Effective remedies extracted from complex plants challenge scientists to imagine other miracle cures lurking in the bushes. In the
early twentieth century, Parke Davis became one of the first drug
companies to sponsor a systematic search of the jungle for new remedies. The 1960s fascination with the psychedelic plants known to
aboriginal peoples also brought ethnobotany to the attention of scientists. More recently, the destruction of the rain forest has led to a
certain panic over the potential extinction of three-quarters of the
world's plant species, with a presumed loss of thousands of potential
remedies. The *Journal of Ethnopharmacology*, founded in 1979, provides a forum for investigators. Several projects, both botanical and
anthropological, are underway to survey, identify, and analyse the

medical potential of plants, some of which are already used by the peoples of Amazonia.

In Canada, botanist Thor Arnason of the University of Ottawa has identified and studied the pharmacological properties of plant products known to the native peoples of North America. Like the classicists who study antiquity, he observes that success depends on the interpretation of myriad dialects and on oral traditions; much information has already been lost. For example, early accounts of European settlement tell how the encampment of Jacques Cartier at Stadacona (Quebec) in the winter of 1535–6 was healed of 'great disease,' probably scurvy, by a so-called white cedar or spruce tea given them by the natives. By the winter of 1605–6, when Samuel de Champlain founded the habitation at Port-Royal (Annapolis Royal, Nova Scotia), the remedy could no longer be identified, although Champlain had heard of Cartier's experience. Evergreen needles contain vitamin C, but dialect discrepancies over the precise plant name mean that Arnason has been unable to trace the exact cure.

Advent of Metals

Copper had been mentioned in the Hippocratic treatises, but it was not until the late fifteenth century that metals were widely used as medical therapy. By then, the Greco-Roman element 'earth' was thought to have expanded to include new elements, mercury, salt, and sulfur. Among the proponents of metals was Theophrastus Bombastus von Hohenheim, who called himself Paracelsus. Born in the German mining community of Einsedeln, he deplored the fact that minerals were not used in pharmacy. Influenced by alchemists, he thought that plants and minerals contained specific healing properties called arcana. For every disease, he maintained, a specific remedy must exist, and he proposed that diseases be classified by the drugs that cured them, a notion that has currency today in the concept of the therapeutic trial. Paracelsus expounded his ideas with elaborate demonstrations, including public burnings of the works of Galen and Avicenna. Such behaviour did little to help him find and keep employment, and he wandered over Europe for much of his career.

To the twentieth-century student and many earlier observers, Paracelsus's writings seem confused and incoherent. For his bombastic style, he has been portrayed as a ridiculous villain whose legacy is easily dismissed. Recently, however, scholars in history, medicine, and even public administration have reconsidered his work to find that his impact may have been greater than previously thought, if only because he dared to challenge the established authority of ancient writers.

New substances, including mercury, sulfur, and antimony, became the wonder drugs of the late Renaissance. In the early sixteenth century, Girolamo Fracastoro recommended mercury to treat the 'new' European epidemic of syphilis. Mercury causes gastrointestinal disturbances, gum swelling, salivation, and neurological toxicity, but it does appear to have been an effective treatment for syphilis.

Similarly, antimony compounds produce nausea, vomiting, purging, and cardiovascular collapse. This toxicity led to a ban on antimony at several medical faculties, including Heidelberg and Paris. In the form of tartar emetic, however, the drug was said to cure almost everything, and the ban was overturned by popular demand after it was credited with saving the French king, Louis XIV, from typhoid fever in 1657. In the nineteenth century, high-dose tartar emetic was used for pneumonia; clinical statistics testified to its efficacy, but toxicity led to its disappearance once again. One of my own research projects, with Dr Pierre René of Montreal's Royal Victoria Hospital, demonstrated that – its toxicity notwithstanding – tartar emetic has bactericidal properties.

Classification and Therapeutic Change

The earliest classifications sorted drugs into poisons and antidotes. Other classifications were based on physical properties (Dioscorides) or physiological effects. For example, poppy juice (containing opium) and nightshade (containing atropine) were both classified as sleep-inducing narcotics, although the latter is no longer thought of in that context. Willow bark, which contains salicylic acid, was an 'astringent' that dried secretions, explaining its effect on gout. Substances that produced vomiting were emetics. Those that caused diarrhea were laxatives, cathartics, or purges, depending on their ferocity. Sudorifics made patients sweat. Stimulants woke them up. Diuretics made them urinate. The classification followed the description of the physiological effects, whether or not the effects were the reason for administering the drug. To a certain extent, we still view drugs in this way, but now we tend to explain the side effects through the rationale.

For example, digitalis was first thought to be a diuretic because it reduced peripheral swelling and increased urinary flow. It is now a heart-strengthening drug or cardiotonic, but still it reduces edema and increases urinary output. In other words, the rationale has changed, but the benefits are constant. In his treatise of 1785, William Withering brought digitalis into medical orthodoxy, described its harmful effects, and reported on his experiments with it on poor patients. He had learned of foxglove, he said, from a secret remedy belonging to 'an old woman in Shropshire, who sometimes made cures after the more regular practitioners had failed.' Sadly, the identity of this woman is unknown, although some say that her name was Hutton. Medical history holds many other unknown progenitors, while experiments conducted on disadvantaged people continue into our time (see chapter 6 on Tuskegee; chapter 13 on Nazi science and Willowbrook).

As recently as the early nineteenth century, the pharmacopoeias of Europe and North America contained drugs that are now considered poisons: mercury in the form of calomel; antimony in the form of tartar emetic; jalap, a powerful cathartic; strychnine; opium and laudanum for pain and sleep; alcohol as a stimulant. Combined with restrictive diets, vicious enemas or clysters, and various means of bleeding, such as phlebotomy, leeches, and cupping, this style of interventionist therapy has been called drastic, or heroic. Not everyone took it lying down – hence, the famous artistic and literary lampoons of Thomas Rowlandson, James Gilray, Honoré Daumier, and G.B. Shaw. The word 'heroic,' which normally signifies admiration, became a pejorative term in medicine. Originating from the vigorous last-ditch attempts to save lives, it now implies overdrugging, overdosing, and overreacting.

Medical therapeutics has undergone a greater change in the last century and a half than in the preceding two thousand years. Why? A number of reasons can be offered. No doubt, the fashion of period and place had an influence. In postrevolutionary France, for example, things associated with the old order were rejected because they were old. Reflecting this ideal, the physiologist François Magendie hoped that physicians would abandon the complex derivatives of the past in favour of new, chemically pure drugs. In eight editions of the formulary for the Hôtel-Dieu hospital in Paris between 1821 and 1834, he recommended purified chemicals over the older 'simples' (the plant-based precursors): morphine over opium, quinine over cinchona bark. He referred to his animal tests of new alkaloids, such as codeine and bromide. Some scientists favoured therapeutic nihilism, but the degree to which it was actually practised is difficult to determine.

Three other reasons may account for the decline in drastic remedies. First was the rise of surgery after the advent of anesthesia and antisepsis. Why give a pill forever if an operation will cure the problem in an instant? Second, the wide acceptance of germ theory in the 1880s (see chapter 4) and the discovery of hormones soon after caused doctors to turn from attacking disease symptoms to finding a set of 'magic bullets,' aimed at the causes of disease. Third, pressures from homeopathy and other medical competition may have pushed medicine toward less drastic therapy. Using a computer-assisted analysis of prescription records from two urban hospitals, John Harley Warner elucidated a change in doctors' prescriptions between 1820 and 1885: side-effect-ridden 'heroics' were replaced by more gentle therapies. Among other factors, Warner related the change to issues of professional identity between doctors (allopaths) and unorthodox practitioners whose remedies were less harmful and more attractive to patients.

Magic Bullets: Antibiotics, Hormones, and Twentieth-Century Optimism

When microorganisms became accepted as a cause of disease, research focused initially on producing vaccines to heighten natural immunity; only secondarily were agents sought to attack bacteria. Cinchona (or Jesuit bark) to prevent and treat malaria had been around for centuries, long before the *Plasmodium* organism had been visualized; its 'rationale' was as a 'tonic' that heightened resistance to the noxious atmospheres thought to cause malaria. Discovery of the parasite in 1880 by the future Nobel laureate Charles Laveran provided a new rationale for the therapeutic effect of quinine. The conscious quest for agents to kill germ invaders yet leave a living, healthy patient has been called the search for the magic bullet.

The first two magic bullets were developed by Paul Ehrlich: the dye, trypan red, for experimental trypanosomiasis in 1903; and the arsenic-containing Salvarsan, for human syphilis in 1910. Ehrlich worked with dyes that had a special affinity for bacteria, hoping that they would selectively carry a toxin into the invading cell. His 1909 Nobel Prize was awarded for his theoretical work on immunity, although his work on drugs is better known.

Sulfa drugs also formed part of the magic bullet agenda. Gerhard Domagk, working for the Bayer laboratories in Elberfeld, Germany, developed the first sulfa drug, Prontosil, having proved that it was effective against streptococcal infections in rats. Domagk's first human trial was conducted on his own daughter, who suddenly developed septicemia in December 1933. The girl recovered. Domagk was awarded the Nobel Prize in 1939, but he was arrested and jailed by the Gestapo for having attracted undue foreign approbation. He did not receive his award until 1947, when the prize money was no longer available. Few present-day physicians have heard of Domagk, possibly because of the wartime hostilities with Germany and possibly because he worked for a big pharmaceutical firm.

The most famous magic bullet is penicillin. Schoolchildren are taught the story of Alexander Fleming who was culturing bacteria and rejecting plates that had been infected with mould. But historians, including the Montreal mycologist Jules Brunel, have shown that Fleming's 'discovery' that penicillium mould kills bacteria had been published earlier by others (notably, Bartolomeo Gosio of Rome in 1896, and E. Duchesnes of Lyons in 1897). Brunel also reported that elderly Québécois had long used moulds on jam as a therapy for respiratory ailments. Fleming recognized the significance of his findings but did not pursue applications, nor did he cite his predecessors. The Oxford researchers, Howard W. Florey and Ernst Chain, extracted, purified, and manufactured penicillin, which was released in 1939 a decade after Fleming's observation. Fleming, Florey, and Chain shared the Nobel Prize in 1945.

Hormones and vitamins do not kill invading organisms, but they too can act as magic bullets when they specifically target and replace deficiencies. (On vitamins, see chapter 13.) The isolation and elaboration of several hormones early in the twentieth century contributed to a rising medical optimism (see chapter 3). Frederick G. Banting, a practitioner in London, Ontario, became convinced from his reading that a pancreatic disorder was the cause of diabetes mellitus. In the summer of 1921 he borrowed laboratory space from J.J.R. Macleod at the University of Toronto to work with medical student Charles Best on experimentally induced diabetes in dogs. The rapid isolation and purification of the hormone was the elegant work of biochemist J.B. Collip. Within a short time, insulin was the first hormone to be developed as specific replacement therapy for this common and previously fatal disease. The 1923 Nobel committee overlooked Best and Collip and gave the prize to Banting and Macleod, who shared it with the other two.

Hormones were soon applied to the treatment of tumors, fuelling the growing quest for substances that could not only replace deficiencies but cure all disease. Several hormone discoveries and treatments followed in succession. P.S. Hench and E.C. Kendall of the Mayo Clinic found the hormone of the adrenal cortex in 1949; in keeping with the buoyant mood of the time, their Nobel Prize was awarded the following year. Soon after their achievement had been announced, an awestruck clinician rushed up to historian E.H. Ackerknecht to tell him that he was a lucky man: all diseases would soon be wiped out and the only professor left in the medical faculty would be the historian (Ackerknecht 1973, 2)! One of the byproducts of this overwhelming enthusiasm would be an effect on history itself – toward further ridicule of the past.

Clinical Trials

Historical comparisons with untreated human groups of the past had long been made to introduce new treatments. Deliberate clinical testing began in the early nineteenth century in parallel with the statistical methods of numerical medicine (see chapter 4). Animal trials, much used by Magendie and Bernard, continued to precede trials on humans.

In response to the many pharmacological discoveries of the early twentieth century, committees were formed to develop standards to ensure that results could be ascribed only to the drug and not to other extraneous factors (e.g., British MRC Therapeutics Trial Committee 1931). The active recruiting of concurrent untreated 'controls' was a conscious development of this century: first, self or alternate controls (ca. 1900); later, randomized (ca. 1940). The practice of 'blinding' observers as well as subjects increased after 1940 as a means of dealing with the powerful placebo effect. The MRC-funded study of streptomycin in tuberculosis (*British Medical Journal* 2 (1948), 769–88) is often cited as the first randomized con-trolled trial (RCT). By 1972, however, Archie L. Cochrane had com-plained that despite years of RCTs, most medicine was still being conducted without evidence of its efficacy. In his name, an interna-tional collaboration has endeavoured to collate all available RCT information in various areas of practice.

Standardization meant that drugs were carefully tested on 'the seventy-kilogram man'; effects on women, pregnant women, and racial minorities were often ignored. The zeal to investigate trod on patients' rights, sometimes with disastrous results (see chapters 6 and 13). More recently, projects to define ethical standards in research have been addressed.

Late-Twentieth-Century Scepticism: Is There No Magic Bullet?

The mid-century optimism was premature, if understandable. Aside from their many side effects, magic bullets created magic microbes. Drug-resistant malaria and gonorrhea, and multi-drug-resistant sta-phylococcus (MDRS) stalk the literature if not the wards, and we worry about penicillin-resistant syphilis. Dreadful nosocomial infec-tions lurk in the antibiotic-ridden ferment of hospitals, where few but resistant strains can survive. In his *Medical Nemesis* (1975), Ivan Illich suggested that the medical establishment had become a seri-ous threat to health. More recently, the blunt title of Allan Brandt's history of venereal disease, *No Magic Bullet,* expressed the post-modern disillusionment with the earlier hopes for universal disease eradication.

Antibiotics have certainly saved individual lives, but did they really prolong life expectancy? Few historians were prepared to assess the possibility that the new drugs, which were so effective in isolated cases, might not be as effective for the collective. People live longer now than they did two hundred years ago, but how much of that enhanced longevity is actually due to drugs? For example, we now know that mortality from the leading killer, tuberculosis, began to decline before the advent of vaccination and antituberculous drugs. In other words, hygiene, diet, wealth, and lifestyle probably counted as much for the decline, if not more. The late-twentieth-century rise of the disease in North America coincides with a decline in wealth, living conditions, and nutrition (see chapter 7).

Thalidomide

The story of thalidomide provides a powerful example of innovation gone awry. A highly effective sedative developed in the late 1950s, thalidomide was on the Canadian market for less than a year before overwhelming evidence from other countries blamed it for gross limb abnormalities in infants (phocomelia). Its removal in Canada on 10 April 1962 came five months after German doctors had linked it to birth defects. The first affected Canadians were born in Saskatoon in February and June 1962 (*Canadian Medical Association Journal* 87 (1962), 412, 670). Because the drug was teratogenic in the early weeks of pregnancy, the scope of the tragedy was not known until nine months later. In total, 125 affected children were born in Canada; probably many more pregnancies were wasted. The living victims were of normal intelligence and eager to work, but they received no compensation until September 1992 when they were thirty years old. Because the drug had been properly licensed, the government was held liable, not the pharmaceutical industry and not the medical practitioners who had prescribed it. Ironically, and perhaps not inappropriately, thalidomide is being reintroduced for the management of graft-versus-host disease, an iatrogenic disorder.

Thalidomide is an extreme example of therapeutic disaster; even its victims understand that their deformities were unintended. But it should not be forgotten. Thalidomide reminds us that good intentions do not prevent medicine from being harmful; it helps to account for the complicated licensing procedure in this country, which is said to be among the most stringent in the world. The thalidomide story also renews and explains the public's continued mistrust of the medical establishment. The negative image guarantees a market for the dissenting literature and for products of the largely unregulated folk-medicine and health-food industry, an industry whose net worth is difficult to determine.

Rational Derivatives and the Pharmaceutical Industry

Magic bullets were extracted from the living tissues of animals, plants, and moulds, and they could also be synthesized in the laboratory. They were designed to repair the biological causes of infections and deficiencies. But in the early twentieth century, many other diseases were defined in a chemical sense. Attempts to 'design' rational remedies have been based on an understanding of the precise biochemical error producing the disease. For example, in Parkinson's disease, chemicals that appear to be deficient in the brain become the medicines administered by doctors. Other examples abound: histamine antagonists to reduce gastric acid secretion; ß-blockers to prevent transmission of certain nervous impulses; calcium channel blockers for ischemic heart disease. In the majority of these cases, the 'designer drug' emerged out of trials as the most effective and least toxic of a series of related compounds created in a laboratory to solve a chemical problem.

Since the late 1800s, when specific chemical agents were isolated and characterized, the need for standardization and synthesis of natural substances favoured the development of a drug industry. For more than a century, drug companies have engaged in and supported research with funds and laboratories. In Canada, the pharmaceutical industry is now worth nearly $2 billion. Not only does it have power over the sales and distribution of remedies, but it controls more than 70 per cent of the funds spent on drug research even when that research is done in universities. Privately funded research is often extremely productive. Like Domagk of sulfa fame, James Black, Gertrude B. Elion, and George H. Hitchings worked for big pharmaceutical firms – specifically, Burroughs Wellcome and SmithKline and French. They shared the 1988 Nobel Prize for the development of '*rational* methods for designing' treatments: cimetidine, propanolol, 6–mercapto-purine, 6–thioguanine, allopurinol, and trimethoprim.

Medical and public reaction to drug companies is ambivalent. Their discoveries are welcome, but their big profits and grants are sources of discomfort. Beneficiaries worry that drug-funded research is ethically compromised or that accepting sponsorship is a form of advertising. Critics also point to the financial gain from selling drugs, claiming that the industry is not motivated to prevent disease; chronic illness is good for business.

In the 1970s various procedures, such as Ontario's 'parcost' system, were implemented to allow pharmacists to replace expensive brand-name drugs with the least expensive substitute, often a pirated copy with the same composition. These policies were unpopular with the drug industry because they ignored its investment in developing drugs. The situation created problems with our international trading partners. In 1987 Canada's patent laws were amended with Bill C-22 and again in 1993 with Bill C-91, to satisfy the demands of the General Agreement on Tariffs and Trade (GATT). The new laws guarantee patent owners a longer period of exclusive sales of their product. In return, the pharmaceutical industry was obliged to increase its research and development spending within Canada. It has complied, and private funding of academic research has increased.

But because of, or in spite of the changes, drug prices have risen to take a larger slice out of the tax dollar, since a large proportion of the drug spending is for seniors and welfare recipients. Sensitive to the criticism of money making during a time of fiscal restraint, the Pharmaceutical Manufacturers Association of Canada, headed by former federal cabinet minister Judy Erola, began an aggressive campaign of public information in 1993–4. It argued that research into newer and better drugs for the management of chronic illness would control health-care costs by keeping people out of hospital. In 1995 the thirty-seven member companies donated $4.9 million to charity and invested almost $700 million in research and development.

The pharmaceutical industry also exercises considerable, though not exclusive, control over drug information. Doctors are usually unable or ill-equipped to examine the research literature. As a result, they tend to learn about new drugs from roving representatives or from advertisements in medical journals. Continuing Medical Education initiatives of medical schools and professional bodies are working to improve the situation by keeping the onus for disseminating news of innovations and dangers in the hands of supposedly impartial practitioners.

The Life Cycle of Innovations in Treatment

By 1954 Ernest Jawetz had shown that medical approval follows a pattern. At first, the use of a new remedy rises quickly in a period of optimism; then some untoward side effect is noted, and the approval wanes rapidly to a low based on mistrust and fear; finally, use stabilizes at a moderate level (*Annual Review of Medicine* 5 (1954), 2). These swings have been called 'from panacea to poison to pedestrian.' The Jawetz model certainly fits the life cycle of chloramphenicol, which was developed in 1948 as an effective antibiotic. By 1967, it was found to produce aplastic anemia in one in every 30,000 patients treated. Sales fell dramatically, and its manufacturer, Parke Davis, was forced to merge with Warner Lambert. Since then, chloramphenicol use has risen slowly to a stable but lower level.

Jawetz's curve has been applied to the natural history of other remedies, including digitalis, which suffered a long period of unpopularity. For digitalis, the margin between therapeutic and toxic is narrow; levels high enough to be of benefit are close to those causing side effects. Only when dosage could be stabilized was medical approval stabilized too (Estes, 1979).

Legislation is intended to level off peaks and troughs, but the Jawetz curve is unlikely ever to become a straight line. Drug testing may eliminate the precipitous drops due to unexpected side-effects, but gradual decline in a drug's use will always occur as one remedy is replaced by safer and more effective products or as the disease in

Table 5.1
Top treatments used or sold in various practices, 1795-1995

1795	1850s	1880s	1931	1995
Opium	Quinine	Cupping	Codeine	Diltiazem (Cardizem)
Blisters	Opium	Opium	Acetylsalicylic acid	Omeprazole Mg (Losec)
Senna	Venesection	Tartar emetic	Sod. bicarbonate	Nifedipine (Adalat)
Aloes	Tartar emetic	Chloroform	Acetphenetidin	Fluoxetine HCl (Prozac)
Tartar	Calomel (mercury)	discontinue order	Elix. pepsin comp.	Lovastatin (Mevacor)
Cinchona	Blisters	Bromide/ergot	Sodium bromide	Beclomethasone (Beclovent)
Licorice	Ipecac	Aconite	Glycerin	Enalapril (Vasotec, Apo-Enalapril)
Enemata	Cupping	Chloral hydrate	Sodium salicylate	Simvastatin (Zocor)
Mercurials	Iron	Enemata	Nux vomica	Ciprofloxacin (Cipro)
Jalap	Jalap	Milk	Ammonium Cl.	Sertraline (Zoloft)

Sources:
1795: based on a practitioner's prescriptions: Estes, J. Worth, 'Drug Use at the Infirmary, the Example of Dr. Andrew Duncan, Sr', in Guenter B. Risse, *Hospital Life in Enlightenment Scotland: Care and Teaching at the Royal Infirmary of Edinburgh* (Cambridge: Cambridge University Press 1986), 351–4
1850s and 1880s: based on a practitioner's prescriptions: Jacalyn Duffin, *Langstaff: A Nineteenth-Century Medical Life* (Toronto: University of Toronto Press, 1993), 75
1931: based on survey of >120,000 pharmacy prescriptions in four states. E.N.: Gathercoal, *The Prescription Ingredient Survey* (American Pharmaceutical Association, 1933), 22
1995: based on national sales: Pharmaceutical Manufacturers Association of Canada, *Annual Review* (Ottawa: PMAC, 1996–7), 23

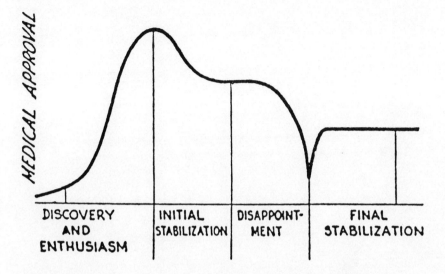

Graph depicting the phases in a drug's use. From Ernest Jawetz, *Annual Review of Medicine* 5 (1954), 2

question becomes something else (see chapter 4). Dips in the curve are generated not only by the recognized side effects but also by what disease happens to be in fashion and who the target population comprises.

The most used or most sold drugs have changed markedly in the last two centuries (see table 5.1). At the time of writing, the list is dominated by agents for the treatment of atherosclerotic heart disease, high cholesterol, chronic lung disease, stomach ailments, mental disorders, and arthritis – all chronic problems, many the product of diet and lifestyle, conditions that can be treated unto death. The list is yet another sign of an aging society in which neither patients nor practitioners are particularly enamoured of the concept of disease prevention.

Suggestions for Further Reading

Ackerknecht, Erwin H. *Therapeutics from the Primitives to the Twentieth Century.* New York: Harper, 1973

Arber, Agnes Robertson. *Herbals, Their Origin and Evolution: A Chapter in the His-*

tory of Botany, 1470–1670. Cambridge and New York: Cambridge University Press, 1986

Brandt, Allan M. *No Magic Bullet: A Social History of Venereal Disease in the United States since 1880.* New York: Oxford University Press, 1987

Brody, Howard. *Placebo and the Philosophy of Medicine.* Chicago and London: University of Chicago Press, 1980

Brunel, Jules. 'Antibiosis from Pasteur to Fleming.' *Journal of the History of Medicine and Allied Sciences* 6 (1951), 287–301

Clendening, Logan. *Source Book of Medical History.* 1942. Reprint, New York: Dover Publications and Henry Schuman, 1960

Estes, J. Worth. *Hall Jackson and the Purple Foxglove: Medical Practice and Research in Revolutionary America, 1760–1820.* Hanover, N.H.: University of New England Press, 1979

Gehan, Edmund A., and Noreen A. Lemak. *Statistics in Medical Research: Developments in Clinical Trials.* New York: Plenum Medical Book Co., 1994

Haller, John S. *American Medicine in Transition, 1840–1910.* Urbana and London: University of Illinois Press, 1981

Illich, Ivan. *Medical Nemesis: The Expropriation of Health.* London: Calder and Boyars, 1975

Kremers, Edward. *Kremers and Urdang's History of Pharmacy.* 4th edn., ed. Glenn Sonnedecker. Philadelphia: Lippincott, 1976

Kudlien, Fridolf, and Richard J. Durling, eds. *Galen's Method of Healing: Proceedings of the 1982 Galen Symposium, Christian-Albrechts Universität.* Leiden and New York: E.J. Brill, 1991

Leake, Chauncey D. *An Historical Account of Pharmacology to the Twentieth Century.* Springfield, Ill: Charles C. Thomas, 1975.

Lederer, Susan E. *Subjected to Science: Human Experimentation in America before the Second World War.* Baltimore: Johns Hopkins University Press, 1995

Lilienfeld, Abraham. '*Ceteris Paribus:* The Evolution of the Clinical Trial.' *Bulletin of the History of Medicine* 56 (1982), 1–18

McKeown, Thomas. *The Role of Medicine: Dream, Mirage, or Nemesis?* 2nd edn. Oxford: Blackwell, 1979

Majno, Guido. *The Healing Hand: Man and Wound in the Ancient World.* Cambridge, Mass.: Harvard University Press, 1975

Mann, Ronald D. *Modern Drug Use: An Enquiry on Historical Principles.* Lancaster, England: MTP Press, 1984

Parascandola, John. *The History of Antibiotics: A Symposium.* Madison, Wis.: American Institute of the History of Pharmacy, 1980

– *Sources in the History of American Pharmacology.* Madison, Wis.: American Institute of the History of Pharmacy, 1983

– *The Development of American Pharmacology: John J. Abel and the Shaping of a Discipline*. Baltimore: Johns Hopkins University Press, 1992

Peitzman, Steven J. 'When Did Medicine Become Beneficial? The Perspective from Internal Medicine.' *Caduceus* 12 (Winter 1996), 39–44

Porter, Roy, and Mikulas Teich, eds. *Drugs and Narcotics in History*. Cambridge and New York: Cambridge University Press, 1995

Riddle, John M. *Dioscorides on Pharmacy and Medicine*. Austin: University of Texas Press, 1985

Rosenberg, Charles E., and Morris J. Vogel, eds. *The Therapeutic Revolution: Essays in the Social History of American Medicine*. Philadelphia: University of Pennsylvania Press, 1979

Sullivan, Robert B. 'Sanguine Practices: A Historical and Historiographic Reconsideration of Heroic Therapy in the Age of Rush.' *Bulletin of the History of Medicine* 68 (1994), 211–34

Warner, John Harley. *The Therapeutic Perspective: Medical Practice, Knowledge, and Identity in America, 1820–1885*. Cambridge, Mass., and London: Harvard University Press, 1986

On Canada

Arnason, Thor, Richard J. Hebda, and Timothy Johns. 'Use of Plants for Food and Medicine by Native Peoples of Eastern Canada.' *Canadian Journal of Botany* 59 (1981), 2189–325

Bliss, Michael. *The Discovery of Insulin*. Toronto: McClelland and Stewart, 1982

Cadotte, Marcel. 'A propos de la description par Jacques Cartier d'une "grosse maladie" survenue au cours de son deuxième voyage au Canada.' *Union medicale du Canada* 113 (1984), 651–5

Collin, Johanne, and Denis Beliveau. *Histoire de la pharmacie au Québec*. Montréal: Musée de la Pharmacie du Québec, 1994

Connor, J.T.H. 'Minority Medicine in Ontario: A Study of Medical Pluralism and Its Decline.' PhD dissertation, University of Western Ontario, 1989

– '"A Sort of Felo de Se": Eclecticism, Related Medical Sects and Their Decline in Victorian Ontario.' *Bulletin of the History of Medicine* 65 (1991), 503–27

Crellin, J.K. *Home Medicine: The Newfoundland Experience*. Montreal and Kingston: McGill-Queen's University Press, 1994

Desrosiers, Georges. 'Les observations médicales de Jacques Cartier et Samuel de Champlain.' *Union médicale du Canada* 99 (1970), 677–81

Li, Alison. 'J.B. Collip, A.M. Hanson, and the Isolation of the Parathyroid Hormone, or Endocrines and Enterprise.' *Journal of the History of Medicine and Allied Sciences* 47 (1992), 405–38

Macbeth, Robert A. 'Louis Hébert: Le père de la Nouvelle France.' *Annals of the Royal College of Physicians and Surgeons of Canada* 30 (1997), 37–41

Marks, G.S. 'The History of Pharmacology in Canada.' *Trends in Pharmacological Sciences* 15 (1994), 205–10, erratum 349

PMAC annual reports and other publications. 302-1111 Prince of Wales Drive, Ottawa K2C 3T2; tel 613-727-1380; FAX 613-727-1407.

Report of the Thalidomide Task Force. 3 vols. Ottawa: War Amputations of Canada, 1989

CHAPTER SIX

On Being a Doctor:
History of Health-Care Delivery*

That any sane nation, having observed that you could provide for the supply of bread by giving bakers a pecuniary interest in baking for you, should go on to give a surgeon a pecuniary interest in cutting off your leg, is enough to make one despair of political humanity.

G.B. Shaw, *The Doctor's Dilemma*, 1911, 1

The Doctor-Patient Contract

Doctors can be doctors only when someone else agrees. A contract has always existed between physician and patient, although usually it was not recorded in writing. This contract assumes doctors have expert *knowledge* that will fill patient *expectations*. When these expectations are met, patients grant doctors the privileges of *authority* and professional *control*, which are exemplified by autonomy over examination, licensing, and discipline. Privileges continue as long as the contract is filled to the satisfaction of both parties.

When doctors fail to meet expectations, penalties ranged from the ancient extremes of amputation of both hands as recommended by the Code of Hammurabi, ca. 1700 B.C., to crucifixion as recommended by Alexander and described by Plutarch (*Life of Alexander,* ch. 72) and Arrian (*Anabasis* 7, 14). The less drastic penalties of our

*Educational objectives for this chapter are found on p. 395.

own time include fines, revocation of the licence to practise, and jail. Professional authority is still a privilege, not a right. But doctors have sometimes forgotten the negotiated nature of their contract and construed their autonomy as a right.

The history of the medical profession is a history of this contract and how it has been negotiated and changed. Simply meeting its terms does not necessarily guarantee adulation or even respect. The profession has passed through periods of ascendancy and decline.

An Image

The 1891 oil painting by Sir Luke Fildes called *The Doctor* is a magnificent example of nineteenth-century strength and pathos. The caring physician sits beside a suffering child whose distraught parents hover in the background. He comforts with his presence, even if he offers little in the way of medicine. Is the message conveyed by this moving picture still valid in our own time?

On Fildes's *Doctor*

Few would dispute the values symbolized by Fildes: patience, tenderness, wisdom, even courage, as the physician exposes himself to disease. The bearded doctor is distinguished and wise; he has come to the patient's home without special equipment, and he gives all the time that the family needs. The parents are displaced by his authority. Indeed, they willingly cede their place. An accord is implicit in the shared culture of the family and the doctor. It is probable (though not evident in the painting) that he has treated the child with mercury, antimony, bloodletting, or other measures no longer indicated today. Whether she lives or dies, the parents will owe him money; whether or not he accepts their payment, is another matter, but he certainly has their account in his ledger at home. Failure to save the child's life will bring sorrow to the family, but it is unlikely to bring a subpoena for malpractice.

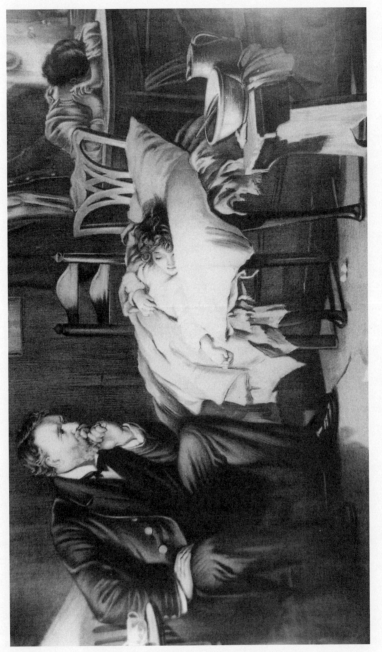

The Doctor, by Luke Fildes, 1891 (detail). Colour engraving based on original in the Tate Gallery, London. Gift of Dr J.W. Kerr, Faculty of Health Sciences, Queen's University

Can all the ideals portrayed by Fildes be retrieved in the health-care system of today? Now the doctor may not share the cultural, religious, or racial origins of the patient. The family is apt to have brought the child to the unfamiliar setting of a brightly lit emergency room, bustling with sparkling white coats, electronic gadgets, and strange sounds, where the doctors, almost half of whom will be women, have no time to sit and ponder. Furthermore, the family will not wish to be displaced from the bedside in unquestioning acquiescence with the doctor's opinion.

True, many schools educate their students in the importance of reviving the house call, honing communications skills, and providing reassurance for those confronted with the terrifying aspects of a modern hospital. But as much as doctors and patients alike may wish to emulate this empathy, patient expectations now go well beyond those of the stricken family in Fildes's painting of a century ago.

People now want and expect to be cured. They want 'the best,' even if it means immediate heart surgery or intrauterine correction of fetal defects. Newspapers report on families who have lost loved ones simply because of the long wait for procedures. We seem to be unable to provide the curative technology without sacrificing much of what is perceived to be valuable in Fildes's picture. When and how did the change happen?

History of the Elements of the Doctor-Patient Contract

Expectations of patients have changed dramatically since medical writing began some 3,500 years ago, but most of the changes are recent. In antiquity, being a successful doctor meant being able to predict the outcome of an illness. Alleviation of suffering was also important, but knowledge of the condition and its prognosis for death or healing constituted medical triumph. Most patients accepted the potential limitations of treatment, and the physician was just one among many different advisers, who included soothsayers, oracles, and priests. During the dominance of Christianity, the perfect practitioner was one who combined knowledge of disease with deference to God's will. Nevertheless, by the middle of the fourteenth century, most European jurisdictions required some form of

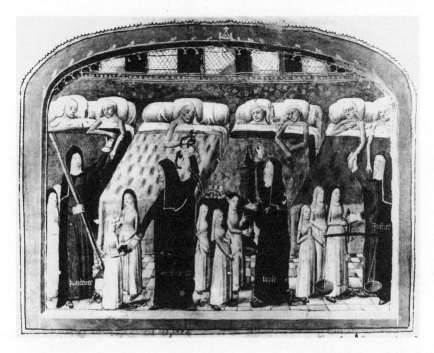

A medieval hospital scene. Care was the objective of religious sites of healing; cure, a gift of God. From the fifteenth-century French manuscript by Jehan Henry, 'Livre de vie active.' Musée de l'Assistance Publique, Paris

a licence, to be obtained through examination by a guild, a public authority, or a university (see table 6.1).

Medical *knowledge* changed before patient expectations. After the so-called scientific revolution, European doctors began to scientificize illness and to make claims for their superior abilities as healers. From the sixteenth century, religion and medicine were formally separated and the independent power of doctors began to grow. Charters of autonomy were granted to physicians and to guilds of barber-surgeons, first by cities, then by nations. Being a professional was defined by membership in a body of practitioners who held the privilege of examining, licensing, and disciplining their own.

Society may have acknowledged the advantages of the new scientific learning, but expectations of what a physician could actually

Table 6.1
Some milestones in the medical professionalization of Europe

Date	Authority	Licence requirement or limitation
Mid-12th C	Roger II of Sicily	Public examinations of practitioners
1215	Fourth Lateran Council	Clergy forbidden to cauterize or incise
1219	Bologna	Examination of archdeacon
1231	Frederick II of Sicily	Salerno masters have right to examine
13th C	Montpellier	Barber-surgeon guild
1260	Collège St Côme	Paris surgeons' guild
1418	Montpellier	Barber-surgeon guild examinations
1423	London	Brief merger of surgeons and physicians
1518	London	Royal College of Physicians
1540	England	Company of Barber Surgeons
1617	London	Apothecaries separate from physicians
1699	Louis XIV of France	Dentists examined by surgeons

accomplish changed little. Some were amused by the credibility gap. Playwrights such as Shakespeare and Molière, and caricaturists such as Rowlandson, Cruikshank, and Daumier poked fun at pompous doctors, portraying them as expensive, ineffective, and incomprehensible purveyors of drastics that killed as readily as they cured. Physicians and barber-surgeons still competed with a variety of other healers, including wise-women, quacks, charlatans, and the adepts of alternative theories. The history of medical professionalization is the shift from pluralistic health care to a monopoly of a powerful orthodoxy.

Other professional societies were formed at both local and national levels. Their goals were to act as professional lobbies and to preserve and advance standards of medical knowledge through meetings, publication, and licensing. For example, in nineteenth-century United States, doctors resented the financial threat and personal success (as much as they mistrusted the knowledge) of their 'unorthodox' colleagues, the homeopathics, eclectics, Thomsonians, and midwives. The American Medical Association was founded in 1847 partly as a professional lobby to protect the market share of doctors against homeopathists.

In Canada, medical practice has been regulated by regional licensing bodies since the seventeenth century. Before medical schools

Table 6.2
Founding of Canadian medical schools

1822–9	Montreal Medical Institution	
	(became McGill U)	Montreal, Que.
1824–6	Rolph and Duncombe	St Thomas, Ont.
1829	McGill U	Montreal, Que.
1843–91	Toronto School (merged with U of T)	Toronto, Ont.
1843–53	King's College (at U of T)	Toronto, Ont.
1843–90	Ecole de Montréal (merged with Laval)	Montreal, Que.
1850–?	Upper Canada / Trinity College	Toronto, Ont.
1852	U Laval	Quebec City, Que.
1854	Queen's U	Kingston, Ont.
1854–74	Victoria U, Cobourg	Toronto, Ont.
1866–90	Victoria U, Cobourg (merged with Ecole)	Montreal, Que.
1868	Dalhousie U	Halifax, N.S.
1870–1903	Trinity (merged with U of T)	Toronto, Ont.
1871–1905	Bishop's (merged with McGill)	Montreal / Lennoxville, Que.
1878–1920	Laval succursale (became U de M)	Montreal, Que
1882	U of Western Ontario	London, Ont.
1883	U of Manitoba	Winnipeg, Man.
1883–95	Women's Medical College	Kingston Ont.
1883–1906	Woman's Medical College	Toronto, Ont.
1891	U of Toronto	Toronto, Ont.
1913	U of Alberta	Edmonton, Alta
1920	U de Montréal	Montreal, Que.
1926–44	U of Saskatchewan (premed only)	Saskatoon, Sask
1944	U of Saskatchewan (full program)	Saskatoon, Sask
1945	U of Ottawa	Ottawa, Ont.
1950	U of British Columbia	Vancouver, B.C.
1966	U de Sherbrooke	Sherbrooke, Que.
1969	McMaster U	Hamilton, Ont.
1969	Memorial U	St John's, Nfld
1970	U of Calgary	Calgary, Alta

were founded, a degree from elite institutions in Europe was sufficient for a licence. American graduates and other candidates were subject to examinations. In the early nineteenth century, with the founding of Canadian schools (see table 6.2), examination eventually became compulsory for all.

Since 1911, the licence of the Medical Council of Canada (founded 1906) has been portable across all provinces. Special examinations are required of foreign medical graduates who come to the United States or Canada (called ECFMG, first held in 1958).

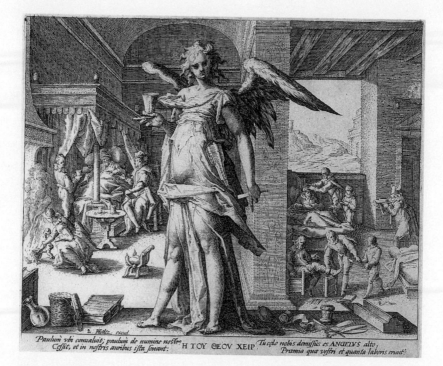

The physician as angel (*above*) and as devil (*opposite*). Both anonymous Dutch, 1587, after Hendrik Goltzius. These are the second and fourth images in an allegory of the medical profession from the patient's perspective. The doctor changes from a god hearing a prayer for help, to an angel dispensing medicine, to an ordinary man who hurts as he tries to help, and finally to a devil seeking payment. Philadelphia Museum of Art

Professional colleges, operated by physicians, continue to regulate practice within each province; they exercise the power to license, investigate, and discipline practitioners. Other associations lobby for doctors' financial well-being. With the goal of disseminating knowledge and protecting the interests of physicians, the Canadian Medical Association emerged from a variety of provincial and municipal precursors, some of which still exist. Its constitution was ratified in 1907, and its journal was begun in 1911.

Patient expectations began to rise in the mid-nineteenth century

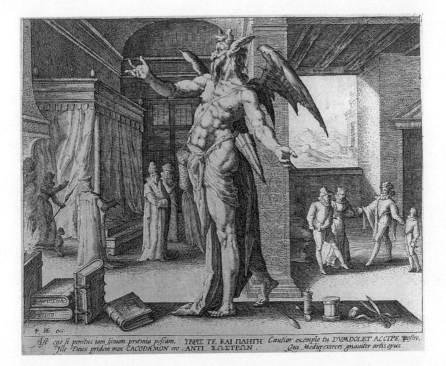

Aft ego si penitus iam simon premia poscam,   YBPIΣ TE, KAI ΠΛΗΓΗ   Cautior exemplo tu DVMDOLET ACCIPE, nostro,
'Ille Deus pridem max CACODÆMON ero. ANTI   Σ.Ω.ΣΤΡΩΝ .   Qui Medice exerces gnauiter artis opus.

with the major discoveries of anesthesia and antisepsis. Diseases that had been accepted as fatal or chronic could now be painlessly repaired (see chapter 10). Anesthesia has been cited as the most important technology in shaping the modern contract. Patients 'now expected a "technical fix" for every pain'; but by acquiescing to medical expertise, they lost individual autonomy over their well-being (Pernick 1985, 233). The advent of antibiotics in the 1930s and 1940s had a similar effect (see chapter 5). Now that a cure was sometimes possible, it quickly became an imperative.

Between 1850 and 1950, the medical profession could point to a succession of surgical and medical giants, who were hailed as national institutions within their homelands. The great books of these great men sustained Fildes's country doctor through his bedside vigils year after year. In the early twentieth century, simply being a doctor was automatically a reason to be accorded admiration and respect.

Medical power and prestige increased further with the advent of specialties in the late nineteenth century. The first autonomous specialty board appeared in the United States in 1924; more than twenty such boards, representing more than fifty subspecialties, operate there. In Canada, the Royal College of Physicians and Surgeons was founded in 1929 to train, examine, and license specialists.

The Mace of the Royal College of Physicians and Surgeons of Canada

A gift of the Royal College of Surgeons of England in 1964, the mace symbolizes the 'corporate power' of the college and is carried by the executive member-at-large during academic processions. The original was stolen in 1992, but a replacement was quickly commissioned and was completed in 1993. Canadian specialists take their power and its symbols very seriously.

Some sectors of society continue to venerate the medical profession, but veneration is no longer a given. Practitioners are not necessarily trusted, nor do they possess the same control over practice that they once enjoyed. While society has come to expect miracle cures from medicine, its expectations of medical professionals have declined to 'low': doctors are sometimes said to be dangerous, unsympathetic, and cruel. Why?

Twentieth-Century Changes in the Doctor-Patient Contract

First, it is now widely known that medical knowledge has sometimes been 'wrong.' Errors in our century may be no more frequent than those in earlier times, perhaps less; now, however, they are more conspicuous. Some procedures touted as panaceas have waned or been abandoned; examples include tonsillectomy, and surgery for visceroptosis (see chapter 10). Some practices were hounded into quackery: the once respectable Brinkley procedure, begun in the

A Less Respectful View

Mistrust of authority is reflected in the writings of current historians, whose works on 'great doctors' seldom fail to address shortcomings that previously might have been passed over as virtues or quirks. Galen, we are told, fled Rome during a plague. Similarly, Thomas Sydenham fled London during an epidemic. William Withering first tested digitalis on the poor. Edward Jenner's courageous demonstration of vaccination would not meet present-day standards of ethics. William Osler perpetrated practical jokes. William Halsted used cocaine. Alexander Fleming was given more credit for penicillin than he deserved. The Canadian surgeon Norman Bethune drank and womanized. Frederick Banting hit his wife.

1890s, purported to rejuvenate by 'transplantation' of monkey or goat gonads; by 1930, charges were brought against John R. Brinkley of Kansas, despite patient testimonials in his defence. Most drugs have undesirable side effects, but some have resulted in serious harm, for example, thalidomide, chloramphenicol, and phenacetin (see chapter 5). The same is true for intrauterine devices and breast implants.

Doctors who administer dangerous treatments have generally been protected from blame. In most cases, it is the drug companies, manufacturers, and, occasionally, governments who bear the legal responsibility. Will doctors continue to make unfortunate decisions? Yes. Will they always enjoy relative insulation from blame? Will they readily acknowledge their errors? We do not know.

Second, the nature of medical knowledge is changing as much as its content. Some claim that 'knowledge is increasing,' but the increase is in information – not knowledge. The *Index Medicus* provides references to the medical literature of the preceding year; in 1879 it was a single volume, five centimetres thick. Its slim size pales in comparison with the more than thirtyfold expansion required to hold the nineteen volumes of the 1997 edition. How can any doctor profess to 'know' the tens of thousands of medical periodicals filled with so-called new knowledge? Ideas that are true at the beginning of a medical education are sometimes false by the end. Faced with a labyrinth of conflicting information, how do doctors learn when to reject what they have been taught in favour of something new? In having so much more information about different things, do today's doctors really know more than Fildes's? Is it better knowledge? And has it come with no cost?

Third, medical heroes may continue to hold authority in some countries, but they are no longer fashionable in North America. In France, a recent campaign put the faces of the country's famous oncologists on billboards, exhorting the *citoyens* to give generously. This project would not succeed in Canada, where cancer doctors are relatively unknown; the pleas of patients are more effective.

Mistrust of heroes is not confined to medicine. Our age has become suspicious of class distinctions, authority, and anything scientific. Like medicine, science too has been 'wrong.' Science brought the atom bomb, Love Canal, ozone depletion, Chernobyl, pollution, and the much-disputed problem of global warming. Inspired by environmental ethics, patients say that they don't want to poison their systems with drugs.

Doctors are human. Sometimes they make fatal mistakes – because their knowledge was used for crime, perhaps, or in the service of political and cultural ideology. In experimentation, the rights of disadvantaged groups have on many occasions been cast aside. For example, the Tuskegee study of untreated syphilis in black men continued until the 1970s, long after effective treatments were known; not until May 1997 did the survivors receive a formal apology from President Bill Clinton for the U.S. government's role in that project. Sobering recent histories dissect the actions of Nazi doctors, who somehow managed to reconcile racial extermination with their Hippocratic oath to 'do no harm' (see chapter 13). Abuses of medical power and privilege should never be forgotten.

Fourth, cure, which gradually became an important expectation, is now considered a right. As a result, the contract between doctor and patient suffers from a double-bind. On the one hand is the cultural mistrust of medicine, science, and authority; on the other, a belief that every person has the right to a technological fix. How can doctors cure patients using the very knowledge and skills that patients tend to suspect? Recognizing these problems in the 1990s, Ontario initiated a 'demand-side' approach in a program called Educating Future Physicians (EFPO), which defined twelve complementary and sometimes conflicting roles for doctors.

Injured? Need a Lawyer? Call 1–800–XXX-XXXX

Billboard on many eastern U.S. interstate highways, 1990s

Doctors have been sued for failing to cure an incurable disease, as if someone must be held to blame for natural decay. Medical protective fees in the United States have risen to unprecedented levels. Even in Canada, where contingency fees are illegal and malpractice suits less frequent, premiums have been rising steadily in parallel with costs. In 1976 Canadian Medical Protective Association disbursements in damages and legal fees were about $4.5 million; by 1981 they had more than doubled to just over $10 million; in 1991, they were in excess of $60 million; and by 1995 they had doubled again to $120 million, a twenty-six-fold increase in twenty years. Over the same period, the rise in the Canadian consumer price index was less than threefold.

Health-Care Systems

Finally, a third party has entered the doctor-patient contract. Illness could easily ruin patients and their families. The problem of paying the doctor found various solutions over the years, each reflecting the political and cultural ideals of place and time. In the 1700s charity clinics were served by prominent doctors, while wealthy patients paid according to approved fee schedules, which were modified to fit the medic's reputation. Benevolent societies were organized to care for the sick, sometimes in workhouses that closely resembled jails. With the rise in technology and expectations of success, insurance schemes grew; many were run by doctors.

Table 6.3
Founding of health-care systems

1883	Germany	Compulsory health insurance for workers in wage category
1888	Austria	"
1891	Hungary	"
1893	France	Free medical care for the poor
1911	Britain	National Health Insurance Act
1916	Saskatchewan	Municipal doctors' scheme (salaries)
1947	Saskatchewan	Hospital services insurance
1948	Britain	National Health Service
1962	Saskatchewan	Medical services insurance
1968	Canada	National medicare program launched
1984	Canada	Canada Health Act

As inequities in access to medical care became a problem for governments, a variety of programs emerged (see table 6.3). Some covered all costs, while others covered only hospital and/or doctor care and excluded dentistry, drugs, physiotherapy, and other forms of practice. At first, special consideration was given to people with certain devastating diseases, such as tuberculosis or cancer. Later, systems were extended to national scales, ranging from health-insurance programs (in which the citizen pays a premium, the doctor receives a fee for service, and the government is the broker) to state medicine programs (in which the doctor is salaried, and health care is funded from taxes and provided 'free').

The purpose of these systems – be they private or public – is threefold: first, to remove the onus for payment from the sick or the poor; second, to ensure that health-care services are remunerated; and third, to prevent disease. The first two goals are often met; the third, however, is not. 'Health-care system' is a euphemism for managing and paying the wages of disease.

The first compulsory national health-insurance plan appeared in Germany in 1883 under the direction of the statesman Otto von Bismarck. Workers whose earnings fell within the specified range were obliged to pay premiums for coverage of health-related services, including dental, hospital, and medical care. Those whose wages fell below the range were obliged to seek charity; those who earned more were recommended to private coverage. Nationalized health plans have been demonized, especially by Americans, as the thin edge of a communist wedge; however, Bismarck's aim was the opposite: he reasoned that providing health care for workers within a capitalist system would thwart the growing labour movement by eliminating one of its chief complaints. The German system received wide attention because the country's well-funded laboratories were a leading destination for physicians (see chapter 3).

France enacted free medical care for the poor in 1893. The National Health Insurance Act of Britain was passed quickly in 1911 under the leadership of the future prime minister, David Lloyd George. It did not provide for hospital coverage, except for tuberculosis patients, and it forced employers to pay premiums for workers; the unemployed were excluded. The Russian Revolution created a decentralized system of clinics in which paramedical professionals, called *feldshers*, played a prominent role and fees for service were abolished. These sweeping changes so intimately connected with a totalitarian regime heightened suspicions in the United States.

Fear of Health Care: The Radio Debate on State Medicine, 12 November 1935

A publicly funded medical service 'would socialize if not communize one phase of American life,' stated Morris Fishbein, editor of the *Journal of the American Medical Association.* 'We shall become a nation of automatons, moving, breathing, living, suffering and dying at the will of politicians and political masters.'

American Medical Association Bulletin, November 1935, reprint, 7

In 1948 further reforms were implemented in Britain prompted by the 1943 report of the distinguished economist William Henry Beveridge. Health care was to be only one item in a comprehensive program of welfare 'from the cradle to the grave.' Beveridge intended state services to complement but not stifle individual initiative. British doctors who participated were paid a salary and limited to certain sites of practice. Negotiations resulted in compromises, and a parallel private system quickly became the sanctuary of elite physicians – the 'Harley Street set' – who served the wealthy. Many attempts to introduce health-care legislation in the United States have met with failure.

Most European countries, as well as Australia, New Zealand, and other developed nations now have health-care systems administered by the state. These countries may not enjoy better health, but First World jursidictions without nationwide medical care must face some depressing statistics. In the United States, for example, at least 35 million citizens have no insurance at all. The majority of those who died in a 1990 measles epidemic in Texas were unvaccinated black or Hispanic children living in poverty. In private systems, the public and the medical profession have relatively more difficulty dealing with the nonmedical determinants of illness: war, pollution, poverty, illiteracy, and lifestyle. Efforts to address these issues have been left to less-effective remote bureaucracies, such as the United Nations and the World Health Organization, or to the efforts of extraprofessional groupings of highly motivated individuals.

Prevention on a Grand Scale

Physicians for Social Responsibility (PSR) was founded by a small group in the Boston area in 1961. In the late 1970s it grew into an worldwide organization dedicated to eradicating nuclear war: International Physicians for the Prevention of Nuclear War (IPPNW). Founded in 1981 by two cardiologists, the Russian Evgueni I. Chazov and the American Bernard Lown, IPPNW included a wide variety of experts, led by Australian-born pediatrician Helen Caldicott of Harvard and Toronto psychiatrist Frank Summers, presidents of the American and Canadian PSR, respectively. While visiting Queen's University in Kingston in 1985, Chazov and Lown learned that the IPPNW had won the Nobel Prize for Peace.

Canada has been a world leader in health-care delivery. During the Second World War, the country embarked on measures to prevent another economic disaster like the Great Depression of the 1930s. All political parties endorsed the concept of funding health care. Unlike the majority of their American colleagues, Canadian medical professionals were interested in the decentralized plans of their Russian ally. Following the election in 1944 of the Co-operative Commonwealth Federation government of Tommy C. Douglas in Saskatchewan, that province became the first to enact hospital and medical coverage. The plan began with provincewide hospital coverage and a pilot project of full medical services in the town of Swift Current. A handful of doctors participated, but most opposed the changes until they realized that they were earning more than they had in the past. In 1962 medical coverage was extended to the entire province, and doctors went on strike for twenty-three days. In 1964 a royal commission, chaired by Emmett Hall, recommended a national system modelled on the Saskatchewan plan. The initial legislation was passed in 1966, and the program was launched in 1968. Like other countries, Canada soon saw more of that peculiarly twentieth-century phenomenon, the doctors' strike (see table 6.4).

Despite criticism from many practitioners and some Americans, the Canadian health-care system is the envy of the Western world; however, it is also the second most expensive (next to the United States). The system has changed the doctor-patient contract. Even when physicians fill most expectations, keep up to date, and do not make mistakes, control over practice no longer belongs entirely to them, but to the third party who pays. Access to care is also called a 'right,' but it is shaped by the pressures on the government of servicing a huge national debt.

Questions are now being asked about physician incomes, patient entitlements, and the allocation of costly instruments and procedures. Economists and policy makers point to the tremendous savings that would result from concentrating our efforts on the prevention of heart disease, stroke, and lung disease, rather than waiting to deal with their consequences. Others cite the global inequities of spending millions of dollars to prolong the lives of elderly, sedentary, and well-heeled North Americans while thousands of children die every year from malnutrition and simple infections. These population-based arguments have little resonance for the caregivers and families of individuals who are already sick. The

Table 6.4
Doctors' strikes or threatened strikes: A partial list

COUNTRIES OF THE WORLD
Australia, 1984
Bulgaria, 1922–3
Britain, 1911 (threat)
Czech Republic, 1995
Denmark, 1981
Finland, 1984
France, 1995, 1996
Germany, 1904 (Leipzig), 1982 (West), 1996 (threat)
Hungary, 1914
India, 1987, 1992, 1995
Israel, 1983 (118 days)
New Zealand, 1992 (resident doctors)
Russia, 1905, 1917–18, 1992 (threats)
Spain, 1995
USA, 1969 (Charleston, S.C.), 1975 (New York City; California hospitals), 1990
  (California housestaff)

CANADA
Alberta, 1986 (medical abortionists' work action), 1998
British Columbia, 1983 (threat), 1990 (foreign MDs' hunger strike), 1992
Manitoba, 1932–4 (Winnipeg), 1990
Newfoundland, 1982 (threat)
Nova Scotia, April 1984 (threat)
Ontario, June 1982 (1 day), June 1986 (25 days), 1996
Quebec, 1991 (threat)
Saskatchewan, 1962

---

discrepancy underscores a fundamental problem in trying to alter the medical model of disease in the context of North American democracy (see chapter 4).

Suffering individuals cannot accept the reasoning that procedures which are available for some should not be available to all. The traditional, medical-model obligation to the individual must be reconciled with providing optimal care for the majority at minimum cost. Some specialists move to the United States hoping for bigger incomes and greater freedom; others hold press conferences with bereaved families to protest delays.

Doctors complain about loss of autonomy and control, and they express nostalgia for the respect enjoyed by their less-effective nineteenth-century predecessors. But the past was not as rosy as it may seem. Practitioners worked long hours for relatively low wages, and they knew by name and face the identity of their charity cases. The weeping parents in the background of the Fildes painting could be indebted to the doctor for the rest of their lives.

Striking doctors display few of the qualities that earned the social standing of their predecessors. They act against their patients as well as the system, and they abrogate public responsibility by refusing to accept financial restructuring. Striking doctors lose public esteem, and their gains in financial concessions come at a moral cost. The unemployed and people on low incomes may tolerate the huge salaries of sports 'heroes,' but they do not sympathize with the strikes of imperfect physicians – medical 'villains' – whose earnings continue to be well above the national average.

Those who now control the purse strings recognize that the more doctors there are, the more they cost. Provinces have taken steps to limit physician numbers and earnings. Quebec capped the income of general practitioners in the early 1980s, and later in the same decade British Columbia tried to deny billing rights to newcomers. In Alberta, the number of doctors increased by 20 per cent in the early 1990s, while the population remained stable. The Alberta government made drastic cutbacks in hospital funding and refused to prosecute the illegal private clinics that were wielding expensive technologies. Ontario decreased the number of medical students and residents simultaneously, stressing access to postgraduate training.

Limits on earnings and sites of practice are a form of charity, but they lack the personal appeal of the one-on-one benevolence of the past. Doctors do not readily accept the concept of anonymous enforced charity. The twenty-five-day doctors' strike in Ontario in June 1986 was over the right to bill the patient for the remainder of the fee not covered under the system – a right that had been outlawed two years earlier by the Canada Health Act. The doctors' goal of full billing was labelled 'extra billing' by legislators and the media. The government won the issue, instigating a global rollback of fees – a legislated charitable donation. In a leading ethics journal, Eric Meslin characterized the strike as a double failure for the profession: it lost its case; and having reneged on a moral duty to provide health care, it lost sympathy and credibility. Epidemiologists discovered that the death rate actually decreased during the strike, and policymakers added this statistic to other arguments for limiting physician practice.

Despite the rhetoric of medical lobby groups, striking doctors cannot convince the public that they are motivated by concern for patient well-being. Instead, they appear to be preoccupied with incomes, especially those of their senior members rather than those of younger doctors or fellow professionals in nursing, midwifery, and rehabilitation. For example, on several occasions the Ontario Medical Association has proposed disincentives against new graduates; and it has long resisted the notion of mandatory retirement at age sixty-five, a concept that applies to most other government-funded workers.

A Thought Experiment

An associate dean at Queen's University once dreamed of giving every new medical student a copy of the Fildes picture, 'because,' he said, 'that's what medicine is really all about.' If students could keep that image foremost in their minds, they might remember the attributes that earned the respect enjoyed by their professional predecessors. Another colleague, in the Community Health and Epidemiology Department, agreed and recommended that the picture should have an empty thought-bubble above the doctor's head; students could imagine what he might be thinking. Some suggestions showed a marked preference for the present:

'I wish I could get an X-Ray.'
'Why did I leave my tracheostomy set at home?'
'Will the family pay my bill?'
'If only we had clean water.'

In a postwar attempt to block the public health-insurance initiatives that were launched in the United States, the American Medical

Association distributed copies of Fildes's painting to every physician in the country under the headings 'Keep Politics Out of this Picture'; and 'Do You Want Your Own Doctor or a Job Holder?' In 1947, the image also appeared on a U.S. postage stamp. The campaign worked. But neither the Americans, who succeeded in keeping out the so-called threat of socialized medicine, nor their Canadian neighbours, who 'failed,' can claim to have preserved the ambiance so movingly portrayed by Fildes.

Suggestions for Further Reading

Berlant, Jeffrey L. *Profession and Monopoly: A Study of Medicine in the United States and Britain.* Berkeley: University of California Press, 1975

Chivian, Eric, Susanna Chivian, Robert Jay Lifton, and John E. Mack, eds. *Last Aid: The Medical Dimensions of Nuclear War.* San Francisco: W.H. Freeman, 1982

Cook, Harold J. *The Decline of the Old Medical Regime in Stuart London.* Ithaca: Cornell University Press, 1986

Coulter, Harris L. *Divided Legacy: A History of the Schism in Medical Thought.* 3 vols. 1975–82. Esp. vol. 3, *The Conflict between Homeopathy and the American Medical Association.* Richmond, Calif.: North Atlantic Books, 1982

De Ville, Kenneth A. *Medical Malpractice in Nineteenth-Century America: Origins and Legacy.* New York: New York University Press, 1990

Digby, Anne. *Making a Medical Living: Doctors and Patients in the English Market for Medicine, 1720–1911.* Cambridge: Cambridge University Press, 1994

Forsyth, Gordon. *Doctors and State Medicine: A Study of the British Health Service.* Philadelphia and Toronto: Lippincott, 1966

Freidson, Eliot. *Profession of Medicine: A Study of the Sociology of Applied Knowledge.* New York: Harper and Row, 1970

Ham, Christopher. *Health Policy in Britain: The Politics and Organization of the National Health Service,* 3rd ed. London: Macmillan, 1992

Herman, John R. 'Rejuvenation: Brown-Sequard to Brinkley: Monkey Gland to Goat Gonads.' *New York State Journal of Medicine* 82 (1982), 1731–9

Hodgkinson, Ruth G. *The Origins of the National Health Service: The Medical Services of the New Poor Law, 1834–1871.* Berkeley: University of California Press, 1967

Jackson, Stanley W., ed. 'The Hippocratic Oath.' *Journal of the History of Medicine and Allied Sciences* 51 (1996), 403–500

Jones, Helen. *Health and Society in Twentieth-Century Britain.* London and New York: Longman, 1994

Jones, James H. *Bad Blood: The Tuskegee Syphilis Experiment.* New York: Free Press, 1981

Kater, Michael H. *Doctors under Hitler.* Chapel Hill: University of North Carolina Press, 1989

Kawakita, Yoshio, Shizu Sakai, and Yasuo Otsuka, eds. *History of the Doctor-Patient Relationship. Proceedings of the 14th International Symposium on the Comparative History of Medicine – East and West, Japan, 1989.* Tokyo: Ishiyaku EuroAmerica, 1995

Kett, Joseph F. *The Formation of the American Medical Profession: The Role of Institutions, 1780–1860.* New Haven and London: Yale University Press, 1968

Lederer, Susan E. *Subjected to Science: Human Experimentation in America before the Second World War.* Baltimore: Johns Hopkins University Press, 1995

McVaugh, Michael R. *Medicine before the Plague: Practitioners and Their Patients in the Crown of Aragon, 1285–1345.* Cambridge: Cambridge University Press, 1993

Numbers, Ronald L. *Almost Persuaded: American Physicians and Compulsory Health Insurance, 1912–1920.* Baltimore and London: Johns Hopkins University Press, 1978

Pernick, Martin S. *A Calculus of Suffering: Pain, Professionalism, and Anesthesia in Nineteenth-Century America.* New York: Columbia University Press, 1985

Porter, Roy, ed. *Patients and Practitioners: Lay Perceptions of Medicine in Pre-Industrial Society.* Cambridge: Cambridge University Press, 1985

Rosen, George. *Fees and Feebills: Some Economic Aspects of Medical Practice in Nineteenth-Century America.* Baltimore: Johns Hopkins University Press, 1946

– *Specialization of Medicine with Special Reference to Ophthalmology.* New York: Arno Press, 1972

Rosen, George, and Charles E. Rosenberg, *The Structure of American Medical Practice, 1875–1941.* Philadelphia: University of Pennsylvania Press, 1983

Shorter, Edward. *Bedside Manners: The Troubled History of Doctors and Patients.* Harmondsworth, England: Viking Penguin, 1986

Solomon, Susan Gross, and John F. Hutchinson, eds. *Health and Society in Revolutionary Russia.* Bloomington: Indiana University Press, 1990

Starr, Paul. *The Social Transformation of American Medicine.* New York: Basic Books, 1982

Warner, John Harley. 'Power, Conflict, and Identity in Mid-Nineteenth-Century American Medicine.' *Journal of American History* 73 (1987), 934–56

Weisz, George. 'Medical Directories and Medical Specialization in France, Britain, and the United States.' *Bulletin of the History of Medicine* 71 (1997), 23–68

Wolinsky, Howard, and Tom Brune. *The Serpent on the Staff: The Unhealthy Politics of the American Medical Association.* New York: Putnam, 1994

On Canada

Badgley, Robin F., and Samuel Wolfe. *Doctors' Strike: Medical Care and Conflict in Saskatchewan.* Toronto: Macmillan, 1967

Bernier, Jacques. *La médecine au Québec: Naissance et évolution d'une profession.* Quebec: Presses de l'Université Laval, 1989

Canadian Medical Protective Association. *Newsletter* 2, no. 2 (1987); 11, no. 3 (1996)

Crichton, Anne, David Hsu, and Stella Tsang. *Canada's Health Care System: Its Funding and Organization.* CHA Press: Ottawa, 1994

Duffin, Jacalyn. 'The Guru and the Godfather: Henry E. Sigerist, Hugh MacLean, and the Politics of Health Care Reform in 1940s Canada.' *Canadian Bulletin of Medical History* 9 (1992), 191–218

Duffin, Jacalyn, and Leslie A. Falk. 'Sigerist in Saskatchewan: The Quest for Balance in Social and Technical Medicine.' *Bulletin of the History of Medicine* 70 (1996), 658–83

Gelfand, Toby. 'Medicine in New France.' In *Medicine in the New World: New Spain, New France, and New England,* ed. Ronald L. Numbers, 64–100. Knoxville, Tenn.: University of Tennessee Press, 1987

Gidney, Robert D., and W.P.J. Millar. 'The Origins of Organized Medicine in Ontario, 1850–1869.' In *Health, Disease, and Medicine: Essays in Canadian History,* ed. Charles G. Roland, 65–95. Toronto: Hannah Institute for the History of Medicine, 1984

– *Professional Gentlemen: The Professions in Nineteenth-Century Ontario.* Toronto: University of Toronto Press, 1994

Godfrey, Charles M. *Medicine for Ontario: A History.* Belleville, Ont.: Mika, 1979

Hamowy, Ronald. *Canadian Medicine: A Study in Restricted Entry.* Vancouver: Fraser Institute, 1984

Jecker, N.S., and E.M. Meslin. 'United States and Canadian Approaches to Justice in Health Care: A Comparative Analysis of Health Care Systems and Values.' *Theoretical Medicine* 15 (1994), 181–200

Lewis, David Sclater. *The Royal College of Physicians and Surgeons of Canada, 1920–1969.* Montreal: McGill University Press, 1962

McPhedran, N. Tait. *Canadian Medical Schools: Two Centuries of Medical History, 1822–1992.* Montreal: Harvest House, 1993

Meslin, Eric. 'The Moral Costs of the Ontario Physicians' Strike.' *Hastings Center Report* 17 (August 1987), 11–14

Naylor, C. David. *Private Practice, Public Payment: Canadian Medicine and the Politics of Health Insurance.* Kingston and Montreal: McGill-Queen's University Press, 1986

– ed. *Canadian Health Care and the State: A Century of Evolution.* Montreal :
    McGill-Queen's University Press, 1992
Neufeld, Victor R., et al. 'Demand-side Medical Education: Educating Future
    Physicians for Ontario.' *Canadian Medical Association Journal* 148 (1993),
    1471–7
Shephard, David A.E. *The Royal College of Physicians and Surgeons of Canada, 1960–
    1980: The Pursuit of Unity.* Ottawa: Royal College of Physicians and Surgeons of
    Canada, 1985
Shortt, S.E.D. 'Physicians, Science, and Status: Issues in the Professionalization
    of Anglo-American Medicine in the Nineteenth Century.' *Medical History* 27
    (1983), 51–68
Taylor, Malcolm G. *Health Insurance and Canadian Public Policy: The Seven Decisions
    that Created Canada's Health Insurance System and their Outcomes.* 2nd edn.
    Kingston and Montreal: McGill-Queen's University Press, 1987

CHAPTER SEVEN

Plagues and Peoples: Epidemic Diseases in History*

> Behold, a pale horse and its rider's name was Death, and Hades followed him; and they were given power over a fourth of the earth, to kill with sword and with famine and with pestilence.
>
> Revelation 6:8

Epidemics have destroyed populations and significantly altered economic, social, intellectual, and political aspects of life. With apologies to W.H. McNeill, whose title I borrow, this chapter will explore themes common to epidemics, emphasizing their impact on human life.

The Plague of Athens (ca. 430 B.C.): What Was It, and Does It Matter?

Panic and breakdown of social order typify human reactions to epidemic illness. The Greek historian Thucydides, in his *History of the Peloponnesian War* (Bk. 2, 47–54) told how a lethal contagious disease afflicted the Athenians while Spartans lay siege to their city. The symptoms included fever, painful skin rash, and great thirst. No treatment was effective. Physicians, who were quickly exposed to many cases, died first; even birds and animals disappeared. Among

---

*Educational objectives for this chapter are found on pp. 395–6.

the dead was Pericles, the ruler of Athens and builder of the Parthenon. Thucydides too had been sick, but he reported that the few survivors were considered immune. Opinion on the origin of the disease was divided. One rumour held that it came from Africa, but some thought it was new, stemming from starvation and the strife of war. Still others said that Spartans had poisoned the wells. Religious people were convinced that it was divine punishment for unrevealed sins; however, oracles and priests were no better than doctors at relieving the suffering.

Thucydides' account is the sole surviving record of this disaster. The absence of other testimony raises many questions, including the possibility that the historian simply invented his tale. Doctors, however, have long been intrigued by the plague of Athens, finding the vivid description quite credible – even irresistible. They have sought to discover the precise retrospective diagnosis; contenders include smallpox, typhus, and anthrax. Whenever a new infectious disease is described, it seems that sooner or later someone connects it to the plague of Athens. Recent essays have postulated toxic shock syndrome, legionnaires' disease, AIDS, and Ebola fever as the 'real' diagnosis. But most would-be diagnosticians fail to account for the bioecological reality of rapidly mutating germs. The improbability (if not impossibility) of applying a modern diagnosis to the plague of Athens is a 'Heisenberg uncertainty principle' in medical history. The riddle will likely continue to defy solution.

This ancient disease may not be reduced to our own terms, but Thucydides' story has come to exemplify the timeless extracorporeal side effects of any epidemic. During the plague, social structure decayed, crime was rampant, and codes of behaviour were abandoned. Family members shunned their ailing relatives and often neglected the dead; bodies were thrown on pyres built for others – a sacrilege as well as a crime. The epidemic passed, but Athens lost that war and did not regain its former power.

The Great Dying, or Black Death: Bubonic Plague (1348 and After)

The most famous epidemic in Western history was the fourteenth-century bubonic plague of Europe. Known at the time as the 'great dying,' it was given its gothic and resilient name, Black Death, in 1832 by the German physician-historian J.F.C. Hecker. Earlier outbreaks of plague had occurred, including a sizable epidemic during the reign of the Byzantine Emperor Justinian in the sixth century A.D.; however, none matched the scope and horror of the fourteenth-century epidemic. According to witnesses, European plague travelled from Asia in ships and seemed to begin with the arrival of Genoese vessels at the Sicilian port of Messina in October 1347. From there, the disease marched rapidly north, fanning across Europe to reach Moscow by 1351. The symptoms were fever, swollen and oozing nodes (buboes), dehydration, and death.

Social practices were overturned in the manner described by Thucydides. People abandoned their urban homes to wander in the country; sick family members were left to die. Corpses were shunned, and officials forced criminals to heap bodies into mass graves. In this atmosphere, the Florentine writer Giovanni Boccaccio, whose father had died of plague, wrote the *Decameron* – one hundred risqué but diverting stories told by a group of young men and women sheltering from the epidemic. Boccaccio's introduction is a famous record of the first wave of plague.

We now understand that plague is spread by direct inoculation of *Yersinia pestis*, a bacterium that infects the flea, *Xenopsylla cheopis*, which parasitizes humans only when its usual host, the black rat, has become scarce. Under certain conditions, plague can become pneumonic (involving the lung), then, it is spread by droplets from human to human. But this etiological framework was unknown until the 1890s, with the work of A.J.E. Yersin on the bacillus and of P.L. Simond on the flea.

In the fourteenth century, many hypotheses for the cause of plague were expounded, each of which subtended control measures. A new form of medical literature, the 'plague tractate,' arose to express these ideas. According to the surgeon Guy de Chauliac, the Paris faculty of medicine attributed plague to atmospheric alterations resulting from a rare conjunction of planets in the constellation Aquarius in March 1345. Others saw it as divine punishment for the corruption of priests; this argument gained credibility with the successive waves of plague during the Great Schism (1378–1417), when the church split over rival popes – one in Rome, the other in Avignon. Still others blamed minorities, strangers, and travellers.

Whatever its remote origin, plague was perceived to be contagious. Many doctors fled, and those who stayed used a variety of remedies, all viewed with scepticism. Physicians sometimes wore 'protective covering,' consisting of a gown, gloves, and a mask with mica goggles and a beaklike snout to contain healthful, fragrant herbs. Since travellers were potential carriers of the disease, states enacted laws of quarantine (from the French *quarante*, meaning 'forty' days), the first of which can be traced to the town of Ragusa (now Dubrovnik) in 1377. The number forty related to Christ's self-denial marked by the Christian period of Lent. Ships were required to wait forty days before unloading cargo or releasing passengers. Some cities passed harsher rules to restrict travel and freedoms. If plague appeared in a dwelling, all occupants might be confined there under 'house arrest' until they died or the disease passed. These rules the wealthy tried to avoid.

Foreign travellers were not the only people blamed for plague; minorities who lived in the midst of the illness (and suffered from it too) were also suspected of having provoked it. Village idiots, 'witch' women, and Jews were tortured for confessions and burned alive. The semi-religious flagellants atoned by zealous mortification of their own (and others') flesh; they enjoyed a surge in popularity that threatened organized religion. Other responses included the 'infectious' tarantism, or dancing mania. These practices are now seen to resemble forms of mass hysteria, fed by hopes for protection, salvation, absolution, and control.

One-quarter to one-third of the population of Europe is thought to have died in the first wave of plague, and many more succumbed in further outbreaks that occurred over the centuries. Once isolation became standard practice, special 'pesthouses' were built. The devastation extended beyond the immediate human carnage. Grain was left to rot in the fields, seed was scarce, and years of famine ensued with other attendant illnesses. It has been argued that the lack of peasant labourers contributed to the collapse of the feudal system and the rise of an urban middle class. For their inability to cope with plague, clerics and medics alike lost credibility. Education,

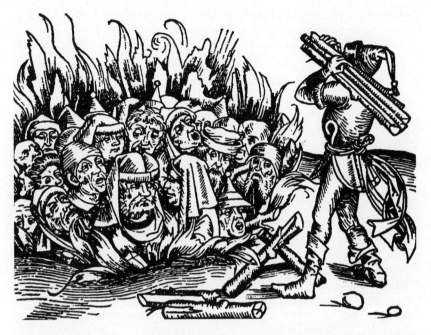

Woodcut depicting the burning of Jews in response to plague. From Hart-mann Schedel, *The Nuremberg Chronicle* (*Buch der Chroniken*), 1493, facsimile. New York: Landmark Press, 1979

which had previously been dominated by the church, became anti-clerical – or at least a-clerical. In medicine, the authority of Galen was challenged, because his copious writings had not described the disease. The effects of plague even extended to the artistic portrayal of naked and dead bodies. In her essay 'The Black Death and the Silver Lining,' historian Faye Getz has shown how later students of plague emphasized the positive outcomes, as if the catastrophe had somehow 'caused' the Renaissance; she speculates on why these writers looked for good in so much bad.

Social Construction: Definition and Examples

To the extent that plague was equated with foreigners and minorities, it was 'socially constructed' (see also chapter 4). The social posi-

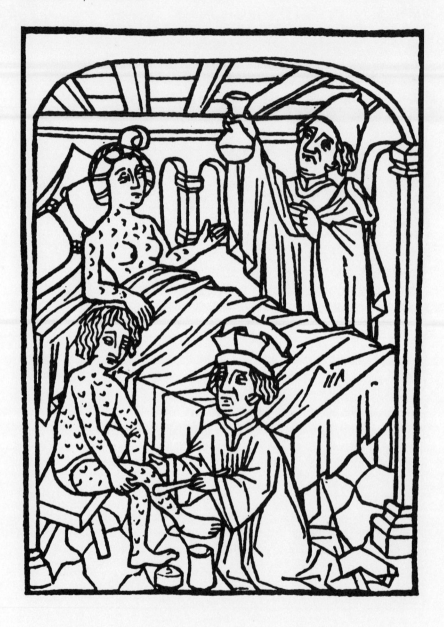

People being treated for the 'French disease.' From B. Steber, *A malafranzos*, 1498, facsimile by K. Sudhoff and C. Singer, 1925, 263

tion of sufferers entered into the medical concept of the disease. Treatment, therefore, included the persecution or elimination of dangerous strangers and practices. Social construction has not been confined to plague.

Syphilis

Social construction is amply demonstrated in syphilis. The origins of this disease are controversial. A virulent outbreak, apparently without precedent, afflicted the French armies and their Spanish mercenaries during a siege of Naples in the mid-1490s. As a result, some maintain that syphilis was transported to Europe from the Americas five hundred years ago by the crew of Christopher Columbus. Syphilis was called the 'great pox,' but it has also been called the 'French disease' by the Italians, the 'English disease' and the 'Spanish disease' by the French, and the 'Neopolitan disease' by the Spaniards.

In the early sixteenth century, the Italian physician Girolamo Fracastoro suggested that contagious diseases were caused by 'seeds' transmitted by people and objects. He concluded that these seeds must be alive, a *contagium vivum*, able to divide and multiply; without this property, he reasoned, they would diminish to negligible quantities through transmission. Fracastoro also understood that the new French disease was spread by sexual contact: he knew that the first lesions appeared on the genitalia, and he cautioned his readers not to 'succumb to the attractions of love.' The name 'syphilis' is taken from his allegorical poem of 1530, in which the cause was 'sin': the shepherd, Syphilus [*sic*], worshipped a king instead of a god, and the angered deity punished him with the disease. Probably through euphemism, the great pox came to bear the shepherd's name.

The skin manifestations of fifteenth-century syphilis were excruciatingly painful, and infection led rapidly to death. Fracastoro advocated mercury ointments and fumigations, applied until toxicity appeared in the form of sweating, salivation, and sore gums. Mercury probably was of some benefit, and it persisted as therapy until the twentieth century. Because spontaneous remissions occur in the course of syphilis, any remedy might appear to be effective. Numerous other methods were recommended, including guaiacum, the bark of a North American tree, which inspired confidence because it shared the presumed geographic origin of the infection. Later, the arsenic compound Salvarsan was formulated by Paul Ehrlich (see chapter 5).

Recognition of the modes of transmission of syphilis led to an alteration in sexual practices and the disappearance of public baths. Many controls were directed against presumed carriers, especially prostitutes and foreigners. Syphilis continues to be sensitive to the 'magic bullet,' penicillin, but the disease has not been eradicated, nor has it been controlled. The medical model treats infection inside the organism; however, prevention and eradication rely on the more difficult task of interfering with behaviour.

Leprosy

Public health standards for water and waste management are the product and legacy of earlier epidemics. Quarantine, for example, continues to have currency, especially for island jurisdictions such as the United Kingdom, Australia, and Newfoundland. Influenced by contemporary ideas about disease transmission, legislative measures can incorporate social prejudice. Sometimes these historically determined controls seem to make little biological sense, and they are better explained by social, cultural, psychological, and religious practices.

Leprosy, for example, is less infective than the responses to it would imply. As we know it, the disease is only mildly contagious. Regulations probably had more to do with protecting the healthy rich from having to confront the dreadful mutilations of the disfigured poor. In the Old Testament, leprosy denoted physical and moral impurity and punishment for sin. Sufferers were forced to live in colonies, to wear special clothes, and to carry bells warning of their presence. The Order of Lazarus, founded in the twelfth century and named for the man whom Christ raised from the dead, built special hospices to isolate and care for sufferers. The 'lazaretto' catered to people with problems other than leprosy or plague, but it became synonymous with 'leprosarium' and 'pesthouse.' Some historians maintain that biblical and medieval leprosy comprised a variety

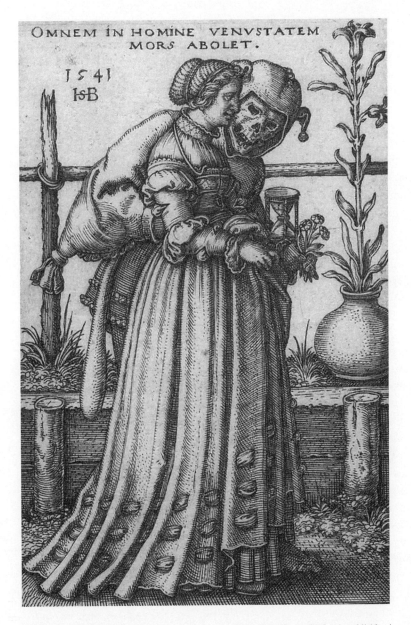

Young Woman Accompanied by Death as a Jester by Hans Beham, 1541. A post-syphilis *memento mori*. National Gallery of Canada

of disorders that differed from the condition, which is now attributed to the bacillus described in 1871 by G.H.A. Hansen. Nevertheless, the old controls persisted. A colony was established in New Brunswick in the mid-nineteenth century and more recently the care of Africans with leprosy was a mission of Cardinal Paul-Emile Léger of Montreal. Other centres still operate in both rich and poor countries, including Japan, Thailand, India, Senegal, Cameroon, and the United States (Hawaii and Louisiana).

Plagues and Numerical Medicine: Cholera and Typhus

With the advent of positivism in the early nineteenth century, numerical medicine soon influenced concepts of epidemic diseases (see chapter 4). The British reformers William Farr and Edwin Chadwick applied statistics to population health and uncovered powerful correlations between poverty, class, and disease. Their observations created a tension among middle-class reformers: some 'blamed the poor for their own misery and opposed public intervention'; others saw disease as a product of 'miserable conditions of life and sought solutions in public action' (Eyler 1980, 2). But the former 'laissez-faire' approach was more popular, especially with bureaucrats who balanced budgets and with physicians who focused on disease rather than prevention. For example, the German physician and statesman Rudolf Virchow argued for education, employment, and social programs to promote health in a population ravaged by cholera and typhus, but he lost his job in an 1849 backlash against reform.

Public health measures are informed by scientific research and predicated on the impulse to help the sick and protect the well. Sometimes, however, they have been both discriminatory and ineffective, causing more disease than they prevented. The nineteenth-century experience with cholera and typhus illustrates these points.

In the early 1830s, cholera swept across Europe from the Baltic in the second of seven great pandemics. Its global mortality is impossible to determine. British military action, colonial trade, and Russian wars may have triggered the spread out of its usual endemic focus in India. Characterized by massive diarrhea leading to death, sometimes within hours, cholera is spread by the *Vibrio cholerae*, which was eventually

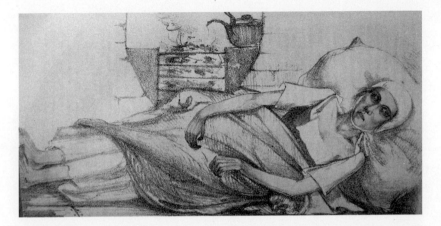

Blue stage of spasmodic cholera. This sketch of a girl who had recently died was published to educate physicians on how to recognize the new scourge. Her face, hands, and feet were hand-tinted in a blue-white wash. *Lancet*, 4 Feb. 1832, opp. 669

identified in 1884 by Robert Koch. The hardy vibrio can live in cool water; contamination cycles are maintained when sewage comes into contact with drinking water during floods, earthquakes, and war.

But cholera's link to drinking water was not established until twenty-two years after its European debut. In 1854 the English doctor John Snow carefully tracked victims to identify London's Broad Street pump as the source of an outbreak. Many doctors remained unconvinced: cholera seemed to be a disease of immigrants, the poor, and the dirty. Images portraying the link between foreigners and death were common.

Cholera came to Canada and the United States on immigrant ships in 1832. Sick newcomers were confined to sheds without fresh water or sewage facilities. Healthy immigrants were herded into the same buildings to be 'quarantined' side by side with those who were already sick. Management of the sheds was a charity, funded by rich and middle-class citizens, who were motivated by sympathy and a desire to keep the sickness at bay. Six thousand people died in Canada's first encounter with cholera. The figures endorsed the view

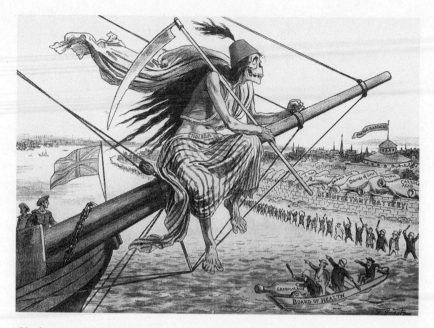

Cholera on the bowsprit, by Graetz. *Puck* magazine, 18 July 1883. 'The kind of "assisted emigrant" we can not afford to admit.' Disease is personified by the death's-head immigrant in Turkish garb. Bert Hansen Collection, New York, N.Y.

that the dirty poor were the most susceptible. Successive waves of cholera were handled in the same way.

Typhus, which is characterized by fever and rash, is now considered to be caused by the louse-borne agent *Rickettsia prowazeckii*. It had been endemic in Europe since antiquity, and severe epidemics occurred at various intervals, related to environmental conditions. An eighteenth-century outbreak in Nova Scotia decimated French troops, local Mi'kmaq, and the settlers in Halifax. From 1816 to 1819, typhus affected 700,000 of the 6 million living in Ireland. With the social instability and political revolutions of the late 1840s, it flared again and crossed the Atlantic, ravaging passengers in the crowded holds of ships. In 1847–8, more than nine thousand immigrants died en route as they fled the Irish potato famine.

> ### Cholera at Quebec, 1832
>
> The dreadful cholera was depopulating Quebec and Montreal when our ship cast anchor off Grosse Ile on the 30th August 1832, and we were boarded a few minutes later by health officers ...
>
> At Quebec ... the almost ceaseless tolling of bells proclaimed a mournful tale of woe and death. Scarcely a person visited the vessel who was not in black, or who spoke not in tones of subdued grief. They advised us not to go on shore if we valued our lives, as strangers most commonly fell the first victims to this malady.
>
> Susanna Moodie, Roughing It in the Bush
(1852; reprint, Toronto: McClelland and Stewart, 1984), 19, 30

The authorities used the quarantine station on Grosse Ile, in the St Lawrence River near Quebec City, to keep typhus from the established communities. Immigrants were housed in the island's inadequate buildings, without water or fresh clothing, where the conditions guaranteed that those who did not already have typhus would soon contract it. Six thousand died on the island, and at least an equal number in hospitals or sheds at Saint John, Quebec, Montreal, Kingston, and Toronto. Some would have died in any case, but others were killed by the laws that confined them to the crowded sheds. Furthermore, typhus – like cholera – spread well beyond the immigrant group. With the advent of AIDS, Canadians have looked back on these tragic episodes with a sense of shame: a commemorative plaque was raised at Grosse Ile in 1989, and the island has been declared a national historic site.

Prevention without Cause: Smallpox

The history of smallpox shows that knowledge of the biological cause of a disease is not essential for its control or even for its eradication. Endemic in Europe since antiquity, smallpox killed kings and

---

Literary Vignette: Typhus at Grosse Ile Quarantine Station, 1847

And then he was trotting back along the deck and down the hatch into the hold ... The smell was staggering. A single oil-lamp hung from the ceiling, and in the dim light Lauchlin saw the stalls and the narrow passages between them. Within the stalls were rows of bare berths stripped of their bedding and hardly more than shelves. In an open area, scores of unshaven men and emaciated women huddled together, some weeping. Children lay motionless. An old man sat on the floor leaning his back against a cask and gasping for breath ...

Lauchlin ... stepped back, now seeing as his eyes adjusted to the light all the other people collapsed on the bare boards. They shook with chills, their muscles twitched, some of them muttered deliriously. Others were sunk in a stupor so deep it resembled death. On the chest of a man who had torn off his shirt, Lauchlin could see the characteristic rash; on another farther along, the dusky coloring of his skin.

Andrea Barrett, *Ship Fever* (New York: W.W. Norton, 1996), 178–9

---

peasants alike. Early modern records indicate that at least 20 per cent of the population had been scarred or blinded by variola. European explorers and traders brought the disease to North America, where it exploded with disastrous effects among the susceptible aboriginals who lacked the relative natural immunity of the intruders. Not only an accident of contact between peoples of two continents, smallpox was sometimes transmitted deliberately on soiled blankets in an early form of biological warfare.

No cure for smallpox exists, although many remedies have been tried. Effective prevention, however, long antedated our concept of its transmission. Folk methods relied on two generally accepted principles: first, smallpox was inevitable; second, survivors were immune. If a mild case occurred in a community, families would feed the scabs of the lesions to their children, hoping to provoke immunity

Smallpox Vignettes

The Death of Louis XV, 1774

[On May 7] ... the king's illness took a turn for the worse. He was racked by a high fever, his face changed. That evening he lapsed into delirium again ... the scabs and dried pustules became black ... and an inflammation of the throat prevented him from swallowing. Within hours, scabs formed on his eyelids and blinded him ... His face swollen by scabs was the color of bronze ... On May 10 ... he remained conscious until noon ... [but] at three fifteen he expired. Immediately the courtiers ran out of the bedroom where the body had already begun to decompose.

Eyewitness account by Emmanuel, duc de Couÿ
(cited in Olivier Bernier, *Louis the Beloved: The Life of Louis XV* [Garden City, N.Y.: Doubleday, 1984], 248–9)

Smallpox in North America

Could it not be contrived to send the smallpox among these disaffected tribes of Indians? We must use every strategem in our power to reduce them.

British officer Jeffery Amherst to Col. Henry Bouquet, 1763

I will try to inoculate the — with some blankets that may fall into their hands and take care not to get the disease myself.

Bouquet's reply (both cited in Heagerty 1928, 1:43)

None of us had the least idea of the desolation this dreadful disease had done, until we went up the bank to the camp and looked into the tents, in many of which they were all dead and the stench was horrid; those that remained ... were in such a state of despair and despondence that they could hardly converse with us ... From what we could learn three-fifths had died of the disease.

Journal of David Thompson, 1780s (cited in Heagerty 1928, 1:45–6)

with only minor suffering. Others introduced the pus from smallpox vesicles directly under the skin, a technique known as variolization. But deliberately acquired smallpox could be just as relentless, disfiguring, and dangerous as the natural variety.

Of unknown origin, variolization was brought to Western Europe in the early eighteenth century by two Greek doctors, Iacob Pylarino and Emmanuel Timoni. Timoni published in Constantinople, where the technique was observed in 1717 by the wife of the British ambassador, Lady Mary Wortley Montagu. Having herself been disfigured by the disease, she determined to inoculate her own child. Montagu's role in the dissemination of the practice is debated, but by 1722 the children of the English royal family had been inoculated, and by the 1740s variolization was common in Britain.

Folk wisdom about cowpox (vaccinia) was the inspiration for the discovery of the physician and naturalist Edward Jenner. As a student he had learned that milkmaids who had contracted the mild pustular eruption from infected cows considered themselves immune to smallpox. Common knowledge for milkmaids was news to the young doctor, who pondered its significance for several years. Historians link Jenner's subsequent investigations to the famous advice he had been given two decades earlier by his former teacher, John Hunter. In reply to Jenner's queries about the anatomy of a hedgehog, Hunter had written, 'But why think, why not try the experiment?' (2 August 1775, Royal College of Surgeons). To test the cowpox hypothesis, Jenner conducted an experiment that would probably fall short of current standards of ethics. He inoculated eight-year-old James Phipps with vaccinia, waited six weeks, then inoculated the boy with fluid from active smallpox – the standard practice in variolization. Young Phipps did not react to variola, and Jenner published his results in 1798. If the boy had died, would Jenner have told the tale?

Fortunately for Master Phipps, for Jenner, and for the rest of the world, the empirical observation was correct: infection by vaccinia prevents subsequent infection by variola. Vaccination soon became standard prevention, but the availability of vaccine lymph was unpredictable, and no legal, medical, or social mechanisms enforced its use. Meanwhile, smallpox had become endemic to the New World.

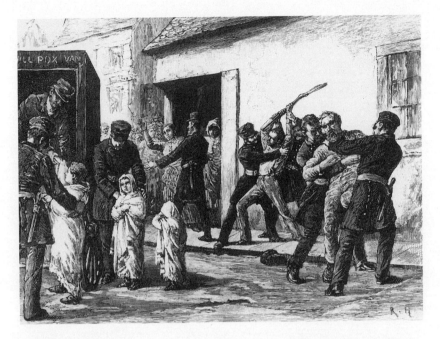

Riot during the 1885 smallpox epidemic in Montreal. Robert Harris illustration in *Harper's Weekly*, 28 November 1885. Bert Hansen Collection, New York, N.Y.

The National Archives of Canada holds an autographed copy of the book of instructions that Jenner sent with his gift of vaccine lymph to the 'Chief of the Five Nations' in 1807.

Despite sporadic vaccination, smallpox outbreaks often occurred among native and immigrant populations. The 1885 epidemic in Montreal killed more than three thousand people. Riots broke out over control measures; some feared that vaccination could spread the disease. The conflict was fuelled by class and linguistic tensions between anglophones, who held power and promoted vaccination, and francophones, who were less affluent and were largely unvaccinated for reasons of finance, neglect, or fear. The last Canadian smallpox epidemic occurred in Windsor, Ontario, in 1924.

In the mid-1960s, the World Health Organization (WHO, founded in 1948) launched a plan to eradicate smallpox by tracking all cases, isolating and supporting sufferers, and vaccinating every person exposed. The task was said to be impossible, but workers persevered in the face of disease, famine, and war; some were killed. The last natural case was identified in a twenty-three-year-old hospital cook, Ali Maow Maalin of Somalia, in December 1977. In August the following year, Janet Parker, an unvaccinated staff photographer, contracted the disease in the Birmingham University laboratory where she worked. Her death and the subsequent suicide of the laboratory director, Henry Bedson, were the last known wages of this great disease.

On 9 December 1979 the WHO formally declared that smallpox had become the first human disease to be eradicated. At the time of writing, scientists are deliberating over the ultimate destruction of the remaining samples of variola virus, which are held by the Centers for Disease Control in Atlanta, Georgia. Some argue for their preservation, questioning the ethics of exterminating a 'living species' and citing the importance of biodiversity. They argue that 'friendly' variola might be needed to combat a possible epidemic caused by an enemy, or by an inadvertent escape from a forgotten freezer in, for example, the former Soviet Union. Untroubled by this possibility, advocates for destruction invoke the huge mortality that could result from any accident in the largely unvaccinated population and cite the large supply of vaccinia as ample protection against oversight or attack. Nevertheless, the 'execution' of variola, originally planned for December 1993, was moved to June 1995, when it was stayed once again until perhaps the year 2000 (J. Maurice, *Science* 267 [1995], 450).

The eradication of smallpox was a triumph of medical science, but the methods had been in place for two hundred years, long before germ theory or antibiotics. It was facilitated by the fact that humans are the only host. No particular knowledge about the causative organism was required. Similarly, the effective prevention of childbed fever, established by Ignaz Semmelweis in Vienna, did not require germ theory (see chapter 11).

If knowledge of a microbial cause is not essential for prevention of some infectious diseases, what then was the impact of germ theory, vaccines, or antibiotics on epidemics? Their impact is difficult to demonstrate. Some would argue that these innovations create as many problems as they solve – witness the side effects of the 1976 influenza vaccine (see below) or the current anxiety over the emerging strains of multi-drug-resistant staphylococcus. Despite the best of intentions, iatrogenic epidemics are nothing new.

Decline (and Rise) of Tuberculosis: Scientific Triumph or Coincidence?

In the late nineteenth century, tuberculosis was the single most important cause of adult death, a distinction it held for more than a century. Many changes had taken place in the medical conceptualisation of this disease. Formerly characterized by its symptoms of wasting, fever, and cough, its anatomical basis was described by R.T.H. Laennec in the early nineteenth century (see chapter 9). Another French doctor, J.A. Villemin, later demonstrated that tuberculosis could be inoculated, and Robert Koch identified its bacterial cause as he established germ theory (see chapter 4). Despite Koch's discovery, notions of heredity persisted, for the disease seemed to run in some families while others were resistant. Tuberculosis pervaded all social classes, and it shaped cultural notions of beauty, art, and genius, as Susan Sontag's *Illness as Metaphor* has shown.

Various stringent public health measures, with more or less prejudicial baggage, were enacted to keep the germs of the tubercular sick, or the potentially sick, away from the more powerful non-sick. Sufferers were isolated or quarantined in sanatoria. An effective vaccine using the Bacillus Calmette-Guérin (BCG) was developed in Paris in the early 1920s. Through the work of R.G. Ferguson and Armand Frappier, BCG became part of Canada's tuberculosis-prevention programs, which were expanded from 1948 until the mid-1960s to include schoolchildren, health-care workers, native people, and prisoners. BCG was never adopted in the United States, but it is still compulsory for schoolchildren and health-care workers in France and other European countries.

Surgical therapies for tuberculosis were invented to create a poorly oxygenated environment hostile to the organism. In 1927 the Canadian surgeon Norman Bethune is said to have insisted on an artificial pneumothorax for himself, against the advice of his physicians at the Trudeau Sanatorium (the movie version has him admin-

Literary Vignettes: Romantic Tuberculosis in CanLit

What had happened to Ruby? She was even handsomer than ever; but her blue eyes were too bright and lustrous, and the colour of her cheeks was hectically brilliant; besides she was very thin; the hands that held her hymn-book were almost transparent in their delicacy ...

She lay in the hammock, with her untouched work beside her, and a white shawl wrapped about her thin shoulders. Her long yellow braids of hair – how Anne had envied those braids in old schooldays! – lay on either side of her ... The moon rose in the silvery sky, empearling the clouds around her ... [and] the church with the old graveyard beside it. The moonlight shone on the white stones ... 'How ghostly!' she shuddered. 'Anne, it won't be long now before I'll be lying over there.'

L.M. Montgomery, *Anne of the Island* (1915;
reprint, Toronto: Bantam Books, 1980), 79–80, 105–6

Cissy could not get her breath lying down that night. An inglorious gibbous moon was hanging over the wooded hills and in its spectral light Cissy looked frail and lovely and incredibly young. A child. It did not seem possible that she could have lived through all the passion and pain and shame of her story ...

But a spasm of coughing interrupted and exhausted her. She fell asleep when it was over, still holding to Valancy's hand ... At sunrise ... she opened her eyes and looked past Valancy at something – something that made her smile suddenly and happily. And smiling, she died.

L.M. Montgomery, *The Blue Castle* (1926;
reprint, Toronto: Seal Books 1988), 119, 121

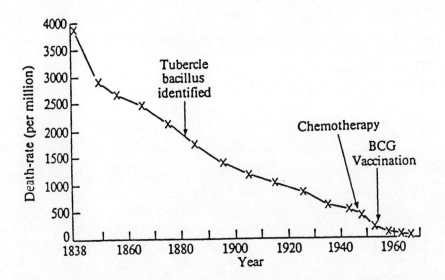

Rate of decline in tuberculosis mortality does not alter with the advent of specific medical interventions. From Thomas McKeown, *Role of Medicine*, 1979, 92

ister it to himself). Antituberculous drugs were greeted with much fanfare; the 1952 Nobel Prize went to the Russian-born American, Selman Waksman, for his discovery of streptomycin. Drugs soon eclipsed preventative measures, but controversies over vaccines and other controls have not vanished. They are intimately linked to social and political ideals in individual countries, and they exemplify the wide gap in the relative status of disease treatment over disease prevention in the medical model.

Tuberculosis mortality declined steadily throughout the twentieth century, and medical scientists congratulated themselves on what they seem to have accomplished. In the late 1970s, however, Thomas H. McKeown challenged this medical self-satisfaction when he demonstrated that tuberculosis mortality had already been waning long before the advent of drugs and that the rate of decline had not altered with the innovations. The germ may have become less virulent or human resistance to it may have grown with a rise in wealth, hygiene, and nutrition.

McKeown identified a similar pre-intervention decline in British mortality from measles, although he acknowledged that diphtheria mortality had fallen with medical intervention. But his observations about tuberculosis were sobering. Antibiotics treat individual illnesses effectively, yet they favour resistant organisms, offsetting relief for individuals with their long-term and possibly harmful impact on humankind. The rise in tuberculosis in the early 1990s was correlated with a parallel rise in poverty and homelessness throughout North America.

Historians have made increasingly sceptical judgments about the medical claims of success in treatment and prevention. In his book *No Magic Bullet*, Allan Brandt showed that wartime control measures against venereal disease included the demonizing and incarceration of prostitutes, who were equated with infective organisms. Jay Cassel and Peter Neary made similar observations about control measures in Canada. Entrenched medical practices die hard.

Influenza and Polio

Two other pandemics swept across North America in the twentieth century: influenza and polio. In mid-1918 as the First World War drew to a close, influenza killed fifty thousand Canadians, many of them young occupants of military barracks or boarding schools. In constrast, the four years of war had claimed sixty thousand lives. Also known as the Spanish flu (some things never change), the disease caused fever, pneumonia, and rapid death. Influenza has since returned in pandemic waves, although not with such virulence. It has been given adjectival labels indicative of the various viral strains: Asiatic (1890), swine (1931), Asian (1957), and Hong Kong (1968). A vaccine was developed in 1943, but it was only moderately effective because influenza changes often, spreads easily in air, and is refractory to other controls. In 1976 rumours of an emerging strain of virulent swine flu reminded authorities of the great tragedy of 1918 and prompted U.S. President Gerald Ford to recommend a sweeping campaign to vaccinate 50 million citizens. This attempt at prevention produced another iatrogenic epidemic – two hundred cases of Guillain-Barré syndrome of ascending paralysis in those vaccinated against the hypothesized influenza epidemic, which in the end never materialized.

Poliomyelitis, an enterovirus infection of nervous tissue with fecal-oral transmission, was endemic in early twentieth-century North America. Its annual outbreaks increased in scope, from a few hundred cases in Canada each year to a maximum of over 8,800 in 1953. The reasons for its rise are still under debate. Also called infantile paralysis, polio worked its dangerous effects on the very young. More than four hundred Canadians died and many more were disabled before the epidemic was arrested by the vaccines of American virologists Jonas Salk (in 1953) and A.B. Sabin (in 1956).

Polio was the impetus for the iron lung and other technologies designed to compensate for damaged autonomic functions. It also provided a powerful justification for the rise of pediatrics as a specialty and the creation of centres of rehabilitation medicine. Naomi Rogers has shown that it took on the identity of its helpless child victims. Its eradication from the American hemisphere by the end of this century has been predicted.

New Diseases

New infectious diseases are not usually as new as they first seem. Rarely are they due to the advent or alteration of a causative organism. Sometimes they have been present for decades at a subliminal level. Frequently, they come to medical attention through social circumstances that favour transmission. Nearly always, the identifying characteristics of those in whom the condition is first recognized – together with our sympathy (or lack of sympathy) for these people – are incorporated into our concept of the disease and what ought to be done about it.

Since 1970, several 'new' epidemic diseases have emerged, although their pathogens have been around for a long time. In 1976 legionnaire's disease was first identified among the participants of an American Legion conference at a Philadelphia hotel. The Centers for Disease Control traced it to a previously unrecognized bacterium, *Legionella pneumophila*, which now has twenty variant species. Toxic shock syndrome, which complicates certain bacterial infections, was originally recognized in young women and – too narrowly (but irreversibly) – was linked to the use of menstrual tampons.

Finally, the AIDS experience has caused us to relive so many of the old responses to epidemics, including the panic described by Thucydides long ago. Retrospective testing of frozen serum has shown that the virus has been causing disease in humans since at least 1959. In 1981, AIDS emerged, simultaneously in California and New York, as an epidemic among male homosexuals. Initially called a 'plague,' modified by 'gay,' 'Haitian,' 'African,' and 'new' – AIDS was understood to be the creation of (and synonymous with) these people. One of its first medical names was GRID (gay-related immunodeficiency). Affecting people of all ages, in all countries, AIDS has caused a few million deaths worldwide; the infected number close to 30 million. Intolerance and fear inform irrational proposals for controls.

Serious questions remain about the origin of AIDS. Molecular biologist Peter Duesberg points out that HIV is still unproved as a cause, because current research has failed to satisfy Koch's postulates (see chapter 4). Medical technology itself has been cited as a causative factor. For example, the historian Mirko Grmek suggested that a window of opportunity for the pathogen was created in the natural disease ecosystem (pathocenosis) following the reduction of other pathogens, such as smallpox, diphtheria, measles, and polio. Others imagine an even more active role for science when they ask if AIDS could have arisen in 1957 from the polio vaccines that were developed by Western scientists in SIV-contaminated monkey cells and tested on Africans. Publicized by freelance writer Tom Curtis in the 19 March 1994 *Rolling Stone* magazine, this hypothesis attracted media interest by implicating the fieldwork of the distinguished scientist Hilary Koprowski. The scientific community quickly dismissed it, however, using historical and epidemiological arguments, rather than the retrospective serological testing of the old vaccines, which Curtis had urged.

Innocent (and Guilty) Victims

The 1976–77 outbreak of Guillain-Barré syndrome in the United States occurred among 'innocent victims' of a clumsy presidential policy. Legionnaire's disease shared the thoroughgoing respectability of its first victims, and it was given prompt, lavishly funded medical investigation. By contrast, toxic shock syndrome was regarded as punishment for 'guilty,' dirty women; however, as marketing trends soon indicated, it was later perceived to be caused by the tampons, not their users.

'Innocent victim' is a term that physicians should never use lightly. Yes, it means that some people are sick through no fault of their own, but it can also imply that others are 'guilty' – responsible for and deserving of their illness. Newborns, hemophiliacs, health-care workers, and the heterosexual wives of bisexual men are called the innocent victims of AIDS. But these differences between sick people are defined by moral estimation of their behaviour, not by the biological effects of the HIV.

Compared with legionnaire's disease, a longer time passed (and more people died) before the United States and Canada gave AIDS the credibility of financed investigation. Medical hubris, blended with entrenched attitudes to the 'sins' of homosexuals and IV-drug users, may also explain why more than a decade went by before anyone asked the still unanswered questions about the role of science in the origins of AIDS.

As with all other epidemics, control measures for AIDS are laden with expectations from the past. In Cuba, for example, people who are seropositive for HIV are indefinitely and forcibly confined, notwithstanding the fact that (1) the 'rest of society' is (or could be) protected with information on how to avoid HIV; (2) seroconversion may take months; and (3) seronegative persons may be equally infective. In Canada, despite demands to the contrary, we do not segregate those with AIDS or HIV seropositivity. Confinement is expensive, and it infringes punitively on the rights of potentially sick people. It could result in the kind of tragedy once seen on Grosse Ile, and in the end it would not prevent the spread of a disease which we already understand how to avoid. Yet the global death toll from AIDS still climbs at an alarming rate: in the United States, it has become the leading cause of death for people between the ages of twenty-five and forty-four. WHO estimates that 2.3 million died of AIDS in 1997; since its onset, 9.7 of 11.7 million deaths were in Africa. Clearly, it is important to prevent more infections and to help the sufferers. The millions of dollars spent on AIDS research are well justified.

But even AIDS statistics pale when compared with malaria and its steady toll of 2 to 3 million deaths, mostly of children, from the half-billion cases each year. With its periodic fever, malaria has been known since antiquity, as 'swamp fever,' 'ague,' and 'paludism' (from the Latin for marsh). The name 'malaria' crept into English from the Italian ('bad air') in the eighteenth century. Malaria was endemic to parts of Europe, where it sometimes killed thousands. During the nineteenth century, it ravaged British colonial troops in India, whence it spread to Canada.

An Inca remedy called cinchona, or Jesuit bark, was brought from Peru to Europe in the early seventeenth century, and its active ingredient, quinine, was isolated in 1820. In 1880, at the height of British imperialism, the parasite was identified by C.L.A. Laveran. Seventeen years later, Ronald Ross elucidated the role of the anopheles mosquito. Ross and Laveran received the Nobel Prize in 1902 and 1907, respectively.

In 1955, despite fears of overpopulation if malaria were to disappear, the WHO launched an eradication program, based on draining swamps and spraying insecticides, including the 1948 Nobel Prize–winning poison, DDT. Unlike smallpox, however, malaria parasitizes other creatures. Moreover, insecticides and the destruction of wetlands conveyed their own harm. Consequently, these methods were revised in 1969, and by 1980 WHO was aiming only for control, not eradication. Meanwhile, malarial resistance to the quinine derivative chloroquine arose, and it continues to spread. This preventable and treatable disease is still endemic to ninety countries containing more than 40 per cent of the world's population.

Why are northern and western populations concerned more with AIDS than with malaria or the numerous other diseases with greater world mortality? For example, measles kills approximately 1.5 million infants annually, and neonatal tetanus kills 0.75 million; schistosomiasis is thought to affect 200 million people each year. The answer may have something to do with the uneven distribution of mortality statistics. AIDS could be 'us'; malaria is definitely 'them.'

Twenty-five hundred years after Thucydides' ineffective but eager doctors perished in the plague of Athens, we seem to have learned very little. Cures, though highly sought after, may not control epidemics. Interventions can cause new diseases or worsen existing ones. Reactions to travellers exposed to Ebola or plague are hauntingly familiar. And social factors have not changed a bit.

Suggestions for Further Reading

Arnold, David. *Colonizing the Body: State Medicine and Epidemic Disease in Nineteenth-Century India.* Berkeley: California University Press, 1993

Beveridge, William Ian. *Influenza: The Last Great Plague.* New York: Prodist, 1978

Biraben, Jean-Noël. *Les hommes et la peste en France et dans les pays européens et méditerranéens.* 2 vols. Paris: Mouton, 1975–6

Brandt, Allan M. *No Magic Bullet: A Social History of Venereal Disease in the United States since 1880.* 2nd edn. New York: Oxford University Press, 1987

Carmichael, Ann G. *Plague and the Poor in Renaissance Florence.* Cambridge and New York: Cambridge University Press, 1986

Eyler, John M. 'Conceptual Origins of William Farr's Epidemiology: Numerical Methods and Social Thought in the 1830s.' In *Times, Places, and Persons,* ed. Abraham M. Lilienfeld, 1–21. Baltimore and London: Johns Hopkins University Press, 1980

Farley, John. *Bilharzia: A History of Imperial Tropical Medicine.* Cambridge and New York: Cambridge University Press, 1991

Getz, Faye. 'The Black Death and the Silver Lining: Meaning, Continuity, and Revolutionary Change in Histories of Medieval Plague.' *Journal of the History of Biology* 24 (1991), 265–89

Grmek, Mirko D. *History of AIDS: Emergence and Origin of a Modern Pandemic.* Trans. Russell C. Maulitz and Jacalyn Duffin. Princeton, N.J.: Princeton University Press, 1990

Hanrahan, S.N. 'Historical Review of Menstrual Toxic Shock Syndrome.' *Women and Health* 21 (1994), 141–65

Hirsch, August. *Handbook of Geographical and Historical Pathology.* 3 vols. Trans. Charles Creighton. London: New Sydenham Society, 1883–6

Hopkins, Donald R. *Princes and Peasants: Smallpox in History.* Chicago: University of Chicago Press, 1983

Kiple, Kenneth D., ed. *The Cambridge World History of Human Disease.* New York: Cambridge University Press, 1993

Kunitz, Stephen J. *Disease and Social Diversity: The European Impact on the Health of Non-Europeans.* New York: Oxford University Press, 1994

Lilienfeld, Abraham M., ed. *Times, Places, and Persons: Aspects of the History of Epidemiology.* Baltimore and London: Johns Hopkins University Press, 1980

McKeown, Thomas. *The Role of Medicine: Dream, Mirage, or Nemesis?* 2nd edn. Oxford: Blackwell, 1979

McNeill, William Hardy. *Plagues and Peoples.* Garden City, N.Y.: Anchor Press, Doubleday, 1976

Markel, Howard. *Quarantine! East European Jewish Immigrants and the New York City Epidemics of 1892.* Baltimore: Johns Hopkins University Press, 1997

Miller, Genevieve. *The Adoption of Inoculation for Smallpox in England and France.* Philadelphia: University of Pennsylvania Press, 1957

Rogers, Naomi. *Dirt and Disease: Polio before FDR.* New Brunswick, N.J.: Rutgers University Press, 1992

Rosebury, Theodor. *Microbes and Morals: The Strange Story of Venereal Disease.* New York: Viking Press, 1971

Rosenberg, Charles E. *The Cholera Years: The United States in 1832, 1849, and 1866.* Chicago: University of Chicago Press, 1962

Sigerist, Henry E. *Civilization and Disease.* Chicago: University Chicago Press, 1962

Sontag, Susan. *Illness as Metaphor.* New York: Farrar, Strauss, and Giroux, 1977

Zinsser, Hans. *Rats, Lice, and History: Being a Study in Biography ...* 1934. Reprint, Boston and Toronto: Little, Brown, 1963

On Canada

Bliss, Michael. *Plague: A Story of Smallpox in Montreal.* Toronto: HarperCollins, 1991

Cassel, Jay. *The Secret Plague: Venereal Disease in Canada, 1838–1939.* Toronto: University of Toronto Press, 1987

Feldberg, Georgina. *Disease and Class: Tuberculosis and the Shaping of Modern North American Society.* New Brunswick, N.J.: Rutgers University Press, 1995

Guérard, François. *Histoire de la santé au Québec.* Montréal: Boréal, 1996

Heagerty, J.J. *Four Centuries of Medical History in Canada and a Sketch of the Medical History of Newfoundland.* 2 vols. Toronto: Macmillan, 1928

Houston, C.S. *R.G. Ferguson: Crusader against Tuberculosis.* Toronto: Hannah Institute for the History of Medicine and Dundurn Press, 1991

Keating, Peter, and Othmar Keel. *Santé et société au Québec: XIXe-XXe siècles.* Montréal: Boréal, 1995

MacDougall, Heather A. *Activists and Advocates: Toronto's Health Department, 1883–1983.* Toronto: Dundurn Press, 1990

Marble, Allan Everett. *Surgeons, Smallpox, and the Poor: A History of Medicine and*

Social Conditions in Nova Scotia, 1749–1799. Montreal: McGill-Queen's University Press, 1993

Neary, Peter. 'Venereal Disease and Public Health Administration in Newfoundland in the 1930s and 1940s.' *Canadian Bulletin of Medical History* 15 (1998), 129–51

O'Gallagher, Marianna. *Grosse Ile: Gateway to Canada, 1832–1937.* Ste-Foy, Que: Carraig Books, 1984

Pettigrew, Eileen. *The Silent Enemy: Canada and the Deadly Flu of 1918.* Saskatoon: Western Producer Prairie Books, 1983

Roland, C.G. 'Sunk under the Taxation of Nature: Malaria in Upper Canada.' In *Health, Disease, and Medicine: Essays on Canadian History,* ed. Charles G. Roland, 154–70. Toronto: Hannah Institute for the History of Medicine 1984

Rutty, Christopher J. 'Middle-Class Plague: Epidemic Polio and the Canadian State, 1936–37.' *Canadian Bulletin of Medical History* 13 (1996), 277–314

Spaulding, W.B. 'The Ontario Vaccine Farm, 1885–1916.' *Canadian Bulletin of Medical History* 6 (1989), 179–83

Wherrett, George J. *The Miracle of the Empty Beds: A History of Tuberculosis in Canada.* Toronto and Buffalo: University of Toronto Press, 1977

CHAPTER EIGHT

Why Is Blood Special? Changing Concepts of a Vital Humour*

Blut ist ein ganz besonderer Saft. (Blood is a very special juice)

J.W. von Goethe, *Faust*, I, 1, 1808

Blood as Magic and Mystery

Blood is important. It has always been important, and it has always *seemed* to be important to everyone. Of the four ancient humours, it alone remains a vital entity, with a status well above that of phlegm or bile of any colour. Most people immediately understand that blood is essential for life. On the other hand, when asked if the spleen, liver, kidneys, or pancreas are essential, they are less certain. People do not think of those organs in the way that they think of blood.

Why has blood always enjoyed a special status? Two reasons. First, it is eminently visible, being the only internal organ that regularly surfaces for perusal; all humans have seen some of their own blood. Every injured person knows that bleeding marks the severity of the wound. Every woman can expect a flow at regular intervals allied to the phases of the moon.

Second, blood is always associated with life. Even children know that when blood is lost in great quantities, death may ensue. In many languages, it is synonymous with life and health. Some cultures, such

---

*Educational objectives for this chapter are found on p. 396.

as the vanished Beothuk of Newfoundland, prepared the dead for burial by colouring bodies with red ochre (containing hematite) to restore the blushlike colour of life. Scholars have analysed how menstruation influenced perceptions of women at various times and places, noting how mythologies and traditions cast suspicion on those who bled regularly without ill effect. For example, orthodox Judaism forbids a man to have sexual relations with a menstruating woman or, following her menses, until she has taken the ritual *mikvah* bath. K.C. Carter speculates that in the nineteenth century, menstruation may have served as a model for regular bloodletting in men to provide healthful 'monthly evacuations.'

In ancient Greek mythology, blood was one of the first miracle drugs. Perseus severed the snake-tressed head of the Gorgon monster Medusa and presented the gruesome trophy to the goddess Athena, who placed it on her shield. Athena gave blood from the Gorgon's head to the healer Asklepios (in Latin, Aesculapius), who used it for amazing cures and to raise the dead. The potent treatment led to his deification as the god of medicine. Asklepios's staff, around which a snake is entwined, is the medical caduceus, the symbol of medicine for more than two thousand years.

Christianity has done nothing to diminish the importance of blood in our culture. Blood is central to the mysteries of the sanctuary: not only is it life and health, it also indicates redemption of sin and eternal salvation. The blood of martyrs symbolizes pain and faith; that of children, the worst of the world's many unjust tragedies. The word 'blood' and its derivatives are mentioned no less than 460 times in the Bible; 'life' is mentioned only slightly more often (487 times). How often does the word 'kidney' appear? Seventeen times. 'Liver'? Thirteen times. 'Bile'? Once. And 'brain,' 'pancreas,' 'lungs,' and 'phlegm'? Never. True, 'heart' is mentioned more often than 'blood' (817 times). The reason relates to the importance of the religious signifiers: if blood was life, heart was love or soul.

Given its ancient connection with life, blood as therapy is also very old; however, blood-medicine was not always convenient. Wine often served as a proxy, taken as a panacea, a stimulant, a depressant, a restorative, a digestive, an hypnotic, or an escape. Rooted perhaps in their visual similarities, the substitution of red wine for blood was further endorsed by the Christian doctrine of transubstantiation: in the mass, wine becomes the redeeming blood of Christ. Renaissance images showed the body of Christ crushed in the 'miraculous press' from which blood trickled into waiting barrels.

The English word 'blood' is neither Latin nor Greek in origin, as are so many of the words used in medical terminology. Medicine makes use of the terms 'hematology' (derived from Greek) and 'sanguinous' (derived from Latin), but words such as these with classical roots are rarely used in regular practice to identify the humour itself. Even the leading journal of the field, published by the American Society of Hematology, is called *Blood*. The word comes from Old English through Nordic and Saxon roots. Language theory holds that as the French-speaking Norman invaders married the Anglo-Saxon women, Latin-derived French words took over the vocabulary of the external environment of masculine authority; however, the words pertaining to the interior domestic female environment, and to emotions and feelings, were retained – with these words we have 'blood.' The derivation may illustrate blood's special importance to women's work rather than its power. For example, the words 'liver,' 'kidney,' and 'heart' also come from Old English, possibly because these organs, like blood, are edible parts of animal bodies. Body parts with Latinized names – such as aorta, colon, duodenum, rectum, vagina, tendon, and cartilage – have little or no culinary interest.

More along Linguistic Lines

Anglophones appear to have a special subliminal respect for the word 'blood.' Think about the psychic power in its many derivatives: cold blood, blue blood, bad blood, fresh blood, blooded, hot-blooded, red-blooded, bloodline, blood red, bloodless, bloodthirsty, blood-curdling, bloody, bloody-minded, bloodshed, bloodshot, bloodstone, blood money, blood poisoning, bloodstain, blood feud, flesh and blood, and lifeblood.

How many similar words can be found for the liver? Liverish and lily-livered – not very impressive words. And for the kidney?

If the linguistic argument for the special power of blood is unconvincing, a psychological analysis is difficult to refute. Most patients who are referred to a hematology clinic have no symptoms at all; they are sent for abnormalities picked up during routine testing; even patients with newly diagnosed leukemia may be symptom-free. Nevertheless, people consulting hematologists are probably more apprehensive than other ambulatory patients. A problem with blood is a problem with life.

Blood as Medical Science

Medical professionals discount magic and mythology, finding them quaint but incredible. As blood has been medicalized and objectified by technology, its mystique with scientists may have waned. But blood and its multiple functions still occupy an exalted state – a position that seeks to reconcile the ancient notions of blood's great power with our understanding of modern science.

Blood Therapy: Transfusion

If blood is life, it is only logical to assume that faltering life might revive with a little extra blood. The first 'transfusion' is often said to have been given in 1492 to the dying Giovanni Battista Cibò, who had been elected pope as Innocent VIII in 1484. His Jewish physician, Giacomo di San Genesio, is said to have tried to resuscitate the ailing pontiff by having him drink the blood of three ten-year-old boys whom he had had killed. The evidence for this peculiar treatment is unreliable, and the story is probably an anti-Semitic fabrication, not unlike the rumours of ritualistic child murder that tracked the customs of Passover.

Oral blood had probably been tried many times before, and without the prerequisite of donor death. Galen held that blood was elaborated from ingested substances; surely consumption of blood would facilitate the process of building more. The mouth offered an appropriate, accessible, logical, and comfortable site of administration, and drinking of blood enjoyed faddish popularity both before and after the discovery of circulation.

Interest in vascular transfusion was stimulated by William Harvey's 1628 treatise *On the Motion of the Heart* (see chapter 3). Soon after, experiments were conducted, using quills, bladders, and silver tubes to remove blood from one animal and give it to another. Indirect transfusion entailed the removal of blood into a container and its subsequent administration into the recipient; direct transfusion took place through a connector between the vessel of the donor animal and the vein of the recipient. These experiments captured the interest of many, including the quiet cleric Francis Potter, the illustrious polymath Sir Christopher Wren (architect of London's St Paul's Cathedral), and the physician Richard Lower, who began to transfuse dogs.

Borrowed Blood

At dinner on 14 November 1666, Samuel Pepys learned of a successful direct transfusion between dogs, which had taken place in London that day. The potential of such an achievement did not escape the diners. Pepys recorded their mischievous reaction in his famous diary:

'This did give occasion to many pretty wishes, as of the blood of a Quaker to be in an Archbishop, and such like. But, as Dr. Croone says, [it] may, if it takes, be of mighty use to man's health, for the amending of bad blood by borrowing from a better body.'

Diary of Samuel Pepys, ed. Robert Latham and
William Matthews (Berkeley: University of California Press,
1970–83), 7:371

In early 1667 the French physician Jean-Baptiste Denis appears to have been the first to attempt intravenous transfusion in humans when he gave lamb's blood to a fifteen-year-old boy to calm his nerves. Not to be outdone by the competition from across the channel, Lower performed his own sheep-to-man transfusion later the same year. Back in France, Denis became a transfusion specialist, but

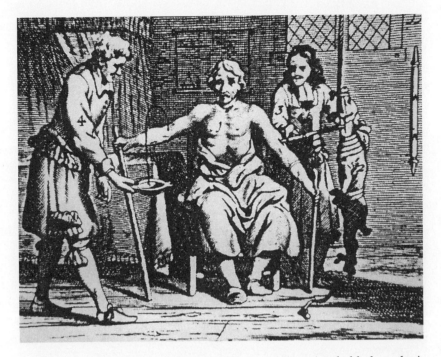

A direct transfusion from animal donor to recipient (probably hypothetical). From J.B. Lamzweerde, *Appendix ad Armamentarium chirurgicum Johannis Sculteti*, Amsterdam, 1671, 28

the next year a man died following a failed attempt to give him a third transfusion of animal blood. Denis was sued – but the court decided that the patient had been poisoned by his wife. The doctor was exonerated; however, the sobering publicity dampened enthusiasm, and transfusion activities were curtailed for nearly a century and a half.

Indeed, blood transfusion was (and still is) a potentially life-threatening intervention, never to be undertaken lightly. Three problems posed serious hurdles: the reactions that were later known as blood-group incompatibility, clotting, and infection. The first two were partially solved early in the twentieth century; the third remains a serious concern.

Transfusion was revived in the early nineteenth century. The

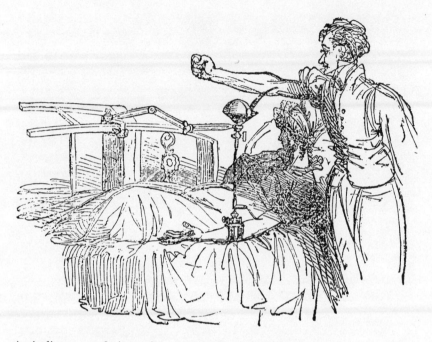

An indirect transfusion using a gravitator and the blood of a family member who is a house officer. James Blundell, *Lancet*, 13 June 1829, 321

perennial problem of obstetrical bleeding became more obvious to practitioners as childbirth was medicalized (see chapter 11). In 1829 James Blundell of Guy's Hospital in London, England, had attempted transfusion for uncontrollable postpartum hemorrhage. Using a syringe, he injected the bleeding mothers with blood taken from the resident housestaff; a few lives appeared to be saved. Patients given this heroic therapy were not expected to live; if death resulted from transfusion, it would have been ascribed to the original hemorrhage.

Another stimulus to transfusion came from the urgent need to save bleeding soldiers. During the Franco-Prussian War of 1870–1, direct transfusions were given on the battlefield, soldier to soldier, by medics in the armies of Austria, Belgium, and Russia. Sterile technique was used, but incompatibility and clotting had yet to be resolved. Storage of blood seemed to be virtually unattainable.

(a) Compatibility

The problem of compatibility began to unravel with the work of Karl Landsteiner, who in 1901 published a short paper on a study of the twenty-two workers in his laboratory. He had found that their blood could be divided into three major groups, A, B, and C (now called O). The following year, two of his pupils discovered the fourth major blood group, AB. Landsteiner's work was ignored until just before the First World War. Now hundreds of blood groups are recognized, the most important being the ABO and rhesus systems. The ability to wash, freeze, and thaw blood safely has made it possible to provide a relatively compatible supply for even the rarest types.

(b) Anticoagulation

Untreated blood will clot within a few minutes. Storage depended on finding a method to inhibit this natural property without harming either the product or the recipient. Testing began on techniques for removing fibrin (the clotting protein) and on anticoagulant drugs. Just prior to the Second World War the Russians took advantage of natural anticoagulation – cadaver blood will not clot because it has already clotted and lysed. Cadaver blood and, for similar reasons, placental blood, were also used for transfusion in India and elsewhere.

At the time of writing, the preferred anticoagulant is sodium citrate, discovered in 1914. It was first applied to battlefield needs of the First World War by an American army doctor, O.H. Robertson, working with a British unit. Using only O^+ donors, Robertson demonstrated that citrate combined with dextrose (to nourish the blood cells) allowed safe storage of blood for up to three weeks. Work on heparin as an anticoagulant for medicine and surgery was the product of Canadian research by Charles Best, Louis B. Jaques, and D.W. Gordon Murray in the early 1930s.

(c) Blood Components

With the problems of compatibility and coagulation under control, hospital blood-banking began. By 1927, plasma was usefully extracted from outdated blood by centrifugation. The Canadian surgeon Norman Bethune helped to establish a mobile unit for plasma transfusion in December 1936 during the Spanish Civil War. Plasma for shock and clotting factors became the mainstay of emergency treatment in the Second World War. Component therapy, the use of specific parts of blood – red cells, platelets, white cells, factors, and plasma – is now standard practice.

In Canada, the blood transfusion service was run by the national Red Cross from 1947. Blood collection, storage, and transfusion was only one of many peacetime services offered by the organization, but in 1998 this role came to an end with new controversies over infection (see Krever below; on the Red Cross, see chapter 10).

(d) Infection

Sterile technique for handling blood has been in place for more than a century; however, infection remains a serious problem and is currently the object of public anxiety. Syphilis, several forms of hepatitis, and AIDS are among the many infections that can be transmitted by blood. Serological testing has reduced the risk; nevertheless, hepatitis remains the most frequent of the transfusion infections. Vaccination against hepatitis B, which received U.S. Food and Drug approval in late 1981, is an important consideration for medical personnel. In countries where donation equipment may not be sterilized properly, donors can transmit infections to each other. And when donors fear infection, supplies falter.

Members of the Christian religious group, Jehovah's Witnesses, base their stand against transfusion on an interpretation of biblical passages forbidding consumption of blood. The same passages are cited as an origin of kosher butchery methods in the Judaic tradition. They also illustrate how the story of the Last Supper and the tenets of the Catholic mass, especially transubstantiation, could be seen as a surprising rupture. Concern over infection, with steady pressure from those who have philosophical objections to transfusion, has stimulated research into blood surrogates such as plasma expanders, hemoglobin, and clotting-factor substitutes.

Blood Is Life, but You Should Not Eat It

Only you shall not eat flesh with its life, that is, its blood.

Genesis 9:4

If any man of the house of Israel ... eats any blood, I will set my face against that person who eats blood, and will cut him off from among his people. For the life of the flesh is in the blood.

Leviticus 17:10–11

Only be sure that you do not eat the blood for the blood is the life, and you shall not eat the life with the flesh.

Deuteronomy 12:23

The shape and image of blood-banking and transfusion have been altered. No longer 'the gift of life,' blood therapy is mistrusted, especially in the United States, where donors may be paid. In France, an inquiry into the policies surrounding blood products indicted several prominent officials on criminal charges between 1991 and 1995. In Canada, a royal commission into the issue of transfusion-related infection, chaired by Justice Horace Krever, began hearings in 1993. It has resulted in allegations of wrongdoing by politicians and Red Cross officials. Entrepreneurial persons have taken advantage of the situation to open private blood banks, where the anxious can stock their own blood for future surgery or a disaster that occurs within convenient reach of the freezer. At the time of writing, Canadian parents are suing for the right to direct donations for the use of their own children. These procedures are inaccessible to many citizens. If they are tolerated, they will replace the previously imperfect but equitable system with a two-tier system. Transfusion experts worry that reporting of risk behaviours could decline with added pressure for family donations.

Marrow transplantation can be seen as the ultimate form of component transfusion. It was developed in Seattle, Washington, under the direction of E. Donnall Thomas, who used the principles of anti-coagulation and intravenous infusion, and the cell-cloning techniques of Canadian researchers J. Till and E.A. McCulloch. Marrow transplant offers new hope for the chronic anemias and malignancies. As a side effect, the iatrogenic problem of graft-versus-host disease has arisen.

Blood in Diagnosis: What Is Normal Blood?

Today's physicians have few opportunities to look at their patients' blood. Blood is visible in surgery and emergencies, but these settings do not allow for contemplation. Nurses, IV teams, laboratory technologists, blood banks, computerized analysis, and printed reports have distanced the doctor from the physical realities of blood. Not so in the past. From antiquity until the mid-twentieth century, bloodletting was standard treatment, and doctors regularly examined their patients' blood for the changes that took place in it upon standing.

Bloodletting seemed to be beneficial in fevers: it lowered the pulse, lessened plethora, and calmed agitation. The let blood soon coagulated and separated into several easily distinguished components, in which could be visualized the four ancient humours: yellow serum above, dark (deoxygenated) blood below, a rim of bright red (oxygenated) blood in the middle, and above it a pinkish-beige layer called the 'buffy coat' and 'web,' which contained white cells and clotting protein. After performing a bloodletting, doctors noted the colour and quantity of each component and were able to link the appearance with diagnosis and prognosis. Dark blood was a poor prognostic sign in pneumonia. A thick buffy layer with a concave configuration (called 'buffed and cupped'), which we would now attribute to an increase of white cells and proteins, was a sign of acute inflammation.

(a) Red Cells: Linking Blood to Air

(i) *Hemoglobin and oxygen.* With his early microscope, Antoni van Leeuwenhoek observed the tiny 'particles' now known as red cells.

Their existence, however, was controversial; those who saw them could not explain their function. Around the same time, both the French chemist Nicolas Lemery and Richard Lower of transfusion fame noticed that iron was a constituent of blood. Lower also described the change in colour of venous blood, from dark to bright red, on exposure to air. Some years later, iron became a treatment for anemia after the 1725 observations of the Russian military doctor Alexei Bestouyev-Rioumine. But neither iron nor the colour change were connected to the little globules, and oxygen had yet to be described.

In 1668 John Mayow demonstrated the life-sustaining properties of some air (see chapter 3), but one hundred years passed before the vital air could be identified. In the 1770s oxygen and 'laughing gas' were isolated by Joseph B. Priestley, an English theologian and chemist, and a sympathizer with the revolutionaries in France. Uncertain of his findings, he explained his discovery to his friend, the French aristocrat Antoine-Laurent Lavoisier, who quickly recognized its importance. With his personal fortune and the help of his wife, Marie-Anne-Pierette Paulze, Lavoisier experimented on respiration, combustion, and oxygen. By 1777 he had formulated a chemical theory of life as a process of oxidation. But the French Revolution put an end to their work: Priestley's church was sacked, and he fled to the United States; Lavoisier was guillotined.

If life had now become the chemical consumption of oxygen, then oxygen had to be linked to blood, because it too had been equated with life since prehistoric times. This vast scientific project began in the late eighteenth century and extended well into our own. Hemoglobin was identified as the 'red pigment' in the globules in 1851 by the German physiologist Otto Funke. His compatriot, Felix Hoppe-Seyler, proved that the pigment could take up and discharge oxygen. Two independent ideas – one ancient, the other relatively new – had been brought together in the red blood cell: blood was life; life was the combustion of oxygen.

An elegant contribution to the characterization of hemoglobin function was the oxygen-transport work of the Danish scientist Christian Bohr, whose son Niels and grandson Aage are both Nobel laureates in physics (1922 and 1975, respectively). Bohr used mathematics

---

A Tragedy Links Blood, Oxygen, and Life

In 1875 the French physiologist Paul Bert sent a hot-air balloon, the Zenith, to 7,900 metres, the highest altitude yet reached by humans. When the balloon descended, two of the three-man crew were dead. Bert concluded that for survival at low pressures, *supplemental* oxygen was needed to ensure adequate uptake by the blood. His insight laid the ground for the theories of partial pressures in the lung and helped resolve the mystery of the well-known but poorly understood condition called mountain sickness.

---

to express the relationship of oxygen to hemoglobin. His oxygen-dissociation curve describes a remarkable property of blood – its variable affinity for oxygen. The curve is sigmoid; the dips above and below a straight line show how hemoglobin picks up oxygen more readily when it is plentiful (for example, in the healthy lung) and releases it more readily when it is scant (for example, in the healthy tissues). These affinities are ingenious, especially compared with those of a mundane transport protein sporting a banal linear relationship to its object. Moreover, Bohr's curve shifts right or left, according to the environment in acidosis or alkalosis, to favour the transfer of oxygen to the host. The curve also illustrates the dangerous 'point of no return' situation that can occur in severe lung damage, where low concentrations of oxygen 'on the shoulder of the curve' can cause hemoglobin to release rather than take up oxygen.

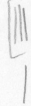
Hemoglobin was the first protein to be chemically identified. Using X-Ray crystallography, Max Perutz, John Kendrew, and colleagues elucidated the primary, secondary, and tertiary structure of the hemoglobin molecule in 1960. Its genetic basis was so well understood that researchers could define the molecular substitutions, in both protein and DNA, that are responsible for many abnormal hemoglobins. For example, in 1957 Vernon M. Ingram demonstrated that hemoglobin in sickle-cell disease involved the substitution of a single molecule. Variations in hemoglobin structure

were related to changes in function. Altered control over the genetic production of hemoglobin explains the common and devastating thalassemias.

This vast restructuring of knowledge into biochemical terminology promises new therapies through marrow transplant and genetic engineering; but at the time of writing, little change has taken place in the therapy of afflicted persons. For sickle-cell crisis, we still provide analgesics, hydration, oxygen, and transfusion; for thalassemia, transfusion. These treatments generate new iatrogenic problems, which require secondary therapies, including chelation of excess iron following multiple transfusion, social support for addiction to analgesic drugs, and management of infections.

(ii) *Morphology and a bevy of fathers.* Extending the microscopic observations of van Leeuwenhoek, William Hewson measured the size and shape of blood cells in different animals. He found that the red globule is usually flat, not spherical, and he recognized that coagulation is a process of change in the plasma, not in the red cells. Hewson died in 1777 of an accidental scalpel wound, which he sustained while performing an autopsy. For his precise observations and his romantic end, he has been called the father of hematology, especially by the British.

Despite Hewson's elegant studies, cell theory was not established until late in the nineteenth century. The vista presented by early microscopes was unreliable. Only after the achromatic lens and compound microscope became available in the 1830s did observers begin to trust their eyes and turn their attention to the cellular components of blood. Gabriel Andral and Alfred Donné, both of France, pioneered quantitation in hematology by linking various illnesses with the number, concentration, size, and shape of red cells. These men too have been called fathers of hematology, mostly by the French.

Andral was the first to suggest that anemia could occur if red cells were destroyed (hemolysis), and he described anemia as a decrease in the number of red cells. He associated anemia with pregnancy and with chlorosis. Once called the 'green sickness of virgins' for the peculiar cast it gave to the complexion, chlorosis had been described in the sixteenth century by Johannes Lange, who recommended marriage as therapy. It has come to be synonymous with what we would now call iron-deficiency anemia, although it also resembles anorexia nervosa. Andral was the first to observe the small size of red cells in chlorosis. Here was a capital discovery: a diagnosis formerly bound to a patient's subjective account of vague symptoms could now be reduced to an accessible, objective test.

Insight concerning red cells sometimes emerged from intensely practical observations. The American George Minot, for example, noticed that fewer than the expected number of red cells were found in patients with the aggressive and uniformly fatal disease, pernicious anemia (also known as Biermer's anemia, for the German physician who described it in 1868). Minot found that red-cell production increased with a diet containing up to half a pound of raw liver daily (*Journal of the American Medical Association* [*JAMA*] 1926). Pernicious anemia is now linked to an inability to absorb vitamin B_{12}. At the time of Minot's celebrated cure, however, the existence of vitamins was still under dispute (see chapter 13). Minot's diet was yet another example of empirical success, advocated before the definition of the chemical errors in the disease: intrinsic factor was described in 1929 by W.B. Castle; vitamin B_{12} was isolated in 1948 by E.L. Rickes and K.A. Folkers.

(iii) *Red-cell chemistry.* Red cells are unusual. They have no nuclei and no mitochondria. They are tiny 'brainless' packages whose 120-day lifespan is dedicated to the transport of oxygen and carbon dioxide between the lungs and the tissues. Their other functions include buffering, but their physiology is largely devoted to maintaining the integrity of their hemoglobin and cell walls to provide safe, efficient passage of their precious cargo (oxygen or carbon dioxide). Enzymes were the key.

Red cells were known to be consumers of glucose, but how they could use sugar without indulging in oxygen was not understood until the work of three German scientists: Otto Warburg, his student Otto Meyerhof, and Gustav Embden. The three researchers uncovered two enzyme pathways: the hexose-monophosphate shunt, which provides energy to repair damaged hemoglobin; and the glycolytic pathway, which generates energy for the cell itself. Warburg and Meyerhof are both Nobel laureates.

In 1911, during this wave of 'chemicalizing' the red cell, H. Günther characterized the porphyrias, hemolytic diseases that result from an absence of enzymes that govern the production of hemoglobin. Soon after, physicians who are fond of using the 'retrospectoscope' invoked porphyria to account for strange behaviours of the past, ranging from the intermittent madness of King George III of Britain to the werewolf legends of Transylvania.

Later in the century, Canadian Maxwell Wintrobe invented useful instruments, such as the hematocrit, and made practical observations about erythrocyte morphology and behaviour in health and disease. Raised by an Austrian-Jewish family in Halifax, he completed his MD at Winnipeg and went on to New Orleans, finally settling on a career in Salt Lake City, Utah. He was the sole author of the first six editions of his authoritative textbook, *Clinical Hematology* (1942–68). Its bibliography could serve as a model of thoroughness and historical sensitivity. Canadians and Americans alike may be understood (if not forgiven) when they cite him as the father of twentieth-century hematology.

The idea that modifications in the biochemistry of red cells could lead to shortened red-cell survival and human illness resulted from the work during the Second World War, when Allied sources of quinine for malaria prevention in the Pacific theatre had been stopped and alternatives had to be found. Some soldiers, mostly black males, developed hemolytic anemia with new antimalarial agents; a similar phenomenon took place in the Korean War when primaquine was used for malaria prevention. In the mid-1950s, using volunteers from the Stateville Penitentiary near Chicago, the American army scientists Alf S. Alving, Paul Carson, R.J. Dern, and Ernest Beutler demonstrated that the red cells of hemolysis patients were inordinately sensitive to the drug because they lacked the X-linked, reducing enzyme glucose-6–phosphate dehydrogenase (G-6–PD). Not only did the discovery explain a new drug problem, but it also provided a scientific basis for favism, an ancient disease related to eating fava beans. Each of the many red-cell enzymes was discovered when a fortuitous accident of nature provided a mutant in whom the enzyme was missing.

(b) White Cells

First described in the eighteenth century, white blood cells were neglected until the nineteenth-century work of the British physician Thomas Addison and the German pathologist and statesman Rudolf Virchow. Addison noticed that 'colourless corpuscles' passed through the walls of blood vessels to form pus in inflammation. In 1845 Virchow described leukemia – literally, 'white blood.' The thick buffy layer in these patients was like pus, but without the usual inflammation; he suggested that it was due to an inappropriate production of abnormal cells at the expense of normal ones (see also chapter 4).

In the late nineteenth century, new staining techniques facilitated white-cell morphology. This technological change was a by-product of a search for new treatments. Paul Ehrlich had been seeking dyes that could act as chemotherapy for infections by bonding with, and specifically killing, bacteria (see chapter 5). In 1880 he described white-cell types, inventing names based on their staining properties, for example, neutrophil, eosinophil, basophil. Ehrlich believed that white cells played a role in protecting the body from invasion by the newly discovered bacteria.

Elie Metchnikoff shared Ehrlich's opinions about the immune functions of white cells. A Russian working at the Pasteur Institute in Paris, Metchnikoff discovered the capacity of phagocytosis. To some, the notion of one kind of cell gobbling up another seemed ridiculous – and befitting the Russian's strange character. The molecular biologist André Lwoff recalled Metchnikoff's visits to his childhood home – lively, but disorderly, with test tubes of blood and other unusual substances poking out of his pockets. But Metchnikoff's insights were in concert with the new immunology, and he was awarded the Nobel Prize in 1908. The ancient idea that 'bad blood' brought disease had been rephrased in a three-dimensional chemical and physical package that was consonant with contemporary science.

From 1890 to 1910, serotherapy (or serum therapy) – the use of blood or blood components containing what we would now call specific antibody – was advocated as treatment for diphtheria, cholera, tetanus, meningitis, and other infections caused by bacterial agents. Emil von Behring and his Japanese colleague Shibasaburo Kitasato, working in Germany, explored the production of antitoxins by exposing animals to specific infections, such as diphtheria, and extracting the sera they elaborated. Once again, the constitution of these sera was unknown, but they were effective.

A study of lymphocytes and their manufacture of antibodies led to a biochemical explanation of immunity and clone theory. Niels Jerne observed a background production of many antibodies, but when the animal was exposed to a specific antigen, large amounts of specific antibody would result. Clone theory arose from an extrapolation of the ideas of Virchow and Jerne. The Australian Frank Macfarlane Burnet made two postulates: first, each cell could react to only one antigen; second, in the course of development, millions of potentially reactive cells arose. Clone theory explains normal immune function and provides a model for some hematologic malignancies – multiple myeloma, chronic myelogenous leukemia, polycythemia rubra vera, and essential thrombocytosis.

(c) Platelets

After the technical problems of light microscopy had been resolved, the existence of the tiny cells that came to be called platelets was under dispute. In 1868 the Italian anatomist Giulio Bizzozero reported that these tiny blood cells originated in bone marrow and represented a separate cell line. Bizzozero distinguished between thrombus formation and precipitation of clotting factors, and he thought that platelets could trigger the clotting cascade. Knowing of Bizzozero's work, the twenty-four-year-old Canadian, William Osler, soon joined the debate. He reported that these bodies were 'sometimes' found in normal persons, and he speculated on their relationship with bacteria.

The Frenchman Georges Hayem devoted much of his career to a series of elegant experiments that linked platelets to hemostasis.

Against his own evidence to the contrary, however, he viewed plate-lets as a by-product of red cells. One historian has speculated that Hayem's error was the result of 'the unimaginative burden thrust on those, who like him, come early to positions of authority' (T.H. Spaet, in Wintrobe 1980, 553). More likely, Hayem's ideas stemmed from preconception – the 'epistemological obstacle' that has allowed many fine researchers to find precisely what they seek. The French look on Hayem, together with Donné and Andral, as yet another father of hematology.

Platelets occupy a huge literature with a rising profile in our soci-ety, in which cerebrovascular and cardiovascular thromboses are the leading causes of death. The genetics and biochemistry of platelet function are used to predict the antiplatelet effects of drugs. One of the largest longitudinal studies of antiplatelet drugs was conducted in Canada and released in 1980. It suggested that aspirin can prevent coronary thrombosis in males. Yet after nearly three decades of research, the role of antiplatelet drugs in prevention of heart attacks and strokes is unresolved.

(d) Plasma and Coagulation

The tendency to bleed has been recognized since antiquity. Writers of the Talmud seemed to know that male bleeders inherited the problem from their mothers, and they exempted from circumcision a third son of any mother who had already lost two boys to hemor-rhage (Yebamot, 64b). Well before classical hemophilia had been characterized in chemical terms, it was used as a model by the Amer-ican geneticist Thomas Hunt Morgan for his Nobel Prize–winning work on sex linkage.

In his immensely popular book, historian Robert K. Massie sug-gested that hemophilia helped to fuel the Russian Revolution with the stresses it produced in the family of Tsar Nicholas II. The tsare-vitch Alexei suffered from hemophilia, which he had likely inherited from his great-grandmother, Queen Victoria, via his mother, Alexan-dra. The relationship between a hemophiliac and his mother is poi-gnant: she is doubly tormented, by her child's pain and by the ancient idea that the problem was passed through her blood. Desperate to help her son, Alexandra turned to Rasputin, a self-styled spiritualist healer (in)famous for his excessive appetites in all things sensual, from cuisine to sex. Rasputin could calm and comfort the boy, and he also appeared to control the bleeding. Against advice, the 'foreign' tsarina continued the consultations; detrimental rumours about her relationship with Rasputin further eroded public respect for the throne.

Bleeding problems were defined by measuring the length of time for a clot to form in whole blood or plasma. Hemophilic blood took a long time to clot, if it did so at all. In the late 1930s, when component transfusion was first implemented, it was discovered that the clotting defect in hemophilic plasma could be corrected by mixing it with normal plasma. Researchers postulated the existence of a vague but essential 'anti-hemophilic factor' (AHF). By more mixing experiments, they learned that not all bleeders were the same.

In 1947 an Argentinian team noted the 'paradoxical fact' that mixing plasma from two different bleeders sometimes resulted in mutual correction. In her classic paper published at Christmas 1952, Rosemary Biggs presented seven bleeders whose serum could correct the defect in other hemophiliacs. She reasoned that these patients must have a different disease, which she named Christmas disease, both for the season and for the 'patronymic' of her five-year-old Canadian 'patient no. 1,' Stephen Christmas, son of the actor Eric.

Mixing studies continue to be the basis of coagulation screening and the means of identifying new clotting factors. In 1953 the railwayman John Hageman was admitted to a Chicago hospital for elective ulcer surgery. He had no history of bleeding, but his blood clotted poorly on a routine test, and his surgery was cancelled. Hageman's defect was corrected in the laboratory by mixing his plasma with either normal or hemophilic plasma. His doctors concluded that the plasma of both normals and hemophiliacs contained something that Hageman did not; it was Factor XII.

Each factor in the seemingly complicated 'coagulation cascade' has been found in the same way: someone comes along with a defect that can be corrected by normal plasma *and* by all other known factor-deficient plasmas. At first, clotting factors were named after the patients who lacked them (Christmas factor, Hageman factor, Fletcher factor, and Stuart factor). Later, they were numbered to reflect our understanding of their place in the reaction cascade. Mixing studies are basic to coagulation research and service. In the future, new factors will be identified in the same way.

The special clotting properties of cryoprecipitate – a blood component collected by freezing plasma – were recognized and made available in 1964. At that time, researchers still did not know whether the tendency to bleed (the so-called absence of AHF) was caused by a defective molecule, an absent molecule, or the presence of an inhibitor. In 1970–1 classical hemophilia was attributed to a defective Factor VIII molecule. As for the hemoglobinopathies, associated molecular substitutions in DNA have now been defined.

Forty years after his diagnosis, a Canadian team published the precise molecular substitution to account for the coagulation problem in Stephen Christmas, but their work could do nothing to prevent his death from AIDS on 20 December 1993. The success of blood products in the management of bleeding disorders led to a temporary revolution in pain management and lifestyle, but it also brought a tragic reminder of the dangers of blood therapy. At the time of writing, more than four hundred Canadian hemophiliacs have died of iatrogenic AIDS, and another thousand are infected with HIV and/or hepatitis.

With transfusion-related HIV or hepatitis B – and likewise in the 1998 furor over compensation for hepatitis C – we hear again the term 'innocent victim' (see chapter 7). Many drugs, diagnostic procedures, and surgical interventions cause sickness, even death; yet the value-added outrage expressed on behalf of those harmed by 'tainted' blood seems to reflect the primal significance of this fluid in our world.

Blood Is Still Special

Hematology was long considered to be a subdivision of internal medicine or pathology, but it has grown to become its own specialty. The annual meetings of the American Society of Hematology host more than three thousand delegates. Canadian specialist examinations were implemented in 1968 for hematological pathology, and in 1971 for clinical hematology.

Despite its lofty stature as a subject of professional activity, blood is still venerated for its magic and mystery. We may no longer deify great healers like Asklepios, but we do 'canonize' them with the Nobel Prize. Blood research is disproportionately represented among the Nobel laureates (appendix A), not only in physiology or medicine, but also in chemistry and peace.

In demystifying blood, new mechanisms are proposed in different, perhaps less magical-sounding words, but the ancient concepts have simply been rephrased; their essential features are unchanged. Galen said that blood exposed to air was charged with the life force. Now, blood is still seen as the equivalent of life, through its links to oxygen and respiration, while its balance, like that of its ancient Greek precursor, is essential for the preservation of health.

Suggestions for Further Reading

Buckley, Thomas, and Anna Gottlieb. *Blood Magic: The Anthropology of Menstruation*. Berkeley: University of California Press, 1988

Carter, K. Codell. 'On the Decline of Bloodletting in Nineteenth-Century Medicine.' *Journal of Psychoanalytic Anthropology* 5 (1982), 219–34.

Dreyfus, Camille. *Some Milestones in the History of Hematology*. New York: Grune and Stratton, 1957

Freireich, Emil A., and Noreen A. Lemak. *Milestones in Leukemia Research and Therapy*. Baltimore: Johns Hopkins University Press, 1991

Holmes, Frederic L. *Lavoisier and the Chemistry of Life: An Exploration of Scientific Creativity*. Madison: University of Wisconsin Press, 1985

Massie, Robert K. *Nicholas and Alexandra*. New York: Atheneum, 1968

Mazumdar, Pauline M. *Immunology, 1930–1980: Essays on the History of Immunology*. Toronto: Wall and Thompson, 1989

– *Species and Specificity: An Interpretation of the History of Immunology*. Cambridge: Cambridge University Press, 1994

Rather, L.J. *Addison and the White Corpuscles: An Aspect of Nineteenth-Century Biology*. London: Wellcome Institute of the History of Medcine, 1972

Risse, Guenter B. 'The Renaissance of Bloodletting: A Chapter in Modern Therapeutics.' *Journal of the History of Medicine and Allied Sciences* 34 (1979), 3–22

Rosner, Fred. 'Hemophilia in Classic Rabbinic Texts.' *Journal of the History of Medicine and Allied Sciences* 49 (1994), 240–50

Wailoo, Keith. *Drawing Blood: Technology and Disease Identity in Twentieth-Century America.* Baltimore: Johns Hopkins University Press, 1997

Wintrobe, Maxwell M. *Hematology the Blossoming of a Science: A Story of Inspiration and Effort.* Philadelphia: Lea and Febiger, 1985

– ed. *Blood Pure and Eloquent: A Story of Discovery, of People, and of Ideas.* New York: McGraw-Hill, 1980

On Canada

Baird, Ronald J. '"Give Us the Tools ...": the Story of Heparin – as Told by Sketches from the Lives of William Howell, Jay McLean, Charles Best, and Gordon Murray.' *Journal of Vascular Surgery* 11 (1990), 4–18

Bigelow, Wilfred G. *Mysterious Heparin: The Key to Open Heart Surgery.* Toronto: McGraw-Hill Ryerson, 1990

Gent, M., H.J. Barnett, D.L. Sackett, and D.W. Taylor. 'A Randomized Trial of Aspirin and Sulfinpyrazone in Patients with Threatened Stroke: Results and Methodologic Issues.' *Circulation* 62 (Dec. 1980), 97–105

Jaques, Louis B. 'The Hemostasis Paradigm in 1934 and in 1980.' *Annals of the New York Academy of Sciences* 370 (1981), 1–4

Marcum, James A. 'The Development of Heparin in Toronto.' *Journal of the History of Medicine and Allied Sciences* 52 (1997), 310–77

Smiley, R.K. 'History of the Canadian Hematology Society/Société canadienne d'hématologie, 1970–1990.' Unpublished paper, Royal College, Ottawa

CHAPTER NINE

Technology and Disease: The Stethoscope and Physical Diagnosis*

Concern for man himself and his fate must always form the chief interest of all technical endeavours.

Albert Einstein, speech at California Institute of Technology, 1931

Technology (derived from the Greek word for 'craft') refers to the tools in the service of an intellectual enterprise. Social and conceptual factors both influence the invention of new technologies. Once established, technologies not only alter practice, but they also change perceptions of illness, patients, doctors, and disease. The last two hundred years have witnessed an unprecedented burgeoning of technology, partly because of the demands of keeping medicine 'scientific,' defining professional identity, and satisfying an innate human love of gadgetry.

The oldest diagnostic instrument is probably the vaginal speculum, which can be traced to Roman antiquity, though a wide variety of surgical tools also have ancient roots. The numerous scientific inventions of the seventeenth century, such as the microscope and thermometer, initially had little to do with the day-to-day practice of medicine. After 1800, however, the emphasis on anatomy caused a reordering of medical knowledge, which fostered technological creation. In this chapter, the discovery and impact of some technologies

*Educational objectives for this chapter are found on pp. 396–7.

will be explored, using the example of the stethoscope as a starting point.

Antecedents to Discovery of Auscultation

Discoveries often seem to have taken place in a flash, a moment of lucky inspiration. Usually, however, they have a long prehistory, during which the inadequacy of old ways – the 'need' – is defined. Conditions that favour scientific discoveries are related to changes in ideas about the body, but they also incorporate factors from society, politics, economics, culture, and philosophy. In this sense, a discovery does not explode on a scene so much as it emerges from a milieu. Consequently, attributing priority is often a delicate matter. The discovery of auscultation and the invention of the stethoscope by René T.H. Laennec illustrate these principles well.

Socio-Political Antecedents

This story involves the French Revolution, the First Empire of Napoleon Bonaparte, and the Restoration of the Bourbon monarchy. These events profoundly altered the personal lives of French citizens and brought changes in the way that society organized the professions and education.

For centuries, medicine and surgery had been separate. Physicians learned in the universities, through lectures and books. Surgeons, on the other hand, were allied into special guilds with the barbers, and they received practical training through apprenticeship (see chapter 10). Since the Middle Ages, hospitals had been places where patients could seek refuge, comfort, food, and care. They were not sites of learning or research. Only rarely were medical or surgical students taught on the wards.

The French Revolution has been described as an uprising of the lower classes – often represented by the peasant women relentlessly knitting as they watched the guillotine in Charles Dickens's *Tale of Two Cities*. But the revolutionaries included an intellectual elite with radical opinions about politics and professional education. Medical revolutionaries, who called themselves *idéologues*, held extraordinary opinions: medicine and surgery could profitably combine; hospitals should be used in teaching; anatomy was important in the clinical setting; and doctors should maintain the health of the populace as well as treating the sick.

In 1789 the French medical faculties were abolished. The Paris school did not reopen until 1794, when it was revived under the enlightened anti-elitist (and short-lived) name, Ecole de Santé (School of Health). But there were no graduates for another five years. Among the new professors were a few of the previously excluded *idéologues,* who immediately put their ideas to work. The old college of surgery was amalgamated with the remnants of the medical faculty; students were taught in the hospitals; and opportunities for the dissection of cadavers were increased, to the extent that supply could scarcely meet the demand.

Intellectual and Philosophical Antecedents

When the revolution began, diseases were elaborate constellations of symptoms (see chapter 4), and their detection had little to do with anatomy (see chapter 2). Because diseases were fabricated from the pattern, sequence, and qualities of the subjective illness as told to the physician, a patient could not have a disease without feeling sick. Meticulous history taking and careful observation of the symptoms were the essential tools of diagnosis. Physical examination was cursory: the facies, the pulse, perhaps palpation of the abdomen and inspection of urine, stools, sputum or vomitus. This emphasis of unassisted observation over reasoning – empirical wisdom over theorizing – characterized the philosophy of knowledge called sensualism (see chapter 2).

Normal anatomy and pathological (abnormal) anatomy had been cultivated for centuries, but the relevance of organic changes to bedside medicine was not obvious (see chapters 2 and 4). In challenging the accepted wisdom that anatomy could not be made to fit in clinical medicine, the newly revived Paris school owed as much to contemporary philosophy as it did to the social and political climate. Hippocrates was resurrected as a founding champion of medical observation, and his wisdom was contrasted with the discredited and 'overly theoretical' views of Galen.

Anatomy conformed to the ideals of careful observation through the senses. French physicians began to imagine that the barrier between symptoms and structure could be broken by painstaking study and description of illnesses both before and after death. Daily ward rounds followed by autopsies became the teaching format of the Paris hospital clinics. New journals were founded to broadcast the 'anatomo-clinical' discoveries.

Jean-Nicolas Corvisart des Marets was one of the new professors in the Paris school. He was a supporter of the revolution, a religious sceptic, and hostile to classical languages and the church. He taught internal medicine in the Charité hospital. In the 1780s he learned of 'percussion' – tapping with the fingers to examine the chest. Resonance indicated healthy aerated lung; dullness indicated fluid or pus. The source was a little-known work, *Inventum Novum* (A New Invention), published in 1761 by the Austrian physician Leopold Auenbrugger. The musical son of an innkeeper, Auenbrugger had been inspired by his father, who tapped on casks in the family cellar to determine their content of wine. Auenbrugger applied the technique to the rigid barrel of the human thorax.

After twenty years of experimenting with percussion in his own practice, Corvisart published his translation and revision of Auenbrugger's treatise. Students flocked to his rounds and crowded into the autopsy theatre to watch him examine patients and cadavers as he gathered evidence for his book. He could predict anatomical findings with surprising success, and students believed that they were witnessing an exciting transformation of bedside medicine. In April 1801 Laennec joined Corvisart's clinic.

Personal Antecedents

René-Théophile-Hyacinthe Laennec came from Quimper, Brittany, in western France. His mother had died in 1786 when he was five years old, and his lawyer-poet father abandoned him to the care of his brother, a physician. Laennec's youth was played out on a background of revolution, terror, and war. Often working alone, he studied music, Greek, and Breton, and at the age of fourteen he enlisted as a surgical aide in the army, planning to follow in his uncle's footsteps. Because the revolution had closed the medical faculty in Nantes, he willingly set out for the capital.

Having already spent seven years in the study of medicine, Laennec excelled in Paris. He supplemented his meagre stipend by working as a student editor on Corvisart's new *Journal of Medicine*, where he published his own discoveries in pathological anatomy. His lengthy article on peritonitis appeared in 1802, during his second year of Paris training. It has since been recognized as the first description of that disease. He also taught private courses in dissection and began a never-to-be-finished treatise on pathology. In 1803 Laennec took first prize in both medicine and surgery, and in 1804 he became a doctor after defending his thesis on Hippocrates.

Despite the academic success, Laennec and his teachers regarded one another with only qualified esteem. Swayed by the political and religious conservatism of his friends, Laennec cultivated the classics and openly supported a return to the monarchy. To find a job in the liberal, atheist climate of postrevolutionary medicine, he needed more than his prizes and his precocious publications. For twelve years he struggled with his research, living from the proceeds of a private clientele. His fortunes did not improve until Napoleon was defeated at Waterloo in 1815 and the throne was restored to Louis XVIII, brother of Louis XVI who had been decapitated in January 1793.

Discovery: Myth and 'Reality'

> I have tried to place the internal organic lesions on the same plane as the surgical diseases with respect to diagnosis.
>
> Laennec, *Traité*, 1826, 1:xxv

In September 1816, just one year after the restoration, Laennec was finally awarded (or rewarded with) an official position in the Necker hospital. During that fall or in the early winter, he made the observation that established his reputation. According to his own account, he was examining a young female in whom he suspected a heart problem, but because of her stoutness, percussion was unhelpful. He thought of placing his ear directly on her chest to learn more about her heart, but decorum dictated restraint. Rolling a notebook into a cylinder, he placed one end on her chest, the other to his ear, and was astonished to hear the beating of her heart.

Years later this tale was embellished by J.A.L. de Kergaradec, a former student of Laennec, who said that just before the consultation, Laennec had been crossing the courtyard of the Louvre, where he saw children playing an acoustic game with a log. When the ear was applied to one end of the log, a pin tapping at the other end could easily be heard.

The 'discovery' at the bedside of the well-endowed young patient was simply the rediscovery of a phenomenon: sound can be transmitted through a mediator. Interpretation of these transmitted sounds consumed Laennec's attention for the next two and a half years, the hospital patients were his focus. His new instrument allowed him to listen at a discreet distance that satisfied both modesty and hygiene.

Laennec's method was clinicopathological correlation. Initially, he busied his students with rolling notebooks into tight 'cylinders,' as he called the first stethoscopes, sealed with gummed paper and string. Then he examined patients by percussion and 'mediate auscultation' (active listening through a mediator). The history and physical findings were carefully recorded. Laennec had to invent words to describe the sounds he heard: rales, crepitations, murmurs, pectoriloquy, bronchophony, egophony. When a patient died, the autopsy was correlated with the clinical findings.

Laennec later named his cylinder 'stethoscope' (from the Greek words for 'chest' and 'to explore'). In less than three years, he had established the anatomical significance of most of the normal and abnormal breath sounds still in use today. His book *De l'auscultation médiate* (On mediate auscultation) was written by February 1819, published in July, translated into English by 1821, and republished in the United States by 1823. A few doctors preferred the pathology in his treatise to the 'gimmick' of the stethoscope, but their opposition soon melted away.

Laennec also described the heart sounds and murmurs, but his interpretation differed from ours. He thought that the first heart sound represented ventricular contraction because of its synchrony with the carotid pulse; he assumed that the second sound must be

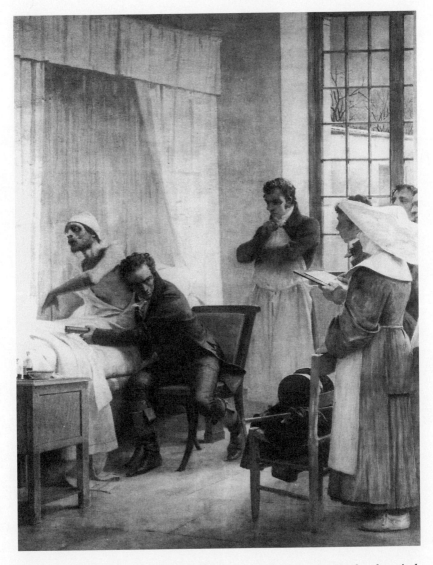

Laennec practising direct auscultation on a patient in the Necker hospital. Laennec preferred to use his stethoscope (which he is holding in his hand) because he was more comfortable at a distance from patients of differing sex and class. Mural by Théobald Chartran, late nineteenth century. Sorbonne, Paris

---

Laennec's Reaction to a Critic

I especially like the disadvantages that [Mérat] finds in a purely mechanical technique, which will tend to turn physicians away from skillful conjectures over the pulse, the facies, and excrement. It is the same as refusing to dash around Paris in a cabriolet for fear of losing the ability to tiptoe over droppings in the street.

Laennec, letter to his cousin,
24 April 1820 (cited in Duffin 1998, 218)

---

due to atrial contraction. Some historians wonder how Laennec could have been 'right' on the lung and so 'wrong' on the heart; however, three more decades of research, including the advent of cardiac catheterization, were to pass before the valvular synchrony of the sounds could be established with confidence.

Laennec enjoyed many favours from his royalist connections: a professorship in the medical faculty, a chair at the Collège de France, and an appointment as court physician. With the growing fame of auscultation, he was soon followed by a throng of foreign students. In response to criticisms, a considerably rearranged second edition of his book was released in May 1826. But three months later, the author was dead of tuberculosis at age forty-five. During his last illness, friends had examined the inventor with his stethoscope, but they concealed the findings to keep up his spirits. His Parisian colleagues did not eulogize him until more than a decade had passed. Most historians ascribe the hostility to religious and political differences, but medical philosophy also played a role.

The Inventor's Doubts

Nicknamed 'cylindromaniac,' Laennec was thought to be overreliant on his new invention; however, close study of his writings does not support the contention. His doubts about anatomical medicine and his ideas about the connection between *psyche* and *soma* brought

ORGANISM

him more disrepute than did his religion or politics. He believed
that a person's mental state influenced health and that the causes of
diseases such as asthma, angina, tuberculosis, and cancer did not
lie in anatomy alone. Something else must precede the physical
change. To explain these illnesses, he cited the psychic trauma of the
Reign of Terror and the Napoleonic Wars. Auscultation and anatomy were limited, he reasoned, because they could detect only some
effects of the myriad causes of disease.

Laennec warned his colleagues against relying too heavily on
organic explanations. To his contemporaries, this 'vitalistic' philosophy from an innovator was paradoxical and reactionary (see chapter
3). By advocating that doctors listen not only to their patients' chests
but to their stories as well, Laennec appeared to reject the very revolution his stethoscope had endorsed. But his personal doubts were
swept away and forgotten in the new-found enthusiasm for his
method.

Impact of the Discovery

The stethoscope was the first diagnostic instrument to achieve rapid
popularity. Within a short time, it was transported over Europe and
to North America by the numerous foreign students. Even Laennec's
enemies adopted the stethoscope, impressed by how easily and accu-
rately it detected signs of internal change. Pierre de Beaubien, a
Montrealer who studied in Paris, referred to the instrument in his
1827 thesis, and he may have been the first to bring it to Canada.

Anatomy had suddenly been made to fit into clinical medicine.
The state of internal organs could now be 'explored' long before the
patient became a cadaver. Laennec began to define lung diseases by
their anatomical lesions rather than by the symptoms. Using Greek
and Latin derivatives, he coined the terms 'bronchiectasis' and 'pulmonary edema,' while 'consumption' soon became 'tuberculosis' (a
name change generally attributed to J.L. Schönlein in the mid-
1830s). Together with the older terms 'emphysema' (puffed up) and
'empyema,' these new words signified diseases in the living rather
than pathological change in the dead.

Medical professionals quickly learned to identify disease by the signs of anatomical lesions, many of which were dragged from the realm of curiosity to diagnostic *sine qua non*. The process extended beyond the chest. Appendicitis, gastroenteritis, cholecystitis, and chlorosis were soon described as separate clinical entities with specific anatomical, microscopic, or chemical definitions. Proponents of neurology and phrenology began correlating behaviour, function, personality, and deviance with lesions in the brain or spinal cord, and with bumps on the head.

Some doctors enthusiastically predicted that all diseases would soon be linked to internal organic changes. This medical philosophy, called organicism, dominated research in the early nineteenth century: diseases were equated with and reduced to their anatomical change, and that change also became the cause. New technologies were devised to serve this new agenda, and the patient's account of symptoms paled in comparison with the objective search for inner change. This process continued into the twentieth century.

Technologies and Technopolies

If a mediator helped in listening to the chest, other instruments might help with percussion, visualization, and measurements of all kinds. Old instruments were redesigned and new ones invented. The durability of each invention relied on its power to demonstrate previously invisible material change to the senses of hearing, touch, and especially sight. Some of these technologies have direct descendants; others disappeared quickly. For example, in 1826 Pierre Adolphe Piorry invented the pleximeter to improve percussion; a small plate and a hammer, it was more cumbersome than useful, and its popularity was short-lived.

Stethoscopes were modified to adapt to differing circumstances, always with an eye to aesthetic form. The rigid cylinder gave way to slender curved models, then to a flexible monaural (one earpiece) stethoscope by 1843, and in 1852 G.P. Camman proposed a binaural (two earpieces) model. After the 1895 discovery of X-Rays, the fluoroscopic stethoscope, called 'see-hear,' or 'stethophone,' allowed examiners not only to hear but also to see inside their patients' chests.

Table 9.1
Advent of some diagnostic technologies*

1590	Microscope	Jansen	Dutch
1614	Thermometer	Santorio	Italian
1670	Microscope	van Leeuwenhoek	Dutch
1807	Light endoscopy	Bozzini	Italian in Germany
1819	Stethoscope	Laennec	French
1826	Pleximeter	Piorry	French
1829	Laryngoscope	Babington	English
1830s	Compound microscope	Donné, Addison	French, English
1851	Ophthalmoscope	von Helmholtz	German
1867	Clinical thermometry	Wunderlich	German
1881	Syphgmomanometer	von Basch	Austrian
1895	X-Rays	Röntgen	German
1897	Bronchoscope	Killian	German
1903	ECG	Einthoven	Dutch
1925	EEG	Pravditchi-Neminsky	Russian
1938	^{131}I in thyroid	Hamilton and Soley	American
1940	Cardiac catheterization	Cournand	French
1952	Radioisotope scanning	Heilmeyer	German
1954	Echocardiography	Edler and Hertz	Swedish
1957	Gamma camera	Anger	American
1962	^{99}Tc	Harper	American
1971	Computerized imaging	Cormack, Hounsfield	American, British

* Dates are approximate and apply variously to invention, patent, use, or publication.

Auscultation relied on the examiner's hearing, but the sounds evoked visual images of internal anatomy: for example, pectoriloquy indicated a cavity in the lung. In this manner, the stethoscope is akin to a speculum. Newer diagnostic instruments also appeal to vision (see table 9.1). Some catered to the sense of sight either directly or indirectly by the use of mirrors. Among these were the first illuminated endoscope (1807), the laryngoscope (1829), the ophthalmoscope (1851), and the bronchoscope (1897). Canulas, fibre optics, and lasers have extended this technology beyond the realm of diagnosis into surgical therapeutics.

Priority is difficult to assign. The microscope is usually described as the invention of the Dutch naturalist and optician Antoni van Leeuwenhoek in 1670, but magnifiers of small objects date back to the family of Zacharias Jansen of Holland in the sixteenth century and to Galileo Galilei of Italy and Robert Hooke of London. Until

Laennec's time, doctors may have been ready to ponder anatomy at the level of tissues, but they mistrusted the microscope. They preferred the naked eye, assuming that less visible changes were inconsequential. With the new anatomical focus of the 1820s and 1830s, efforts were made to improve the microscope. Compound lenses, corrections in spherical aberration, the advent of histological stains (1840), and immersion microscopy (1844) enhanced magnification and improved visualization. The result was a new pathology of microanatomy – tissues, cells, and organelles. The electron microscope, first constructed in 1931 by German physicists Max Knoll and Ernst A.F. Ruska, extended the visualization to the level of molecules. Fifty-five years later, Ruska shared the Nobel Prize in physics for this work.

In December 1895, Wilhelm Conrad Röntgen gave his first formal lecture on the properties of X-Rays. Scholars contend that this powerful discovery has influenced medicine more profoundly than any other technology. The very size of the machines determined a physician-centred locus of practice. The news spread rapidly around the world – for example, just a few weeks later, in February 1896, X-Rays were taken in Kingston, Ontario. Soon the anatomical exploration of the chest could be accomplished by images as well as sound. Ingenious applications of contrast media, including air, barium, and dyes, resulted in miraculously clear definition of tumors, spinal disorders, and vascular lesions. The interior of the brain could be investigated with carotid angiography, developed in 1941 by A.F. Cournand. Some radiographic tests, such as the pneumoencephalogram (1919), were painful and risky for the patient.

Technologies that are the direct descendants of radiography enhanced the visualization of soft tissue and reduced the need for invasive procedures; they contributed greatly to patient comfort even as they extended diagnosis. Echocardiography (1954) was derived from the ultrasound principles used to track submarines in the Second World War; it has proved particularly useful in assessing heart valves. Computerized axial tomography, which provided astonishing detail of lesions as small as one centimetre, was the invention of Allan M. Cormack and Godfrey N. Hounsfield; the first scanner was used at Wimbledon, U.K., in 1971. Many of these achievements won their inventors the Nobel Prize: Röntgen in 1901 (physics); Cournand in 1956; and Cormack and Hounsfield in 1979. The short interval between their discoveries and the Nobel honours indicates the rapid acceptance of these contributions. Some inventions were adopted even before their value had been clearly established – perhaps because they seemed to fill long-recognized needs and because they upheld the image of medicine as 'science' and doctor as 'scientist.'

Still others instruments, such as thermometers and kymographs, translated information of a nonvisual nature into a visual display (see chapter 3). The early thermometers, as invented by Santorio Santorio in the seventeenth century, were too unwieldy for clinical use. But by the 1870s, when Karl Wunderlich and Edouard Séguin used statistical data to write their influential treatises on the visual assessment of body heat, the instrument had been perceived to be of clinical value and had been reduced to a tiny rod that could be slipped into a pocket.

In 1861 Jean-Baptiste A. Chauveau and E. Jules Marey invented a kymographic method of recording pressure changes in vessels and in the catheterized hearts of living animals. Twenty years later, S.S. von Basch devised a sphygmomanometer, and in 1905 Sergei S. Korotkov demonstrated how it could be used with the stethoscope to measure blood pressure. The result was the creation of the new and previously inconceivable disease that now reaches epidemic proportions in an aging population – hypertension.

By 1903, Willem Einthoven had invented an electrocardiograph to translate the electrical function of the beating heart into a visual tracing for easy analysis. This electrical pattern refined the clinical diagnosis of angina and myocardial infarction. Previously detected only at autopsy and debated even then, myocardial infarction emerged from a vague set of earlier diagnoses, including acute indigestion and apoplexy. Einthoven was awarded the Nobel Prize in 1924. His work is often cited as the beginning of modern cardiology.

Like the stethoscope, these diagnostic technologies were invented to 'see' beyond the patient's story into the patient's body to detect a material basis for the symptoms. Insurance companies quickly embraced the technology revolution, welcoming the predictive value of objective signs of disease in subjective states of health. If visual norms could be found, then a range of deviations could be established; physical examination of the healthy became routine. The word 'natural' to denote health was slowly replaced by the more numerical word 'normal' (see chapter 5 and J.H. Warner, 89–91). Instrumentation satisfied the objectives of a knowledge system that increasingly valued numbers. Changing disease concepts drove the search for new technologies; in turn the new technologies drove disease concepts by finding new disorders and discrediting others.

Hospital as Machine

By 1800 the hospital, once the site of charitable care, had become the locus of anatomo-clinical education, providing yet another reason for people of means to avoid it. Nevertheless, with attention to architecture, light, and space, the care and special treatment given in the hospital had transformed it from a religious sanctuary to a purpose-built place of cure. In the vision of the French health reformer J.R. Tenon, the hospital itself was a medical machine – *un instrument qui facilite la curation* (cited in Weiner 1993, 373). As a result, Michel Foucault and others referred to hospitals as *les machines à guérir* (machines for curing).

New diagnoses subtend new treatments. By the mid-twentieth century, new definitions of neurological, respiratory, and cardiac failure had prompted management by special machines that were available only in hospitals (see table 9.2). Attempts to resuscitate near-dead newborns and drowning victims can be traced to biblical antiquity, but poliomyelitis became a stimulus to the further development of intubation, iron lungs, and ventilators, which are now applied to many other situations. The number of patients ventilated for more than twenty-four hours at the Massachusetts General Hospital increased from sixty-six in 1958 to more than two thousand by 1982 (Snider 1989).

Radiation technology not only delineated tumor masses, it became part of the treatment, and machines were invented to deliver controlled doses. At first, techniques relied on brachytherapy (treatment at short distance), with radium and later cesium applied to tumors

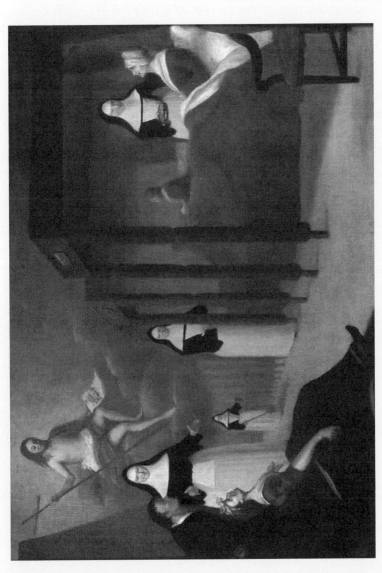

Hospital as a site of healing. Patients in the Hôtel-Dieu in Montreal being cared for by the nuns under the watchful eye of their saviour. Anon., ca. 1710. Musée des Hospitalières de l'Hôtel-Dieu, Montreal

Table 9.2
Advent of some therapeutic technologies*

1881	Neonatal incubator	E.S. Tarnier	French
1898	Radium	Marie and Pierre Curie	Polish-French
1929	Iron lung	P. Drinker	American
1940	^{32}P for polycythemia	J.H. Lawrence	American
1941	^{131}I for hyperthyroidism	S. Hertz, A. Robert	American
1943	Renal dialysis	W.J. Kolff	Dutch-American
1950	IPP ventilators	many models	American-British
1951	Cobalt^{60} teletherapy	H.E. Johns	Canada
1953	Linear accelerator	D. Fry, C. Miller, P. Howard-Flanders	British
1956	Membrane oxygenator	G.H. Clowes	American
1958	Implanted pacemaker	R. Elmquist, A. Senning	Sweden
1975	Ambulatory dialysis	R.P. Popovich	American
1968	Total parenteral nutrition	S. Dudrick	American
1982	Artificial heart	R.K. Jarvik	American

* Dates are approximate and apply to invention, patent, use, or publication.

inside needles, tubes, and plaques. Later, teletherapy (treatment at long distance) was developed, characterized by high-energy beams from X-Ray machines, cobalt units, or linear accelerators.

The analysis of cardiac arrhymias, blood gases, and lung, brain, and renal function implied the need for new methods of managing these newly defined conditions. For example, the clinical definition of ventricular fibrillation subtended a role for defibrillators. Similarly, an understanding of metabolic imbalance, diffusion properties, and anticoagulation revised the treatment of kidney failure. Elegant monitors, catheters, respirators, and pumps occupy the newly vested sanctuaries of healing – units for intensive care, coronary care, respiratory care, renal care, neonatal care, and cancer clinics.

By mid-century, the hospital had become a place for scientific investigation and cure, furnished with expensive equipment and essential to rich and poor alike. The very sick needed the life support that could be provided only there. Those who were not sick at all entered the hospital for diagnosis, which also depended on machinery. The chronically ill, the homeless, and the disabled – the very people who once populated the hospitals – were less welcome. Only with the financial crisis of the 1990s and the parallel reduction in the size and cost of technologies have we begun to question the prevalence of in-hospital investigation and care. Despite the public outcry, the 1990s bed closures in acute care hospitals have yet to be correlated with an anticipated rise in mortality or decline in health.

Distance between Doctor and Patient

> Since I do not foresee that atomic energy is to be a great boon for a long time, I have to say that for the present it is a menace.
>
> Albert Einstein, *Atlantic Monthly*, November 1945

Early detection of disease and diagnostic precision have irrefutable benefits, but they come at a price that critics of modern medicine have called the 'tyranny of the normal.' Prior to the stethoscope, patients could not be sick unless they felt sick. After the stethoscope, it was possible to have a serious disease and feel fine. The patient was no longer the chief authority on his or her own well-being. In our hypermedicalized world, these principles are deeply ingrained. Most people with hypertension have no symptoms at all, but they readily accept a machine's diagnosis even when it obliges them to take pills for many years.

Only the psychiatric diseases have no objective organic or chemical correlatives (see chapter 12). Patients who feel sick but in whom no material sign of disease can be found have 'merely functional' ailments or are mentally disturbed. And they are considered less seriously ill than those who may feel completely well but have technologically defined diseases.

Just as critics of medical ideas deplore the devaluing of subjective accounts of illness, critics of medical technology lament the distance interposed between the doctor and the patient. They complain that medicine treats the data, not the person. Technology also separates the patient from his or her disease, elevating it to the status of a living enemy that must be hunted and destroyed. For example, we speak of the 'war on cancer.' Dissatisfaction with impersonal technol-

ogy generates interest in alternative medicine and holistic explanations. Some critics, like writer Neil Postman, situate the origin of
medicine's loss of empathy in Laennec, but they do not realize that
the inventor opposed the trend that he is said to have launched.

Historian Joel Howell studied the hospital use of blood tests, uri-
nalysis, and X-Rays, and noted an irony: technologies may save time,
but doctors now spend less time with patients than they did before. A
similar irony was observed by historian Edward Tenner: computers
had promised to save paper, but instead, they vastly increased its consumption, as any practitioner familiar with 'pending' lab reports can
testify.

The history of technology is just beginning. It will demonstrate
the ingenious solutions and marvellous potential of medical instruments. It will reveal how each invention created new diseases where
none had been conceived. And it will uncover more fascinating discrepancies between the aspirations of inventors and the applications
that their instruments subsequently find.

Suggestions for Further Reading

On Auscultation, Cardiology, and Early-Nineteenth-Century French Medicine

Ackerknecht, Erwin H. *Medicine at the Paris Hospital, 1794–1848.* Baltimore:
   Johns Hopkins University Press, 1967
Bishop, J.P. 'Evolution of the Stethoscope.' *Journal of the Royal Society of Medicine*
   73 (1980), 448–56
Duffin, Jacalyn. *To See with a Better Eye: A Life of R.T.H. Laennec.* Princeton, N.J.:
   Princeton University Press, 1998
Fleming, Peter. *A Short History of Cardiology.* Amsterdam and Atlanta, Ga.:
   Editions Rodopi, Clio Medica 40, 1997
Foucault, Michel. *Naissance de la clinique.* Paris: Presses Universitaires de France,
   1963
Frank, Robert G. 'The Telltale Heart: Physiological Instruments, Graphic Meth-
   ods, and Clinical Hopes, 1854–1914.' In *The Investigative Enterprise: Experimen-
   tal Physiology in Nineteenth-Century Medicine,* ed. William Coleman and Frederic
   L. Holmes, 211–90. Berkeley and Los Angeles: University of California Press,
   1988

Fye, W. Bruce. *American Cardiology: The History of a Specialty and Its College.* Baltimore: Johns Hopkins University Press, 1996

Warner, John Harley. *Against the Spirit of System: The French Impulse in American Medicine.* Princeton, N.J.: Princeton University Press, 1998

Weiner, Dora B. *The Citizen-Patient in Revolutionary and Imperial Paris.* Baltimore and London: Johns Hopkins University Press, 1993

Weisz, George. *The Medical Mandarins: The French Academy of Medicine in the Nineteenth and Early Twentieth Centuries.* New York and Oxford: Oxford University Press, 1995

On Medical Technology and Its Effects

Baker, Jeffrey *The Machine in the Nursery: Incubator Technology and the Origins of Newborn Intensive Care.* Baltimore: Johns Hopkins University Press, 1996

Bynum, W.F., and Roy Porter, eds. *Medicine and the Five Senses.* Cambridge: Cambridge University Press, 1993

Carlsson, Sten. 'A Glance at the History of Nuclear Medicine.' *Acta Oncologica* 34 (1995), 1095–102

Davis, Audrey B. *Medicine and Its Technology: An Introduction to the History of Medical Instrumentation.* Westport, Conn: Greenwood Press, 1981

– 'Life Insurance and the Physical Examination: A Chapter in the Rise of American Medical Technology.' *Bulletin of the History of Medicine* 55 (1981), 392–406

Howell, Joel D. *Technology and American Medical Practice, 1880–1930: An Anthology of Sources.* New York: Garland, 1988

– *Technology in the Hospital: Transforming Patient Care in the Early Twentieth Century.* Baltimore: Johns Hopkins University, 1995

Kevles, Bettyann. *Naked to the Bone: Medical Imaging in the Twentieth Century.* New Brunswick, N.J.: Rutgers University Press, 1997

Mangione, Salvatore, and Steven J. Peitzman. 'Physical Diagnosis in the 1990s: Art or Artifact.' *Journal of General Internal Medicine* 11 (1996), 490–3

Peitzman, Steven J. 'Science, Inventors, and the Introduction of the Artifical Kidney in the United States.' *Seminars in Dialysis* 9 (1996), 276–81

Postman, Neil. *Technopoly: The Surrender of Culture to Technology.* New York: Knopf, 1992

Reiser, Stanley Joel. *Medicine and the Reign of Technology.* Cambridge and New York: Cambridge University Press, 1979

Rothman, David. *Strangers at the Bedside.* New York: Basic Books, 1991

Snider, Gordon L. 'Historical Perspective on Mechanical Ventilation: From Simple Life Support System to Ethical Dilemma.' *American Review of Respiratory Disease* 140 (1989), S2–7

Tenner, Edward. *Why Things Bite Back: Technology and the Revenge of Unintended Consequences.* New York: Knopf, 1996

Warner, Deborah Jean. 'What Is a Scientific Instrument, When Did It Become One, and Why?' *British Journal for the History of Science* 23 (1990), 83–93

On Hospitals

Abel-Smith, Brian. *The Hospitals, 1800–1948: A Study in Social Administration in England and Wales.* London: Heinemann, 1964

Foucault, Michel, et al. *Les machines à guérir: Aux origines de l'hôpital moderne.* Brussels: Mardaga, 1979

Gerstner, Patsy. 'The Temple of Health: A Pictorial History of the Battle Creek Sanitarium.' *Caduceus* 12 (1996), 1–99

Hickey, Daniel. *Local Hospitals and Ancien Régime France: Rationalization, Resistance, Renewal, 1530–1789.* Montreal: McGill-Queen's University Press, 1997

Martin, Stephen C., and Joel D. Howell. 'Creating University Hospitals: Rationales and Realities.' *Academic Medicine* 70 (1995), 1012–16

Risse, Guenter B. *Hospital Life in Enlightenment Scotland: Care and Teaching at the Royal Infirmary of Edinburgh.* Cambridge: Cambridge University Press, 1986

– *Mending Bodies, Saving Souls: A History of Hospitals.* New York: Oxford University Press, 1999

Rosenberg, Charles E. *The Care of Strangers: The Rise of America's Hospital System.* New York: Basic Books, 1987

Stevens, Rosemary. *In Sickness and in Wealth: American Hospitals in the Twentieth Century.* New York: Basic Books, 1989

On Auscultation, Technology, and Hospitals in Canada

Agnew, G. Harvey. *Canadian Hospitals 1920 to 1970: A Dramatic Half Century.* Toronto: University of Toronto Press, 1974

Aldrick, John E., and Brian C. Lentle. *A New Kind of Ray: The Radiological Sciences in Canada, 1895–1995.* Vancouver: Canadian Association of Radiologists, 1995

Connor, J.T.H. 'Medical Technology in Victorian Canada.' *Canadian Bulletin of Medical History* 3 (1986), 97–123

– 'The Technology of Medicine.' *Canadian Bulletin of Medical History* 6 (1989), 67–70

– 'The Artificial Kidney in North America: Gordon Murray and the Canadian Connection.' *Biomedical Instrumentation and Technology* 23 (1989), 384–7

– 'Hospital History in Canada and the United States.' *Canadian Bulletin of Medical History* 7 (1990), 93–104

Gagan, David. 'For "Patients of Moderate Means": The Transformation of Ontario's Public General Hospitals, 1880–1950.' *Canadian Historical Review* 70 (1989), 151–79

– *'A Necessity among Us': The Owen Sound General and Marine Hospital, 1891–1985*. Toronto: University of Toronto Press, 1990

Hayter, Charles R.R. 'Making Sense of Shadows: Dr. James Third and the Introduction of X-Rays, 1896 to 1902.' *Canadian Medical Association Journal* 153 (1995), 1249–56

– 'William H.B. Aikens: Forgotten Pioneer of Canadian Radiotherapy.' *Annals of the Royal College of Physicians and Surgeons of Canada* 31 (1998), 155–8

Shorter, Edward. *A Century of Radiology in Toronto*. Toronto: Wald and Emerson, 1996

Segall, Harold N. 'The Introduction of the Stethoscope and Clinical Auscultation in Canada.' *Journal of the History of Medicine and Allied Sciences* 22 (1967), 414–17

– *Pioneers of Cardiology in Canada, 1820–1970*. Willowdale, Ont.: Hounslow Press, 1988

CHAPTER TEN

Work of the Hand: History of Surgery*

Any fool can cut off a leg. It takes a surgeon to save one.

George Ross of Montreal

Recurrent Themes

Surgery and medicine are mutually dependent, but they have not always been considered part of the same discipline. The so-called surgical personality originates in the perceived difference between surgical and medical work. The word 'surgery' is derived from the Greek for 'work' and 'hand.' Some cultures looked on handwork as menial and ranked it below that done by the mind. Others, more like our own, have prized it above all other skills. Variations in the relative status of surgery and medicine will be one theme of this chapter.

Surgery may be the oldest of all medical activities. Cave paintings of injured hunters show that prehistoric people responded to the accidental trauma of existence. But not all trauma is accidental. Neolithic peoples used arrows and rocks to injure enemies deliberately, and they devised procedures to treat wounds. The dangerous technologies of war generate a need for compensatory surgical techniques, which then find peacetime applications. This, too, is a recurring theme in surgery's past.

*Educational objectives for this chapter are found on p. 397.

Two other themes can be traced throughout this history. First, the profession of medicine as a whole shaped its structure and values from surgical models. Second, elective procedures – those done by intention and not of necessity – gradually became more frequent through time and are now the result of complex, cautious choice.

Wounds and Fractures: Prehistoric and Ancient Surgery

Prehistoric medicine is said to have involved cooking and mixing foodstuffs, but early traces of this activity are scarce. In contrast, evidence from paleopathology and comparative anthropology testify to the prevalence of surgery. Bark splints for setting fractures have been dated to at least 2450 B.C. Similarly, skulls from the Neolithic period (10,000 to 5,000 B.C.) indicate the great antiquity of the elective procedure of trephination, in which a flap of bone was removed.

Why were early peoples motivated to drill holes in the skull? Answers can only be conjectured. Attention may have been directed to the cranium, perhaps by headache or seizures, or by loss of consciousness following a blow. Observers, who possibly had noticed survival in victims with open fractures, might have decided to open the skull deliberately by boring holes with stone implements. The practice may have been justified by pathophysiological ideas related to the release of pressure or to the dispelling of evil humours or malevolent spirits. Fossil remains with bony healing show that the treatment, if not curative, was at least survivable. Between 3000 and 2000 B.C., trephination was relatively common in South America, Western Europe, and Asia. Today, bore holes are indicted when an epidural or subdural hematoma is suspected, but no evidence tells us if prehistoric surgeons conceived of that condition.

Other sources of information about prehistoric surgery derive from present-day cultures that are isolated from modern technology. For example, biting insects continue to be used as sutures in parts of Africa and South America. The edges of the wound are brought together and an ant is allowed to bite through both 'lips'; when its jaws are firmly locked, the insect's thorax and abdomen are broken off, leaving the head and jaws as a neat staple. Similarly, plant and animal materials are used to bring the edges of wounds together.

Traditionally, Amerindians applied botanical substances to injuries; recently botanists have begun to examine what the active principles might be.

The earliest-known example of medical writing is said to be a Sumerian recipe for a beer poultice dressing that was inscribed around 2100 B.C. on the clay Nippur tablet, which is now in the University Museum, Philadelphia. Surgery also features in the famous Code of Hammurabi of ca. 1700 B.C. Incised on a tall black stone that is now in the Louvre, it describes draconian punishments for surgical 'malpractice.' If a surgeon harmed a free man's slave, he had to replace the slave; if the patient who was harmed was a free man, the surgeon's hand was to be cut off.

In ancient Egypt, some surgeons were members of the elite. The deified architect and physician Imhotep (ca. 2900 B.C.) is thought to have written early surgical texts, but his life is shrouded in mystery. Hesy Ré, chief of dentists and surgeons (ca. 2600 B.C.), was identified by the wooden panels taken from his tomb. Now in the Cairo Museum, they portray him as a scribe or learned man. Other painted objects found in his tomb resemble a series of graduated cylinders.

The most complete treatises from ancient Egypt are papyrus scrolls about the practice of surgery. These documents are usually known by the names of the adventurers who carried them home to Europe or America – for example, the 20-metre-long Ebers papyrus (1550 B.C.) purchased by German professor Georg Ebers in the mid-nineteenth century, and the Edwin Smith papyrus (ca. 1600 B.C.), a 4½-metre scroll, which was found by Edwin Smith in 1862 and now resides in the Malloch Rare Book Room of the New York Academy of Medicine. Neither of these documents was deciphered by the men whose names they bear. Only after the 1930 translation and interpretation by James Henry Breasted of Chicago was the Edwin Smith papyrus shown to be an incomplete surgical text based on even earlier writings (ca. 3000 B.C.). It describes forty-eight case histories, each with a title and instructions for diagnosis and management. It also includes a glossary of ancient terms and stated that some conditions were not to be treated.

As a religious practice, the ancient Egyptians mummified their

---

Case 25 of the Edwin Smith Papyrus

If thou examinest a man having a dislocation in his mandible
... thou shouldst put thy thumb(s) upon the ends of the two
rami of the mandible in the inside of his mouth, (and) thy two
claws (... fingers) under his chin, (and) thou shouldst cause
them to fall back so that they rest in their places ... Thou
shouldst say concerning him: '... an ailment which I will treat.'
Thou shouldst bind it with *ymrw,* (and) honey every day until
he recovers.

The Edwin Smith Surgical Papyrus, trans. James Henry Breasted
(Chicago: University of Chicago Press, 1930), 303–5

---

dead. Mummification led to experimentation in 'surgical' procedures such as suturing. The stitches of one embalmer on the abdomen of a mummy have been dated to at least 1100 B.C. Breasted
argued that papyri recommended suturing for wounds. This opinion
is controversial, however, because sutures in mummies are rare, and
evidence is evanescent elsewhere as a result of the organic decay.
Dexterity in removing organs through small orifices was part of the
embalmer's skill, but its impact on treatment of the living is uncertain.

Evidence for trephination in Egypt is scant, but the ancient Egyptians practised some operations, such as circumcision of males and
possibly also of females. With trephination, circumcision is among
the oldest elective procedures. Phimosis and paraphimosis constituted pathological indications for the operation, which is unique in
its application to the healthy, be they infants or adults. A bas-relief
on a tomb of about 2500 B.C. in Saqqara, near Memphis, seems to
represent an assembly line for circumcision; differences in posture
of the two clients – one being held, the other not – may represent
the effect of anesthetic. The Hebrew religious practice of circumcision may have arisen in Egypt, for it is described in the eighth-
century B.C. Pentateuch of the Old Testament (Genesis 17:10–14;

Exodus 4:25; Leviticus 12:3) and is said to have originated following the exodus from Egypt around 1200 B.C. (Joshua 5:2–8). Female circumcision and infibulation are still practised in African societies. Like their male equivalents, the operators of female circumcision are part of religiosocial orders rather than healers. In Western traditions, elective surgery on healthy female parts found medical indications in the late nineteenth century in the procedures of ovariotomy for psychic disorders and of clitoridectomy for sexual ambiguity.

Effective pain relief has been a preoccupation of most cultures; its absence was long a barrier to elective surgery. Some substances were moderately effective analgesics. The ancient Chinese used henbane, which contains the anticholinergic drug, hyoscine. The ancient Hindus practised fumigation (or 'smoking') of wounds with herbs to soothe them. The Greeks made use of alcohol and opium. Christ on the cross was offered (but refused) a sponge soaked in a mixture to dull his pain (Matthew 27:34).

Even small wounds could be deadly until the recent past. Ancient Greek and Roman treatises contain recipes for wound washing, dressing, and binding. Wine, beer, myrrh, and rust were thought to promote healing. According to Homer, the heroic warriors were surgeons for each other; they bandaged wounds with healing substances, such as rust from their spears, to prevent what the Greeks called suppuration, and what we know as infection. In his book *The Healing Hand*, Guido Majno analysed the anesthetic and antibiotic properties of ancient remedies for pain relief and infection control and found that many were efficacious.

Cautery – or the searing of wounds with hot metal instruments or caustic dressings – was widely practised, especially by the Arabs. The Chinese practice of *moxa*, which applied heat at sites perhaps distant from a wound, was technically speaking not a form of cautery. Heat closed vessels to staunch bleeding, and it probably created temporary sterility. Cautery with red-hot irons was standard treatment for military wounds for centuries – but unless the patient was unconscious, it was exquisitely painful.

Fractures and dislocations resulted from athletics and warfare. Many references in the Hippocratic writings describe an evolving science of orthopedics, which used mechanical apparati, positioning, and gravity for reducing fractures and dislocations. Some Hippocratic texts, especially the *Oath*, seem to frown on specific uses of the knife, such as 'cutting for stone.' But others state that abscesses should be incised and drained, while thoracentesis for empyema (pus in the chest) was clearly described by Hippocrates (*Diseases II*, 47).

Greek and Hindu surgical instruments further extend our knowledge of early practices. Fibulae were safetypin-like devices for wound closure: both sides of a wound were transfixed with a needle (fibula), around which thread was wrapped to approximate the edges. Syringes were introduced by the Greeks for draining abscesses rather than for injection. They were based on the principle of the piston, supposedly invented by a barber in Alexandria around 280 B.C. The Greek word for syringe, *pyulcos*, meant 'pus-puller,' and the earliest reference is in the first-century A.D. treatise *Pneumatics* by Hero of Alexandria. The Romans improved on surgical instruments, fashioning tools from copper alloy. Unlike their Egyptian precursors, they devised dental procedures with special forceps for tooth pulling or filling, and they modelled false teeth in bone and gold for wealthy clients.

Wounds and Fractures: Medieval Surgery

During the Christian-dominated Middle Ages in Europe, disease was seen as divine punishment; care was welcomed, but efforts to cure might be tantamount to hubris. Cure was an act of God or one of his holy agents. The patron saints of medicine, pharmacy, and surgery were the twin healers Cosmas and Damian, who supposedly had been martyred early in the fourth century A.D. They were reported to have effected miraculous cures, including the transplantation of a gangrenous limb with a cadaverous donor leg. Medical schools, hospices, and fraternities, including a Paris college of surgery, were named for these saints.

Religious faith notwithstanding, surgical activities continued. In twelfth-century Salerno, Italy, fresh wounds were thought to fare well if thick white or yellow pus could be made to appear. This pus was later called 'laudable' because it heralded healing. The unlaudable

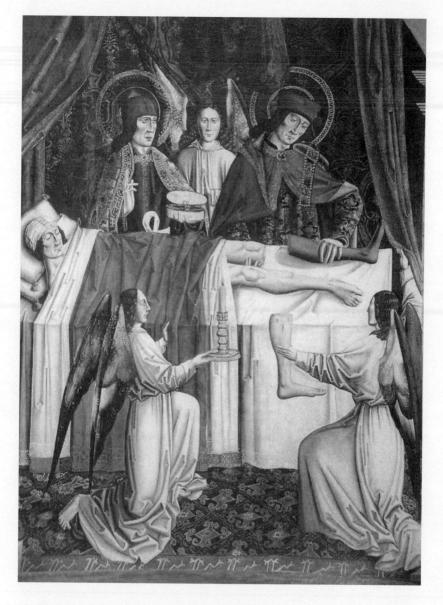

Medical saints Cosmas and Damian in the oft-depicted scene of the miraculous transplantation of a leg from a cadaver donor. Painting by Alonso de Sedano (fl. 1496), Spanish. Wellcome Institute Library, London

variety of pus was thin (serous), pink or red, seeped slowly from the wound, and was associated with spreading inflammation, cellulitis, and gangrene. Like their Greco-Roman precursors, medieval warriors cared for one another on the battlefield; the kit carried into the fourteenth-century battle of Crécy included tiny boxes packed with spiderweb to cover wounds.

In the later Middle Ages, a few surgeons rose to prominence through their teaching and writings. The works of the eleventh-century Islamic surgeon, Abu al Qaim (Albucasis), on bloodletting, cautery, operations, and instruments were translated into Latin in 1137. The 1300 *Chirurgia* of Henri de Mondeville emphasized anatomy and described techniques to dress wounds, relieve pain, and staunch bleeding, including the use of a tight band on a limb that was about to be amputated. De Mondeville taught that wounds could heal without suppuration. The *Chirurgia Magna* (Great Surgery) of Guy de Chauliac, which appeared in 1363, also recognized the importance of anatomy, as it dealt with wounds, fractures, tumors, sores, hernias, ulcers, and cataracts. De Chauliac accepted the theory of laudable pus and devised poultices to encourage its formation. His ideas dominated surgical practice for the next two hundred years; the 1478 French translation was one of the first books ever printed.

The advent of gunpowder prompted further experimentation on wound management. In 1514 Giovanni de Vigo, surgeon to the pope, recommended boiling oil of elder to cauterize this new type of wound. His method caught on quickly; however, the French surgeon Ambroise Paré, discovered quite by accident that the method was superfluous.

Paré wrote on many topics (see chapter 11). His works and other early modern treatises on surgery often contained a 'wounds man' and commentary, illustrating how to manage each injury. Technical details were given for amputation, reduction of fractures, and elective procedures such as trephination. To ensure a wide dissemination of his ideas, Paré wrote in the vernacular rather than in Latin. His humility is said to be revealed in his most famous saying: 'I bandage them, but God heals them.' Paré questioned the long-held belief about laudable pus, but he recommended cautery for other

Paré's Accidental Discovery

My oil ran out and I had to apply a salve made of egg-white, rose-oil, and turpentine. The next night I slept badly, plagued by the thought that I would find the men dead whose wounds I had failed to burn, so I got up early to visit them. To my great surprise, those treated with salve felt little pain, showed no inflammation or swelling, and had passed the night rather calmly – while the ones on which seething oil had been used lay in high fever with aches, swelling and inflammation around the wound.

Ambroise Paré, recalling the 1536 siege of Turin
(cited in Haeger 1988, 108)

problems, including amputation, and his illustrated treatise on instruments described thirty-eight types of cautery irons.

Surgical instruments were sometimes made in the shape of animal heads and named for the creatures they represented. Animal designs are found in Paré, but they date back far earlier. They were a characteristic of the surgical tools of the ancient Hindu tradition of Susruta, the author of *Samhita*, a treatise of unknown antiquity (800 B.C. to 400 A.D.) More than an aesthetic affectation, the designs originated in mythology and appealed to spiritual powers for healing.

Early Modern Operations

Several elective procedures were improved in early modern times, including amputation, cataract surgery, hernia repair, lithotomy, and plastic repair of skin. In amputation, the limb tourniquet was displaced by Paré's recommendation of ligatures for large vessels, but this new technique demanded time, knowledge of anatomy, a relatively clear field, and willing assistants. It was not widely accepted until the early seventeenth century after Fabry von Hilden (Fabricius Hildanus) described the releasing tourniquet, in which a stick twisted into the band could tighten or release pressure. Other tour-

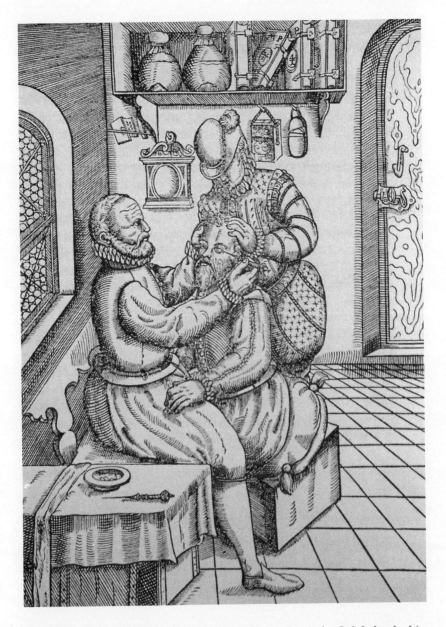

Cataract surgery in the sixteenth century. Georg Bartisch, *Ophthalmodouleia*,
Dresden, 1583, facsimile

niquets were devised by Johannes Scultetus and J.L. Petit, who used screw-clamps.

Lentine cataracts had been 'couched' (from the French *coucher*, to lie down) in ancient India and Rome, according to Susruta and the first-century medical writer Celsus. This procedure involved introducing a needle into the eye at the edge of the cornea to push the clouded lens down and out of the way. A 1559 illuminated manuscript, discovered in the twentieth century, reveals that its author, Caspar Stromayr of Lindau, was an accomplished cataract coucher and herniotomist. The 1583 work of the German surgeon George Bartisch also described both the couching of cataract and removal of the globe of the eye. In 1638 cataract surgery and lens clouding were related to the theory of vision established by René Descartes. Extraction of the lens itself was described in 1753 by Jacques Daviel.

Cutting for bladder stones, or perineal lithotomy, had been mentioned in Celsus. Various approaches and instruments for the procedure were recommended by a special class of wandering lithotomists and barber surgeons. Its rise in popularity in the early modern period has led some to postulate an epidemic of bladder concretions for dietary and environmental reasons.

In the Renaissance, certain plastic procedures were revived, including correction of hare lip deformity and rhinoplasty (repair of the nose). The latter had been known to the Hindu surgeon Susruta, and it was rediscovered and revised by the Italian surgeon Gaspare Tagliacozzi, who published an illustrated treatise demonstrating a technique to replace the nose by displacing a skin pedicle from the upper arm. Operations to repair missing noses were of great importance in the century following the advent of syphilis (see chapter 7). In the eighteenth century, the *Encyclopédie* of Denis Diderot and Jean le Rond d'Alembert glorified the achievements of surgeons with numerous illustrations of elegant instruments wielded by equally elegant practitioners.

Professionalization of Surgery and Medicine

With these surgical innovations, the professional separation of European surgeons from physicians was firmly entrenched. Often illiter-

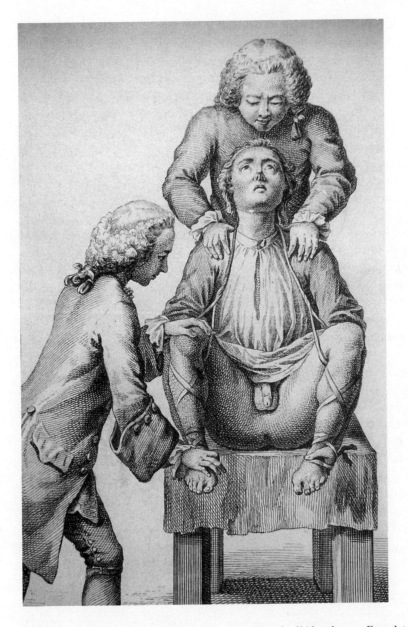

Lithotomy. Denis Diderot and Jean le Rond d'Alembert, *Encyclopédie*, planches, vol. 3, plate 12, 1772

ate and traditionally inferior to physicians, surgeons were part of the barber class, who derived income from shaving, cutting hair, and drawing teeth. Minor operations were incidental. Barber-surgeons learned their trade by apprenticeship, unlike the doctors who read Greek or Latin (usually Galen) at universities and rarely saw patients until after they had graduated. Many famous surgeons, including Paré, Stromayr, and Bartisch, had been trained by barbers; their humble origins hindered their acceptance in learned places.

In 1518 the internist doctors of England formed the Royal College of Physicians to control licensing and the practice of medicine. Soon after, in 1540, barber-surgeons were granted a charter by Henry VIII to form their own guild. The charter protected their right to practise and granted them autonomy over licensing and discipline. Similarly, in other countries, the incorporation of surgeons took place separately from physicians (see table 10.1). By the late eighteenth century, surgeons comprised a range of practitioners, from the village barber to an aristocratic elite, but their practical apprenticeship training continued. These professional organizations created a hierarchy and an environment in which specialties would develop. In twentieth-century Canada, the centuries-old separation of the two disciplines is still reflected in the two branches of the Royal College of Physicians and Surgeons, founded in 1920.

Until the nineteenth century, physicians were mocked for being impractical, bookish, and ineffectual. Their university-based education was considered stagnant: tradition dictated the textbooks, and ambivalence about anatomy reigned. Surgeons, on the other hand, maintained separate schools, where they taught by apprenticeship on living patients and by dissection of cadavers. In France, for example, surgeons rejected the university establishment, which had been allied with the monarchy. Following the revolution, they were central to the revived Paris medical faculty, which emphasized dissection and adopted hospital-based methods of instruction for all students (see chapter 9).

French surgeons rose to even greater prominence during the Napoleonic Wars. Particularly notable was Dominique-Jean Larrey, who was decorated by the emperor for his dexterity as an operator

Table 10.1
Professional organizations for surgery

1260	Confrérie de St Côme et St Damien, Paris
1505	Seal of Cause granted to barbers and surgeons of Edinburgh
1521	Licence by examination of the surgeon-in-chief, Portugal
1540	United Company of Barber Surgeons, London
1603	Academia dei Lincei, Rome
1694	Revival of Collège St Côme, Paris
1731	Académie de chirurgie, Paris
1736	School of Surgery, precursor of Royal Academy of Surgery, Copenhagen
1760	Royal College of Surgery, Barcelona
1787	Royal College of Surgery of San Carlos, Madrid
1800	Royal College of Surgery, London
1929	Royal College of Physicians and Surgeons of Canada

and for his invention of a 'flying ambulance' to carry the injured from the battlefield. In September 1812, at the two-day battle of Borodino near Moscow, Larrey is said to have performed two hundred amputations – one every sixteen minutes. His 75 per cent success rate was said to owe much to the anesthetic and hemostatic effects of the Russian cold.

In the early nineteenth century, a new interest in physiology was kindled, and scholars were receptive to its study by surgical methods. Experimental surgery explored the inner workings of animals, but it could also lead to new operations for sick humans (see chapter 3). Surgery became a tool of scientific inquiry.

Advent of Anesthesia

To relieve pain during surgical procedures, alcohol, opium, and bleeding had been used for centuries. Prior to replacing dislocations, Philip Syng Physick of Philadelphia recommended heavy bleeding in the vertical position until the patient fainted; but this approach was dangerous. The best relief for a person undergoing surgery was rapid loss of consciousness, caused either by the analgesia or by the procedure itself. Surgeons strove for accuracy and speed.

Anesthetic gases had a protracted prehistory, but they eventually

A Vignette: Mastectomy before Chloroform

Next day, my master, the surgeon, examined Ailie. There was no doubt it must kill her, and soon. It could be removed – it might never return ... she should have it done. She curtsied ... and said, 'When?' 'Tomorrow,' said the kind surgeon ...

The operating theatre is crowded; much talk and fun ... In comes Ailie: one look at her quiets and abates the eager students ... Ailie stepped up on a seat, and laid herself on the table ... shut her eyes ... and took my hand. The operation was at once begun; it was necessarily slow; and chloroform – one of God's best gifts to his suffering children – was then unknown. The surgeon did his work. The pale face showed its pain, but was still and silent ...

It is over, she is dressed, steps gently and decently down from the table ... then turning to the surgeon and the students, she curtsies, – and in a low voice begs their pardon if she has behaved ill. The students – all of us – wept like children.

Physician-writer John Brown, *Rab and His Friends and
Other Papers and Essays* (1862; reprint, London: Dent, 1926), 24–8

transformed practice. The earliest advocates were neither surgeons nor physicians; they were chemists and dentists with remarkable personalities. Nitrous oxide ('laughing gas') was known in the late eighteenth century and was used at social gatherings ('frolics') to produce rapid nonsensical inebriation (like glue sniffing in our own time). In 1799 the English chemist Humphrey Davy experimented with a combination of nitrous oxide and oxygen in both animals and humans; he suggested that it might allay surgical pain.

Nitrous oxide was also used by the dentist Horace Wells in late 1844. Wells conducted public demonstrations of 'painless tooth extraction,' but he was mocked with cries of 'Humbug!' when he demonstrated on a person resistant to the effects. His former busi-

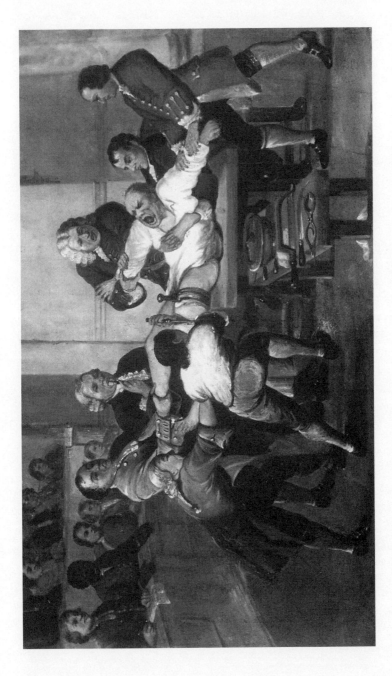

A pre-anesthetic amputation at St Thomas's Hospital, Southwark. Artist unknown. Late eighteenth century. Hunterian Museum. Royal College of Surgeons, London

ness partner, W.T. Morton, used ether with better results. In vexation over Morton's success, Wells became addicted to chloroform. While intoxicated, he threw vitriol at a prostitute and was tossed into a New York City jail, where he committed suicide.

Other Americans also experimented with anesthetic gases. The Georgia surgeon Crawford Long had attended ether parties while a student in Philadelphia, and in the winter of 1842 he experimented with ether for eight minor operations. Negative public opinion put an end to his trials and Long did not publish until a few years later. The chemist Charles T. Jackson of Boston conducted ether experiments on himself and suggested to Morton that he use it as an anesthetic in dentistry. Having disputed priority with S.F.B. Morse over invention of the electric telegraph and the Morse code, Jackson would later become embroiled in another priority dispute over anesthesia, in which he urged Long to stake a claim too.

Following the lead of Wells and Jackson, Morton used inhalation ether as a general anesthetic for tooth extraction on several occasions. Then, on 16 October 1846, at the Massachusetts General Hospital in Boston, he administered ether while the surgeon John Collins Warren removed a tumor from the neck of a young man named Gilbert Abbott. Possibly alluding to the sad experiences of the past, Warren is said to have uttered the understatement, 'Gentlemen, this is no humbug.'

At first, Morton tried to conceal the substance until he had obtained a profitable patent. But he was forced by competition to reveal its composition. By 18 November 1846, Henry J. Bigelow had published his own experience with ether, in the *Boston Medical and Surgical Journal*. The physician and man of letters Oliver Wendell Holmes suggested the word 'anesthesia' for the miraculous new invention. The famous 1882 painting by Robert Hinckley depicts the Abbott operation of 1846 and the Massachusetts General Hospital maintains the 'ether dome' operating theatre as a shrine.

The sixteenth of October 1846 is often but wrongly cited as the date of the first surgical use of anesthesia. Wells, Long, and Morton had used it earlier. But a prestigious endorsement can consolidate acceptance; October 1846 marked the end of anesthesia's long pre-history.

Chloroform was introduced into surgical practice in 1847 by the Scotsman James Young Simpson, who recommended its use in obstetrics (see chapter 11). Controversy swirled around all forms of anesthesia in the late 1840s. The unmistakable danger of gaseous explosions contributed to the debate. But deaths due to anesthesia were slow to be recognized, partly because of the gravity of the pre-operative illness of many patients.

Since antiquity, cutting into the body cavities or the viscera had courted certain death from infection. Once anesthesia became accepted, longer and more complex operations were conceivable, and surgeons began to contemplate opening the sanctuaries of tho-rax and abdomen. But the problem of infection remained. Images from this two-decade period are strange; distinguished surgeons dominate the scene, dressed in elegant frock coats, their hair, mous-taches, and beards blowing in the breeze, their hands bare and only nominally clean.

Antisepsis and Asepsis

Like anesthesia, antisepsis had many precursors and pioneers. In 1847 Ignaz Semmelweis introduced the washing of hands and instru-ments in chlorine water solution to prevent childbed fever, but he did not publish until 1860 (see chapter 11). In 1867 the Scottish surgeon Joseph Lister announced the results of his experiments with carbolic acid in open fractures. By stating the opinion that wound infections were caused by bacteria, Lister based his method on the theory of the French chemist Louis Pasteur (see chapter 4).

News of Lister's principles travelled widely and quickly, but before germ theory was established, opponents pointed to inconsistencies in the various methods used. At first, antiseptics were splashed into wounds or sprayed into the air to kill germs presumed to be lurking there. But surgical wounds were 'clean' from the outset. Preventative asepsis to avoid wound contamination was introduced by Ernst von

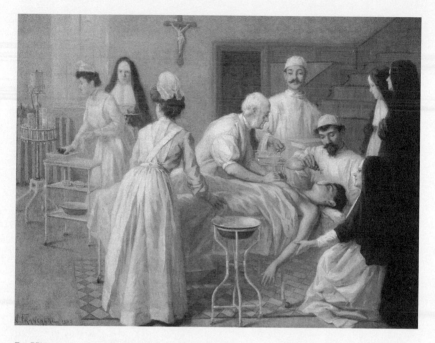

Dr Hingston et la salle d'opération, by F.C. Franchère, 1905. In the religious setting of the oldest hospital in Montreal, the surgeon is attended by nuns as
well as the new professional nurses. He has adopted anesthesia, but his bare
hands reveal his scepticism about antisepsis. Musée des Hospitalières de
l'Hôtel-Dieu, Montreal

Bergmann, in 1877. Rubber gloves were patented the following year.
Lister initially clung to his original views, but by 1896 he too
accepted the advantages of asepsis over antisepsis.

  In Canada, antisepsis was promoted by Thomas G. Roddick of
Montreal and Archibald Edward Malloch of Hamilton. Sceptics
William Canniff and F.J. Shepherd contended that antisepsis
appeared to help wound healing because it drew attention to the
good old rules of cleanliness.

A Montreal Operation with Antiseptic Spray

Dr Roddick assisted [Dr Fenwick] and I looked on. After the operation was over I inquired why they had sprayed the wall instead of the patient – the spray had been going all the time, but it was not turned on the patient – the fact was that it had been forgotten; however the patient did well.

F.J. Shepherd (cited in Howell 1934, 108)

Surgical Optimism and Its Heroes, 1870–1970

After opposition to anesthesia and antisepsis faded away, a period of unbounded optimism ensued – the 'Century of the Surgeon.' New achievements were described in military terms of 'victory' and 'conquest,' and some people imagined that all obstacles to surgical endeavour would eventually be eliminated. No medical heroes have enjoyed greater prestige than the surgeons of the late nineteenth and early twentieth centuries, surgeons who devised daring and previously inconceivable responses to internal pathology. The instruments and procedures that they invented still bear their names, and the list of their contributions flows like a litany of legendary exploits.

The German, Hermann von Helmholtz, invented the ophthalmoscope in 1851. It led to improvements in operative ophthalmology, especially the procedures for iridectomy and strabismus that had been devised by his countryman, A. von Graefe. Theodor Billroth of Vienna embraced aseptic principles and championed gastric and biliary surgery in the 1870s and 1880s; his operating theatre was crowded with students and admirers. The American, Charles MacBurney, also specialized in intestinal surgery, and his 1889 description of acute appendicitis led to eponymic use of his name.

Frederick Treves of London put surgery for appendicitis on the map with an operation on Edward VII only days before his coronation in 1902. The cocaine-and-morphine-using William Halsted, at the urging of W.H. Welch, joined with Osler and Kelly as a founder of Johns Hopkins medical school. Halsted's radical mastectomy, devised in 1890, was intended to remove not only the cancerous breast but also all potential sites of local recurrence.

This new ability to alter internal structures further promoted the anatomical definition of disease (see chapter 4). For example, surgery for appendicitis relied on disease concepts that were less than one hundred years old: peritonitis had been described by Laennec in 1802, while its cause in a ruptured appendix had been suggested in 1812 by John Parkinson. Prior to anesthesia and antisepsis, only a handful of surgeons, such as Willard Parker of New York City, had dared to operate on the belly; their interventions, like the thoracentesis of Hippocrates, were confined to draining abscesses through the abdominal wall.

The new potential for surgical solutions fostered a parallel search for corresponding anatomical problems. For example, the intriguing disease visceroptosis (drooping gut syndrome) was thought to provoke numerous symptoms, including back pain. Various operations to resuspend the sagging organs could relieve the symptoms. As shown by Magdalena Biernacka (MD, Queen's 1998), medical publishing on visceroptosis began in the 1880s and declined temporarily during each of the two world wars while surgeons were otherwise occupied. Its descendant, nephropexy, still figures in the schedules of recognized procedures. Was the disease constructed to satisfy the new possibility of treating it? How did its decline relate to military needs?

Increasingly delicate operations were devised for problems in the most complex of organs, including the brain and the heart. Surgeons were venerated like saints, especially in the United States – for example, J.B. Murphy of Chicago; the brothers C.H. and W.J. Mayo of Rochester, Minnesota, which boasted one of the first departments of anesthesia; George Crile, who pioneered direct blood transfusion; neurosurgeon Harvey Cushing; and cardiac surgeon Alfred Blalock, who worked with Helen Taussig to correct the tetralogy of Fallot and other congenital heart problems. In 1909 Theodor Kocher of Switzerland became the first surgeon to win the Nobel Prize, which was awarded to him for his work on the surgery and physiology of the thyroid gland. Soon after, the French surgeon Alexis Carrel, who spent many years in the United States, won a Nobel Prize (1912) for his technique of vascular anastomosis, a cornerstone of transplant surgery.

Wars continued to have an impact on surgery during this period. The American Civil War is said to have been the first to leave large quantities of documentation pertaining to the epidemiology and care of surgical patients. Reacting to the horrors he had witnessed at the battle of Solferino in 1859, the Swiss businessman and philanthropist, Jean Dunant, founded what became the International Red Cross in 1863–4. It established the Geneva Convention (1864) to guarantee neutrality to wounded soldiers and their attendants. Dunant shared the 1901 Nobel Prize for Peace. The International Red Cross received the same award for war relief in 1917 and again in 1944, although most scholars agree that the agency could have done more for holocaust victims. Created to provide neutral care for the war-wounded, the Red Cross quickly embraced a military structure, which may have hampered its success, as historian John Hutchinson has recently shown.

The brutal injuries of the First World War led to developments in the management of burns and in plastic surgery by Harold Gillies of New Zealand. In the Second World War, experiments with thin skin grafts and remodelling techniques took place at several centres, including East Grinstead in England, where the team of another New Zealander, Archibald McIndoe, included his airmen patients, who called themselves the Guinea Pig Club. Battlefield blood transfusion, piloted in 1917, became commonplace in the Second World War, with the added convenience of component therapy. Safe transfusion was the final breakthrough for cardiovascular surgery of peacetime (see chapter 8).

In 1954, the first successful kidney transplant was performed by Joseph E. Murray on Ron Herrick, the donor being Ron's twin, Richard (reported in *JAMA* 1955). In 1990 Murray shared the Nobel Prize for his transplantation work. In 1967 the South African surgeon

Christiaan Barnard successfully transplanted a human heart. The first recipient lived three weeks, but the media celebrated the achievement with heady excitement. Transplantations of kidney, liver, marrow, lung, and heart have now become standard treatment, while experiments continue with other organs, including pancreas transplant for diabetes. HLA typing has made it possible to match brain-dead donors with recipients on different continents and to establish 'banks' of organs and living donors. Some cities have become transplantation centres, with architectural and human infrastructures revolving around brilliant individuals such as Thomas E. Starzl of Pittsburgh, specialist in liver transplant, and Nobel laureate E. Donnall Thomas of Seattle, founder of a marrow transplant program.

Canada also has its surgical greats. William Canniff, physician, historian, and founding member of the Canadian Medical Association, authored the first Canadian textbook of surgery (1866). The country doctor Abraham Groves of Fergus, Ontario, claimed to have removed the first Canadian appendix in 1883, using a kitchen table as an operating surface. During the Spanish Civil War, Norman Bethune helped to establish one of the earliest mobile plasma transfusions units. The American-born neurosurgeon Wilder Penfield, founder of the prestigious Montreal Neurological Institute, is known for his work in cerebral localization. Innovation in the postwar rehabilitation of soldiers with spinal cord injuries was the result of an interdisciplinary collaboration between neurosurgeon E.H. (Harry) Botterell and physiatrist Albin Jousse in Toronto. Congenital abnormalities of the heart were first collected and defined by the Montrealer Maude Abbott; and both heparin and operative hypothermia were developed in this country and applied to open-heart surgery by D.W. Gordon Murray and Wilfred G. Bigelow, both of Toronto. Later Canadian innovators include William T. Mustard, who devised procedures for congenital heart disease; Wilbert J. Keon, an expert on heart transplantation; and Robert B. Salter, who promoted research during orthopedic training and devised the innominate osteotomy for congenital hip displacement and continuous passive motion for joint healing. The University of Western Ontario in London established a multi-organ transplant service under the direction of internist Calvin R. Stiller, who served as its chief from 1984 to 1996.

Fading Optimism

The uncontested value of coronary-artery-bypass grafts has resulted in grand schemes for ready-and-waiting operating rooms staffed by teams prepared to intervene at a moment's notice. These procedures and transplants are enormously expensive and greatly in demand. But who will pay? With rising health-care costs and a financial recession, the buoyant optimism of mid-century surgery seems to have waned. Even as new surgical techniques become cheaper and, arguably, better than before, operative responses to human ills are being questioned, especially in countries with national health-care programs.

In societies with private health care, such as the United States, rich people can usually afford insurance even if they cannot afford the operation; but the two-tiered system means inadequate or no care for the poor. In Canada, taxation must cover the high costs, yet elaborate procedures are available only in major centres. To control costs, elective surgery in Canada is rationed, not by the patient's ability to pay, but by delay – a situation that generates frustration and fear. Furthermore, surgery itself is criticized on several fronts, including the economics of prevention and epidemiology (see chapter 6).

Sick people and their doctors worry that arguments of cost effectiveness and population health are a bureaucratic pretext for *not* spending money, invoked by a national government with a relatively poor (and declining) record in funding science. Not only does innovation in surgery and bioscience potentially save lives, they argue, it is a manifestation of a 'healthy' society that places high value on thought and creativity. The most imaginative leaps of intellectual energy include surgical solutions for previously invincible problems of sick individuals. Why suppress achievement when it can also relieve suffering?

Epidemiology has also taken the wind out of surgical sails in several different ways, some more effective than others. In the 1970s, epidemiologists worried that surgery would create as many problems as it solved by weakening the gene pool. For example, pyloric stenosis affects a small proportion of neonates; if uncorrected, it leads to death in infancy. People soon realized that the descendants of those with corrected pyloric stenosis would bear an increased risk of the disease, and the operation would be in increasing demand. The implied solution – not to operate on otherwise healthy babies – was totally unacceptable. Our health-care system has yet to collapse under the resultant strain. By the early 1990s, pyloric stenosis actually appeared to have decreased in incidence; epidemiological studies are now devoted to explaining why.

Cost-benefit analyses challenge the effectiveness of tonsillectomy, which in the 1950s was practised on approximately one-third of all children in the United States and Canada. Although the rates have been declining, studies suggest that the procedure may still be over-utilized. A study group in Manitoba asked if higher rates of tonsillectomy can be equated with lower standards of health care. Wide geographic discrepancies in the utilization of other procedures, such as coronary bypass and hysterectomy, have also led epidemiologists to explore how economic factors relate to indications for surgery.

Mastectomy provides another epidemiological example that gave pause to surgical practice. Known since antiquity, breast cancer causes the death of at least 10 per cent of North American women. Operative treatments are almost as old as surgery itself, since the breast – like other appendages – can be amputated without opening body cavities. In the seventeenth and eighteenth centuries, various recommendations were made on how best to achieve the desired result quickly and safely. Several riveting accounts, like the vignette cited earlier, describe the pain of mastectomy without anesthesia.

A certain apathy governed operation for breast cancer, not only because of the undeniable pain, but also because local resection would never cure what might be systemic disease. When surgery got its big boost in the mid-nineteenth century, the notion of breast cancer as a local or surgical disease was reconsidered. Surgeons worried that they might induce metastases by cutting into or close to the tumor. Perhaps, they reasoned, if more tissue and regional nodes also were removed, the patient would stand a better chance. This thinking culminated in Halsted's radical mastectomy, in which the underlying chest muscle was removed. The patient's arm could swell with lymphoedema for her remaining years – a minor annoyance if

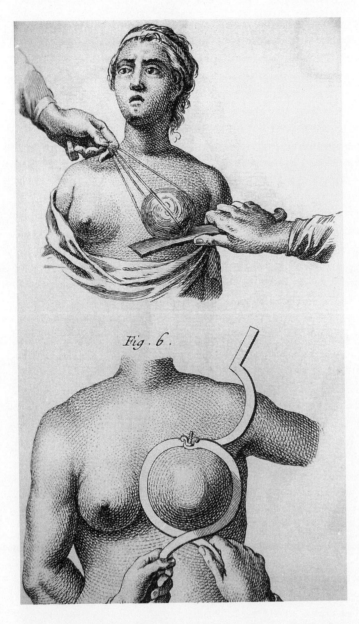

Mastectomy. Denis Diderot and Jean le Rond d'Alembert, *Encyclopédie*, planches, vol. 3, plate 29, 1772

her life should be preserved. Halsted's procedure was the principal surgical response to breast cancer for more than seventy years.

In the 1970s epidemiological surveys suggested that radical mastectomy may prevent local recurrence, but it could not be correlated with increased survival. The result was a gradual shift from radical mastectomies to simple mastectomy. Soon people were asking if removal of the entire breast was necessary to prolong life, especially if the disease was systemic at diagnosis. The concept of 'adjuvant' chemotherapy was introduced, or chemotherapy used together with supposedly curative surgery in the absence of disease. Surgeons were obliged to become statisticians and medical oncologists as well as technical wizards. They also looked to psychiatry to compare the psychological impact of mastectomy with the less invasive and less costly lumpectomy, which had a better cosmetic effect. Unfortunate experiences with artificial breast implants in the 1980s and 1990s again suggested that less surgery may really be more. But did the cheaper, smaller procedures have no cost in survival?

A more rapid change in surgical practice took place in the early 1990s with the advent of laparoscopic cholecystectomy. Within a short five years, the minimally invasive technique completely replaced the open cholecystectomy. Surgeons trained each other in the new skill, motivated perhaps by patients' appreciation of a rapid recovery and by the economic benefit of short hospital stays.

The relative speed with which laparoscopic cholecystecomy replaced its predecessor contrasts markedly with the slowness of lumpectomy to replace mastectomy. Why? Is the difference due to the added attraction of new skills and instruments (present in laparoscopy and absent in lumpectomy)? Or is it because of the fear of malignant recurrence (present in breast cancer and absent in gall bladder problems)? Answers to these interesting historical questions may tell us about the conceptual and social interplay in contemporary surgery.

Life-saving emergency operations are still of prime importance. The tradition of manual dexterity and technical innovation, which now includes microsurgery and laser, has not vanished. With its closer ties to medicine and consideration of economical, ethical, and epidemiological implications, surgery is perhaps more careful, more considered, more precise, and more elegant than it has ever been – even as the huge interventions of mid-century are replaced by smaller procedures.

Suggestions for Further Reading

Cooter, Roger. 'Medicine and the Goodness of War.' *Canadian Bulletin of Medical History* 7 (1990), 147–60

– *Surgery and Society in Peace and War: Orthopaedics and the Organization of Modern Medicine, 1880–1948.* Houndmills and Basingstoke: Macmillan and University of Manchester, 1993

Estes, J. Worth. *The Medical Skills of Ancient Egypt.* Canton, Mass.: Science History Publications U.S.A., 1989

Gelfand, Toby. *Professionalizing Modern Medicine: Paris Surgeons and Medical Science and Institutions in the Eighteenth Century.* Westport, Conn.: Greenwood, 1980

Haeger, Knut. *The Illustrated History of Surgery.* New York: Bell, 1988

Haiken, Elizabeth. *Venus Envy: A History of Cosmetic Surgery.* Baltimore: Johns Hopkins University Press, 1997

Hutchinson, John F. *Champions of Charity: War and the Rise of the Red Cross.* Boulder, Colo.: Westview Press, 1996

McVaugh, M.R. *Medicine before the Plague: Practitioners and Their Patients in the Crown of Aragon, 1285–1345.* New York: Cambridge University Press, 1993

Majno, Guido. *The Healing Hand: Man and Wound in the Ancient World.* Cambridge, Mass.: Harvard University Press, 1975

Milne, John Stewart. *Surgical Instruments in Greek and Roman Times.* Oxford: Clarendon Press, 1907

Pernick, Martin S. *A Calculus of Suffering: Pain, Professionalism, and Anesthesia in Nineteenth-Century America.* New York: Columbia University Press, 1985

Rutkow, Ira M. *Surgery: An Illustrated History.* St Louis: Mosby-Year Book, 1993

Siraisi, Nancy G. *Medieval and Early Renaissance Medicine: An Introduction to Knowledge and Practice.* Chicago: University of Chicago Press, 1990

Wangensteen, Owen Harding, and Sarah D. Wangensteen. *The Rise of Surgery: From Empiric Craft to Scientific Discipline.* Minneapolis: University of Minnesota Press, 1978

On Surgery and Surgeons in Canada

Allan, Ted. *The Scalpel, the Sword: The Story of Dr. Norman Bethune.* Boston: Little, Brown, 1952

Bigelow, Wilfred G. *Cold Hearts: The Story of Hypothermia and the Pacemaker in Heart Surgery.* Toronto: McClelland and Stewart, 1984

Canadian Dental Association. 'A History of Canadian Dentistry.' *Canadian Dental Association Journal* 18, no. 6 (1952)

Cohen, Jack. 'Sir William Hingston.' *Canadian Journal of Surgery* 39 (1996), 422–7

Connor, J.T.H. 'Listerism Unmasked: Antisepsis and Asepsis in Victorian Anglo-Canada.' *Journal of the History of Medicine and Allied Sciences* 49 (1994), 207–39

Dunlop, Marilyn. *Bill Mustard, Surgical Pioneer.* Canadian Medical Lives Series, no. 2. Toronto: Hannah Institute for the History of Medicine, 1989

Gullett, D.W. *A History of Dentistry in Canada.* Toronto: University of Toronto Press and the Canadian Dental Association, 1971

Howell, William Boyman. *F.J. Shepherd – Surgeon: His Life and Times.* Toronto: Dent, 1934.

Lewis, Jefferson. *Something Hidden: A Biography of Wilder Penfield.* Toronto and Garden City, N.Y.: Doubleday, 1981

Lindsay, James. 'Dr. Harold Griffith and the Introduction of Curare.' *Canadian Medical Association Journal* 144 (1991), 588–9

Macbeth, Robert A. 'Canadian Surgery during the French Regime, 1608–1763.' *Canadian Journal of Surgery* 20 (1977), 71–82

MacDermot, H.E. *Sir Thomas Roddick: His Work in Medicine and Public Life.* Toronto: Macmillan, 1938

McPhail, Neil V. 'The History of Vascular Surgery in Canada.' *Canadian Journal of Surgery* 38 (1995), 229–37

Roland, Charles G. 'Bibliography of the History of Anesthesia in Canada: Preliminary Checklist.' *Canadian Anaesthetist's Society Journal* 15 (1968), 202–14

Shephard, David A.E. and Andrée Lévesque, eds. *Norman Bethune: His Times and His Legacy.* Ottawa: Canadian Public Health Association, 1982

Spaulding, William B. 'Abraham Groves 1847–1935: A Pioneer Surgeon, Sufficient unto Himself.' *Canadian Bulletin of Medical History* 8 (1991), 249–62

CHAPTER ELEVEN

Women's Medicine and Medicine's Women: History of Obstetrics and Gynecology*

If men had to have babies, they would only ever have one each.

Diana, Princess of Wales

History may seem to be about the past, but it is really about the present. Chronological lists of persons and events do not constitute good history. Accuracy about dates and events is essential, of course, but history also contains interpretations that reflect our satisfaction or discomfort with our own world. The questions we ask of the past emerge from our present experience. If the history is done well, then the interpretations are explicit and carefully substantiated. As a result, the same historical event can have different meanings, depending on who does the research, what is being studied, and why (see chapter 15).

The historian-philosopher Ray Arney contrasted various histories of obstetrics to illustrate differing interpretations. One scenario reconstructs the past as a series of incremental steps that build progressively upon each other to culminate in our glorious present. Typifying this interpretation is the 1960 graph by Theodore Cianfranci, which shows the history of obstetrics as an exponentially increasing number of wonderful accomplishments. The units of Cianfranci's Y-axis are not identified, but they seem to estimate 'progress

*Educational objectives for this chapter are found on pp. 397–8.

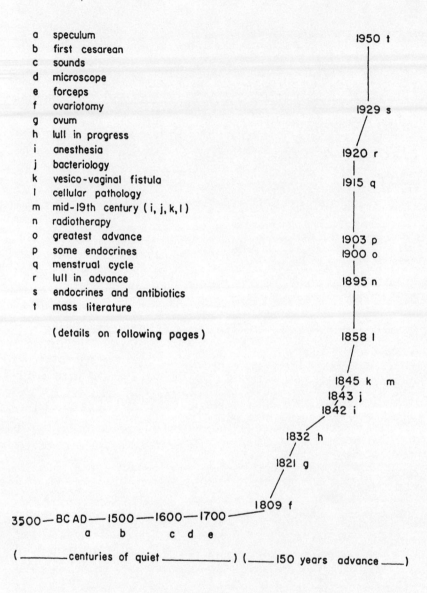

a   speculum
b   first cesarean
c   sounds
d   microscope
e   forceps
f   ovariotomy
g   ovum
h   lull in progress
i   anesthesia
j   bacteriology
k   vesico-vaginal fistula
l   cellular pathology
m   mid-19th century (i, j, k, l)
n   radiotherapy
o   greatest advance
p   some endocrines
q   menstrual cycle
r   lull in advance
s   endocrines and antibiotics
t   mass literature

(details on following pages)

1950 t

1929 s

1920 r

1915 q

1903 p
1900 o

1895 n

1858 l

1845 k   m
1843 j
1842 i

1832 h

1821 g

1809 f

3500 — BC AD — 1500 — 1600 — 1700 —
        a   b   c   d   e

(———————centuries of quiet——————) (——150 years advance——)

Graph displaying the progress of obstetrics and gynecology as viewed by a practitioner. Theodore Cianfranci, *A Short History of Obstetrics and Gynecology*, 1960, viii

points.' An interpretation such as Cianfranci's is called 'presentist,' or 'whiggish' (see chapter 15). Whiggish interpretations not only describe the past; they also valorize it in terms of the present.

Other historians reject Cianfranci's interpretation because they deplore rather than celebrate present-day obstetrics. To typify this critical view, Arney selected the words of the feminist philosopher Mary Daly, who wrote that the 'doctored diseases are increasing' and called obstetrics a 'patriarchal program' of 'gynocide.' Using social constructionism (see chapters 4 and 7), some scholars agree with Daly that femininity has been 'pathologized' (made sick), because doctors control the rhetoric and most doctors have been men.

Medical students can quickly think of arguments to refute Daly's claims: obstetrics cannot be gynocide since maternal and fetal mortality rates dropped dramatically in the last century. In response, Daly might argue that the improved survival is due, not to doctoring, but to better public hygiene and nutrition – the McKeown hypothesis (see chapters 5 and 7). Medical students might counter by saying that doctors did not oppose better survival even if they did not provide it.

But not so fast! Cianfranci's graph should be criticized too. He awarded points for the speculum, forceps, anesthesia, and antisepsis. Yet some techniques that were initially thought safe were subsequently discovered to be harmful; both forceps and anesthetic can harm the baby or the mother. And twice Cianfranci marked a lull in progress, where the slope of his curve is at its steepest. Caught up in endorsing the present, he failed to adjust the graph accordingly, thereby revealing an unwillingness to perceive potential revisions to his hypothesis.

Historians criticize as naive and 'internalist' the whiggish history written by those – often health-care practitioners – who seek to trace the ideas that are familiar in their daily work. Assuming that current practice needs no justification, 'internalists' ignore its social, political, economic, cultural, and technological influences (albeit unintentionally). But those historians who write from an 'externalist' perspective are in turn criticized for doing medical history 'without the medicine' and for being driven by a desire to incriminate present-day practices and practitioners. Inevitably, both histories are presentist. Even if accident or serendipity plays a role, findings in history – just like those in science – are made only when we are conscious of seeking them.

In this chapter the history of obstetrics will be examined from two perspectives: the traditional and the critical. We begin with an examination of women and their bodies as cultural phenomena.

Birthing as Women's Domain

The capacity of the female body to bear children set it apart in prehistoric societies, where statues and paintings exaggerated its secondary sexual characteristics. Because blood loss could be dangerous, menstruation was mystical, and its cyclic predictability signified and defined woman. Some societies viewed menstruation as a curse – and remnants of that assessment survive in our language. In Orthodox Jewish culture, a postmenstrual woman is 'unclean,' until she has taken a *mikvah*, a ritual bath. When women were venerated as deities, their godly tasks were usually feminine: agriculture, procreation, birth, rebirth, and healing. In ancient Egypt, Hathor – a cow – was the earth mother nourishing the world; Isis was goddess of the fertile Nile and of medicine; and Tauret – a hippopotamus – watched over childbirth. The Babylonian goddess Ishtar and the Greek Aphrodite were female patrons of love, and the Roman goddess Juno protected pregnant, birthing, and nursing mothers. Statues depicting the virginal Artemis (Diana) of Ephesus show her chest covered with breastlike eggs or the egglike breasts. Her cult was absorbed into the Christian tradition with the elevation of Mary as the Virgin mother of God.

For most of history, birthing was the exclusive domain of women. When males engaged in caring for women, special provisions were made for gender interfaces. For example, in fourteenth-century China, diagnostic dolls were created to interpose a modest distance between doctor and patient. From then on, and well into the twentieth century, an elite Chinese woman would point to the location of her symptoms on the doll, sparing the physician from seeing or touching her body. (In 1986 a fine collection of Chinese diagnostic dolls was donated to the Osler Library by J.F. Meakins.) Male professionals did not attend births in the West until the seventeenth and eighteenth centuries.

The Obstetrician's View: Medicine for Women

The predominance of women birth attendants did not prevent doctors from theorizing about conception and birth. Women and premature births were the focus of several Hippocratic treatises (*Diseases of Women I, II,* and *III*; *Nature of Woman*; *Girls*; *Nature of the Child*; *Seven Months' Child*; *Eight Months' Child*). In these works can be found the notion of the wandering womb – an etiological hypothesis invoked to explain many symptoms in women; treatments were aimed at luring the uterus back into its proper place. Other ancient authors, including Soranus of Ephesus in the second century, described how babies could reside in and emerge from the womb in a variety of positions. This knowledge predated writing and was handed down from midwife to midwife.

The medicalization of birth was characterized by instrumentation to prevent, terminate, hasten, or relieve deliveries. The ability to make a rapid end to unnaturally lengthy labour – to 'deliver' the woman from her 'travail' – distinguished those who would *intervene* (often doctors) from those who merely attended (often, but not always, midwives). In Cianfranci's graph, the vaginal speculum of the first century A.D. was the only ancient 'contribution': a three-bladed speculum, which opened with a heavy screw, was found during the excavation of Pompeii, having been buried by the volcanic eruption of 79 A.D. In Greco-Roman times, probes, sounds, hooks, and perforators, as well as knives, were used together with surgical instruments. Soranus explained how hooks could be used to extract a dead child. Obstetrical forceps, which were invented in the seventeenth century, may also have been used in antiquity; they are depicted in a marble bas-relief of a birth scene found near Rome – a carving that some scholars describe as a hoax.

Cesarean Birth

Cesarean birth also originated in antiquity, but it was reserved for cases in which the mother was dying or already dead. This terminal or post-mortem surgery was ordered by a Roman law (called the *lex regia* or *lex caesaria*) in order to save the baby for the state. A second-century B.C. Hebrew text (Mishnah, Niddah, 5:1) suggests that Cesarean section may have been performed in Judaic antiquity. Islamic writings and fourteenth-century illustrations show that abdominal deliveries of dying women were known in the Middle East. The fatal operation was conducted without anesthesia, without antisepsis, and without much understanding of tissue planes and suturing. In Europe, in the thirteenth century, the Christian church exhorted doctors to perform the operation after maternal death in order to save the infant's soul by baptism. This practice continued into the nineteenth century in some parts of Europe (Brittany). Early modern treatises on birthing described Cesarean section, but it was rarely used.

Vaginal Birth Too Banal for Heroes?

Asklepios, the Greek god of medicine, was taken from his slain mother's abdomen by his semi-contrite father, Apollo. Similarly, Buddha emerged from the flank of his mother, Maya. Despite the oft-repeated legend, Julius Caesar is unlikely to have been born by Cesarean section, because his mother was alive many years later. In the last scene of *Macbeth*, Shakespeare's hero Macduff reveals that he 'was from his mother's womb untimely ripp'd.'

In 1581 François Rousset published fifteen cases to advocate abdominal delivery while the mother was still alive. He admitted that he had never personally performed the operation, which he labelled *enfantement césarien*, citing a passage from Pliny (*Natural History* VII, 9). Legend holds that the first woman to survive an abdominal delivery was the wife of a sixteenth-century Swiss sow gelder named Nufer, who delivered the child and sewed up his wife. The first documented survival of abdominal delivery in Europe occurred in 1610, but the mother lived only a few weeks. Death so frequently followed the procedure that doctors usually opted to save a mother in obstructed labour by disposing of her child. Only in the late nineteenth century were methods devised to achieve a safer maternal outcome.

A Masterful Understatement on Cesarean Birth

This formidable operation, intended to save mother and child, has been performed during many centuries, with various success. In Britain it has never fully had the desired effect, all the mothers having died.

John Aitken, *Principles of Midwifery*,
2nd edn (Edinburgh, 1785), 84

Early Modern Midwifery

The advent of printing in the late fifteenth century led to a flurry of 'obstetrical' literature. *Rosengarten* (1513), the earliest European obstetrical publication, was written in the vernacular by the German physician Eucharius Rösslin. Purporting to be a handbook for midwives, it explained and illustrated the methods and technology of delivery, including the birthing chair or stool, which took advantage of gravity for the benefit of the mother, although it obscured the view of the attendant. *Rosengarten* was immensely popular and appeared in more than a hundred different editions and translations.

Seemingly written for midwives by either midwives or doctors, midwifery treatises are a curious genre and pose an interesting historical question: Who comprised the intended audience? Male doctors still did not attend deliveries, and the women who did were rarely literate. Recently, historians have suggested that these books may have served voyeuristic purposes of the moneyed and educated elite.

One of the greatest surgeons of the sixteenth century was Ambroise Paré (see chapter 10). His treatise on women's diseases was also written in the vernacular. Without taking credit for his recommendations, he 'innovated' by adopting the traditional ideas of his patients – pessaries for prolapsed uterus, for example, and the

Paré on Podalic Version: Good Guy or Bad?

But that shee may not bee wearied, or lest that her bodie should yeeld or sink down as the Chirurgian draweth the bodie of the infant from her ... let him caus her feet to bee set against the side of the bed, and then let som of the standers by hold her fast by the legs and shoulders. Then that the air may not enter into the womb, and that the work may bee don with the more decencie, her privie parts and thighs must be covered with a warm double linnen cloth.

Then must the Chirurgian, haveing his nails closely pared and his rings (if hee wear anie) drawn off his fingers, and his arms naked, bare, and well annointed with oil, gently draw the flaps of the neck of the womb asunder, and then let him put his hand gently into the mouth of the womb, haveing first made it gentle and slipperie with much oil; and when his hand is in, let him finde out the form and situation of the childe, whether it bee one or two, or whether it bee a Mole or not.

And when hee findeth that hee cometh naturally, with his head toward the mouth of orifice of the womb, hee must lift him up gently, and so turn him that his feet may come forwards, and when hee hath brought his feet forwards, hee must draw one of them gently out at the neck of the womb, and then hee must binde it with som broad and soft or silken band a little above the heel with an indifferent slick knot, and when hee hath so bound it, hee must put it up again into the womb, then he must put his hand in again, and finde out the other foot, and draw it also out of the womb, and when it is out of the womb, let him draw out the other again whereunto hee had before tied the one end of the band, and when hee hath them both out, let him join them both close together, and so by little and little let him draw all the whole bodie from the womb. Also other women or Midwives may help the endeavor of the Chirurgian, by pressing the patient's bellie with their hands downwards as the infant goeth out.

Ambroise Paré, translated by T. Johnson,
1649 (cited in Thoms 1935, 102–4)

birthing chair. He also invented and modified instruments, and he reintroduced the technique of 'podalic version' that had been known to Soranus.

Podalic version is used to deliver a fetus in transverse lie or some other unfavourable position. The attendant introduces a hand into the womb to bring down a foot; a cloth band is loosely tied around the foot, which is then replaced in the womb leaving a length of cloth protruding; the second foot is found, brought down, and bound to the first, which has been relocated with the cloth band. While attendants massage the mother's belly, the child is turned and delivered by gentle traction on the legs. In more than a decade of teaching, I have found that reading Paré's original description of this method to different audiences of students provokes markedly different reactions. Students in women's studies criticize the writing for its cold, clinical objectivity; medical students focus on the frequent references to gentleness and concern for the patient's comfort.

Antoni van Leeuwenhoek's microscope and his announcement that sperm contained 'animalcules' seemed to conform to the ancient Aristotelian views of generation. One observer (Nicolas Hartsoeker, in 1694) drew a tiny, balled-up, bulletlike fetus in the head of a sperm, but he admitted that he had not actually seen it. Women may have carried their children for nine months and endured the effort of pushing them out, but most medical writers assumed that the seed was entirely male. If children sometimes resembled their mothers, it was the effect of gestational environment; babies were the products of their fathers. The discovery of sperm cells simply endorsed the ancient patriarchal (literally!) opinion.

Seeing Is Believing, but Imagination Comes First

Human sperm cells were seen with the earliest microscopes in the seventeenth century. The human egg is several thousand times larger, but – despite earlier postulates – it was not visualized until 1827, by K.E. von Baer. A priority dispute ensued. Once again, we learn that relative size is of little consequence. For something to be found, it must first be imagined and sought.

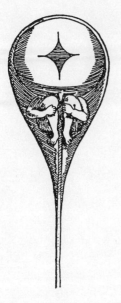

A homunculus hypothesized in a sperm cell. From
Nicolas Hartsoeker, *Essay de dioptrique*, 1694

By the seventeenth century, the man-midwife was appearing in affluent homes. To avoid offending the gentility of his clients, he would make use of new customs, such as the modesty blanket. Why did women allow male practitioners to become involved with birthing at this time? Were the men invited? Or were they extending their market share? Did they and their patients think that their instruments and book learning offered something better than the midwives? Was it coincidental to the recent microscopic proof of males as progenitors? Was it because, as historian Adrian Wilson has suggested, the previously homogeneous female solidarity had been riven along class lines defined by wealth and rising literacy? Did royal patronage or the need for male witnesses to the birth of heirs play a role? Or was this new presence in birthing simply part of the increasing acceptance of doctors in all aspects of health – an early step in the medicalization of our entire culture?

Long after male physicians had entered the birthing chamber, female midwives continued to flourish. Their education, like that of surgeons (see chapter 10) was an apprenticeship entirely separate from the education of physicians. Some midwives were prominent and controversial members of their communities, for example, Anne Hutchinson in colonial America and Mme Victoire Boivin of Paris. A mother of fourteen, Hutchinson is said to have given birth to a hydatidiform mole; consequently, she was accused of witchcraft, excommunicated, and banished, only to be killed during a raid by the native people. Boivin is credited with having recognized the chorionic origin of hydatidiform mole.

Forceps

The story attached to the origin of the forceps is linked to several generations of a seventeenth-century English family, the Chamberlens (also known as Chamberlain), the most famous of whom were Peter and one of his three 'midwife' sons, Hugh. Originally from France, the Chamberlens discovered (or perhaps rediscovered) obstetrical forceps sometime around 1645; yet they kept the instrument as a family secret. When a mother was in obstructed labour, the attendants would send for a Chamberlen, who would arrive with a mysterious parcel. No one was allowed to watch as the baby was delivered, sometimes stillborn, and the mother relieved of her agony. The Chamberlens claimed that they did not publicize their invention because they wanted to avoid tempting unskilled hands; however, their many offers to sell the secret imply that their motive was not patient welfare but greed. The secret soon leaked out, and forceps were rediscovered in the early eighteenth century, when numerous designs were invented for a variety of uses.

Anatomy of the Uterus and Fetus

Once anatomical dissection had become respectable (see chapter 2), doctors who specialized in obstetrics began to study the structure of the gravid uterus. William Smellie of Scotland taught and practised in London during the first half of the eighteenth century, dedicating himself to the service of the poor. His illustrated treatise on midwifery, based on personal experience, described improvements to forceps and their use in breech presentation or in altering the presentation of the fetal head. His directions for measuring the pelvis could predict difficult deliveries.

Chamberlen on His Secret

'Having a better way,' translator Chamberlen wrote, 'I cannot pass without manifesting my dislike' for Mauriceau's method of extracting dead or living children with hooks (chapter 17, 270). Chamberlen referred readers to the preface, where he had written the following:

I will now take leave to offer an Apology for not publishing the Secret I mention we have to extract Children without Hooks ... which is that there being my father and two Brothers living, that practice this Art, I cannot esteem as my own to dispose of, nor publish it without injury to them; and think I have not been unserviceable to my Country, although I do but inform them that the forementionned three Persons of our Family, and my Self, can serve them in these Extremities with greater safety than others.'

Chamberlen in François Mauriceau, *The Diseases of Women with Child*, trans. Hugh Chamberlen (London: Darby, 1683)

A few years later, William Hunter became widely known as a skilled teacher of anatomy in London. He and his surgeon brother, John, assembled anatomical specimens that are the nucleus for the splendid Hunterian museum of London and two collections in Scotland – at Glasgow and East Kilbride. Hunter's *Anatomy of the Gravid Uterus* (1774) featured illustrations by the excellent draftsman, Jan van Rymsdyk. This atlas exemplified the goal of bringing anatomy into bedside practice, but it was not devoid of interpretation. The images are cultural as well as medical documents. In the cut-off thighs and sectioned genitalia, historian Ludmilla Jordanova discerned implicit violence. Pregnancy was given its own structures, rhythms, and anatomical pathology. Shortly it would also acquire a physiology.

Soon after the discovery of auscultation, Jean Lejumeau de Kergaradec was inspired to listen to the pregnant belly. He described the

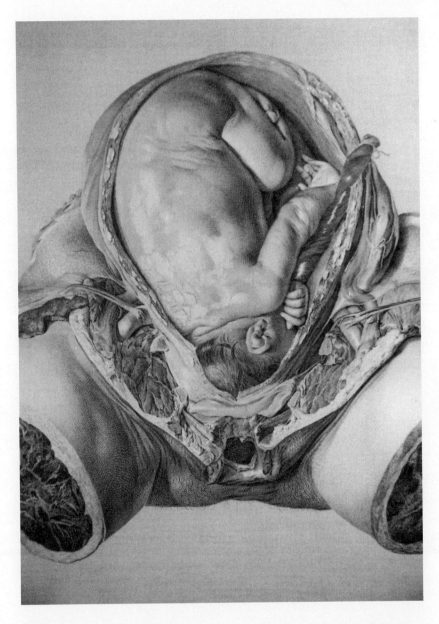

Term infant in utero. The mother died of a placental abruption. Engraving by Jan van Rymsdyk, in William Hunter, *Atlas of the Gravid Uterus*, 1774

fetal heartbeat and the placental 'souffle,' which is the murmur of blood in the vessels of the placenta. Direct assessment of the viability of the uterine contents became possible; with auscultation, the doctor's objective indicator could bypass the mother's perception of movement (see chapter 9).

Control of Hemorrhage

The recognition of pathology in pregnancy and labour prompted a search for systematic methods to correct abnormalities. Then as now, hemorrhage and infection were the major killers of parturient women, while pain was a debilitating obstacle to intervention. Postpartum bleeding could be reduced by ergotamine, a drug derived from *Secale cornutum,* a fungus of rye wheat, which caused contraction of the smooth muscles in arterioles and the uterus. The German H.F. Paulitsky and the American physician John Stearns both advocated ergot (in 1787 and 1807, respectively) for cases of delayed delivery due to ineffectual contractions, retained placenta, antepartum and postpartum hemorrhage, and even anticipated hemorrhage.

Stearns took stock of the side effects of the drug, but he and Paulitsky were disseminators rather than innovators. As a contaminant of rye flour, ergot had been responsible for outbreaks of a disease called St Anthony's fire since at least the ninth century. This poisoning was characterized by severe burning sensation of skin, cramps, and sometimes death from widespread vasospasm. Folk practitioners and midwives seem to have been aware of the antibleeding benefits of wheat rust for many years, possibly through fortuitous observations of labour in affected persons. In 1822 Stearns acknowledged one unnamed predecessor: 'I was informed of the powerful effects produced by this article, in the hands of some ignorant Scotch woman' (cited in Thoms 1935, 24).

Control of Pain

The use of anesthesia in obstetrics was controversial. Early experiments with nitrous oxide were lampooned with the suggestion that

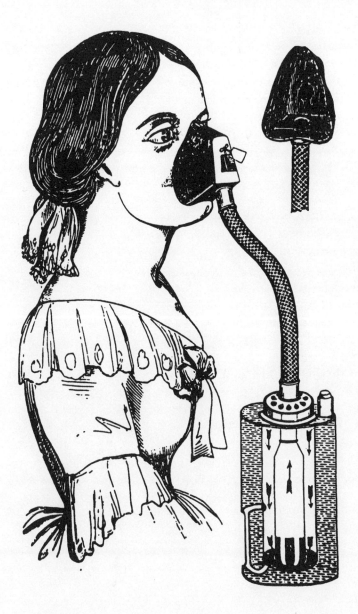

Woman who resembled the reigning monarch inhaling chloroform. From John Snow, *On Chloroform*, 1858, 82

shrews could be turned into hyenas to the relief of their long-suffering husbands. Ether anesthesia was increasingly accepted in surgical practice after 1846 (see chapter 10). The following year, James Young Simpson advocated chloroform inhalation during parturition. But anesthesia for mothers in labour met with staggering resistance, not only out of concern for the infant but for a philosophical reason: doctors, clerics, and other authorities believed that women were meant to suffer in childbirth and that labour pains had intrinsic value. They cited the Bible (Genesis 3:16) to describe women's pain as a manifestation of God's punishment for the 'original sin' of carnal knowledge, which, as it happened, was also the 'original cause' of labour itself. Against them, the proponents of anesthesia argued that only one member of the sinning partnership was suffering. They resorted to scripture too, pointing out that before taking Adam's rib to create Eve, God had put Man to sleep (Genesis 2: 21–2).

The anesthesia debate was resolved for England, at least, when John Snow of Broad Street pump fame (see chapter 7) was invited to administer chloroform to Queen Victoria for two of her many deliveries, in 1853 and 1857. His 1858 treatise contained an image of a refined lady who resembled a youthful and unquestionably sentient version of the British monarch demurely inhaling gas. Soon, educated women pressured their physicians for chloroform.

Only some doctors employed anesthetic, and not every patient could afford it. In the United States, however, the influential Charles D. Meigs of Philadelphia remained opposed. In my research on a nineteenth-century Canadian practice, I found that women who received chloroform during labour were the wives of prominent professionals – the lawyer, the minister, the newspaper editor, and the doctor himself. Did they take an anesthetic because they were more informed than their poorer neighbours and knew to insist upon it? Or did their husbands provide it for them by condoning or paying for it? The record does not say. At any rate, the use of anesthesia doubled the cost of a delivery.

Other historians have shown that women became advocates of the pain relief offered by the new techniques. Various forms of general anesthesia were applied to birthing well into the mid-twentieth century, including the amnesic-analgesic 'twilight sleep' (*Dämmerschlaf*), induced by scopolamine and morphine or other narcotics and first tested on five hundred women in 1906 by C.J. Gauss of Freiburg, Germany. These systemic methods were displaced in two ways. First, regional anesthesia was less risky for the child and less intrusive for the mother. Second, the natural or prepared childbirth methods of Grantly Dick-Read and Fernand Lamaze emphasized education rather than medication for pain management through controlling fear (psychoprophylaxis).

Gradually anesthetists extended their mandate from putting people to sleep to helping them wake up. The field of neonatology was given a boost in the mid-twentieth century with the work of New York anesthetist Virginia Apgar, who devised a quick and reliable method of assessing the status of the newborn baby. Apgar's advisers had diverted her from surgery, in which she had qualified, into anesthesia; thence she went into perinatology and the study of congenital disabilities.

Childbed Fever

By the mid-nineteenth century, hemorrhage, pain, and prolonged labour had been partly controlled by ergot, anesthetics, and forceps. But the deadly problem of childbed (or puerperal) fever remained. Now it is known to be caused by infection of the endometrium by bacteria, especially streptococci. Prior to germ theory, however, childbed fever was an epidemic disease dependent on the environmental miasma, rather than a contagious disease passed from patient to patient. In some practices, childbed fever caused greater morbidity and mortality than hemorrhage. Historians have shown that it was probably less frequent in mothers attended by midwives, who were rarely exposed to dangerous bacteria, than in those attended by doctors, who also attended other patients with infections and used contaminated instruments. The proportion of birthing mothers who died because they were attended by physicians will never be known.

As doctors began to attend more deliveries, the incidence of childbed fever began to climb. Clues lay in statistics revealed by the new method of numerical medicine (see chapters 4 and 7). Several physicians considered puerperal fever contagious. Among them were

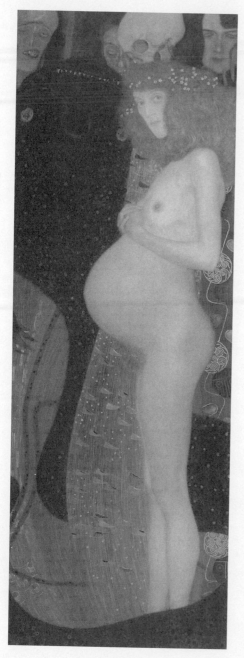

Hope I, by Gustav Klimt, 1903.
National Gallery of Canada

Alexander Gordon and Oliver Wendell Holmes, who in 1795 and 1843, respectively, wrote that the fever was spread from patient to patient by doctors and midwives. Holmes recommended that birth attendants should not perform autopsies on women who had died of the fever. Nevertheless, the dominant theory of miasma persisted.

Maternal mortality statistics suggested similar conclusions to Ignaz Semmelweis, a Hungarian physician working at the Vienna maternity hospital in the nineteenth century. He observed that postpartum fever was less frequent in the wing of the hospital served by midwives than in the wing served by doctors and medical students. The atmospheric conditions – miasmata – were identical in the two wings; the only noticeable difference was that the doctors did autopsies on the women who died of the fever, while the midwives did not. Semmelweis reasoned that a morbid substance was carried on the hands of doctors and students from the cadaver to the tender, traumatized tissues of the next woman in labour. As early as 1847, he introduced a program of hand-washing in a chlorine solution, and he observed an impressive decline in the incidence of the disease.

Despite his success, Semmelweis was criticized, ridiculed, and eventually dismissed. A decade later, he published a repetitive and ranting book, which was not translated into English until 1983. In the interval, his recommendations had spread by word of mouth. The effective recommendations of Holmes and Semmelweis predated germ theory, proving once again that the precise cause of a problem does not always have to be known in order to control it (see chapter 7). Incidentally, Charles Meigs of Philadelphia, who opposed anesthesia, also opposed antiseptic techniques in obstetrics.

Gynecological Surgery: Ovariotomy and Fistula Repair

Gynecological surgery, like all other forms of operative intervention, was promoted by the advent of anesthesia and antisepsis in the mid-nineteenth century. But some operative techniques for women's diseases, such as Cesarean section and the removal of ovaries, already had a long prehistory. The first ovariotomy was successfully performed in 1809 by the Kentucky doctor Ephraim McDowell, who operated on a woman with a hugely swollen belly and severe abdominal pain. Without anesthesia, McDowell removed her ten-kilogram ovary. The woman outlived her doctor by many years. McDowell repeated the procedure for other women, later using alcohol and laudanum for pain relief. Cleanliness was his only precaution for wound dressings, and he later admitted that he had not expected his patients to live.

McDowell's procedure produced relief in desperate patients who were willing to be experimental subjects. By the end of the nineteenth century, however, ovariotomy had become an antidote for many female ailments, including psychiatric disorders. Historians have explored the use of this procedure in lunatic asylums, in Canada and elsewhere. Despite the impression received at this distance, doctors who performed ovariotomies and other gynecological operations claimed that they were acting in the best interests of women, and they called upon their colleagues to sympathize with the tyranny of female biology. Many were venerated by their patients.

Problems of the uterus have always been common, but hysterectomy and amputation of the cervix were scarcely attempted before 1800, and then only through the vagina. An abdominal approach was introduced for malignancy in 1878 by W.A. Freund of Germany. By 1900 the Austrian Ernst Wertheim had treated uterine cancer with radical extirpation combined with oophorectomy and node dissection. The operation, which James Young Simpson once labelled 'utterly unjustifiable,' soon became a standard treatment for cervical cancer, fibroid tumors, and prolapse; however, these conditions were also used as a pretext for surgical birth control. The Pap smear, a cytological screening test devised by George Papanicoulou in 1928, reduced the need for this major intervention, possibly saving many lives, although the benefits of the Pap smear have yet to be assessed in controlled trials.

In the mid-nineteenth century, the American-born surgeon J. Marion Sims became interested in solving the problem of vesicovaginal fistula – a sequela of childbirth – that produced incontinence, chronic infection, misery, and social ostracism. Between 1845 and 1857, Sims experimented with the plastic repair of fistulae, relying on the lateral position for surgery and on three of his inventions: a speculum, silver-wire sutures, and a self-retaining catheter. He also wrote a physiological description of vaginismus and developed a 'uterine guillotine' for amputation of the cervix. His procedures resulted in the cure of morbid conditions that had been overlooked, partly because they were not necessarily life-threatening. At his death, Sims was warmly eulogized, and in 1894 his statue was erected in New York City through donations from admirers on both sides of the Atlantic. But in the 1970s, scholars challenged Sims's ethics: he had perfected his techniques by repeated operations on black slaves. The subsequent 'yes, but' contortions of his professional descendants make interesting reading – and provide yet another fitting subject for the Heroes and Villains game described in chapter 1.

Howard A. Kelly, who was one of the clinical founders of Johns Hopkins medical school, improved on the techniques for vesico-vaginal repair, hysterectomy, and oophorectomy, and he invented the air cystoscope. Kelly also made contributions to gastrointestinal and urological surgery, but he displayed some gender-related ambivalence about the status of gynecological surgery.

Gender Identity and Professional Identity

The vital question which now affects gynecology is this, is she destined to live a spinster all her days? For we see her on one hand courted by her obstetrical ancestor, who seeks to draw her once more into an unholy, unfruitful alliance, destined to rob her of her virility, to be rocked into innocuous desuetude for the rest of her days in the obstetric cradle, sucking the withered ancestral finger in the vain hope of nourishment (with apology for mixed metaphor). On the other hand, we see her wooed by a vigorous, manly suitor, General Surgery, seeking to allure her from her autonomy into his own house, under his own name, obliterating her identity.

Howard Kelly (cited in Garrison 1922, 652)

Attitudes to women were invariably bound up in medical responses to their problems. What is appropriate treatment for women must be consonant with societal expectations. For example, controversy swirled around the advent of sex alteration techniques, widely publicized following the Christine Jorgenson case in 1950. People asked, Should a man become a woman even if he could? More recently, statistics show that the frequency of hysterectomy and other procedures has wide geographic variation even within the same jurisdictions, something Marc Keirse impishly described as the externally 'wandering womb' (*Birth* 20 [1993], 159–61). Different surgeons use different criteria, which depend more on attitude than on biology. As with tonsillectomy, higher rates of surgery may hint at lower standards (see chapter 10).

Just as pregnancy had acquired a physiology, labour and delivery also became subjects of physiological investigation by researchers, such as John Braxton Hicks of Guy's Hospital, London. Gradually, physical and chemical definitions were given to normal labour; problems could be anticipated before they became emergencies. These insights led to the practice, which some deplore, of placing monitors on the bellies of labouring women and on the fetal head. The expressed motive was not to strip women of control over their own physiology but to minimize the faint but real possibility of something going wrong before it could be fixed. As for Pap smears, controlled studies are lacking; some cite economic pressure as a reason for the ubiquity of this practice.

The hormonal chemistry of the menstrual cycle and pregnancy is a twentieth-century concept, but it recalls the lag between the visualization of the sperm and that of the egg. They, too, were subject to the ancient idea that femaleness was the absence of something male. Testicular hormones had been postulated in 1775 by the French physician Théophile Bordeu. Animal experimentation, as early as 1845 by the German physiologist A.A. Berthold, suggested that surgical transplantation of male gonads could replace the effects of castration. But the hormones of the ovary were not postulated until 1923–4 with the work of the American physiologists E.A. Doisy and E. Allen.

The pituitary gonadotrophins and their effects on pregnancy and the menstrual cycle were described simultaneously in the late 1920s by several different investigators, including S.S. Aschheim and B. Zondek, who developed a test for pregnancy in 1928. The Canadian investigator Henry Friesen is well known for his work on prolactin.

Pregnancy tests are now so routine that it is difficult to recall the guesswork, delay, and mystery that surrounded the decoding of subtle signs in the past – absent menses, sore breasts, darkened nipples, a bluish cervix, morning sickness, the inevitably growing womb, and quickening.

Modern techniques have been applied not only to birthing but to conception itself. Controversy over access to diagnostic tests for tubal patency, ovulation, cervical competence, and fetal dates, and over the availability of techniques such as in vitro fertilization and surrogate motherhood, resulted in Canada's Royal Commission on Reproductive Technologies, chaired by the Vancouver geneticist Patricia Baird (report 1993). Understanding the chemical cycles of women has been the *sine qua non* of contemporary birth-control methods, which have played a role in the women's movement, in the sexual revolution of the 1960s and 1970s, and in the patterns of the present epidemic of AIDS and other STDs. Yet recent World Health Organization statistics reveal that birth control is unevenly distributed around the world, and that despite the wonderful new technologies, it is the education of women that can be most highly correlated with their success at limiting births.

Obstetrics and gynecology were the first specialties to make practical use of evidence-based medicine (see chapter 14). In 1979 Archie L. Cochrane awarded the discipline a 'wooden spoon' as the specialty least influenced by randomized controlled trials (RCT). Since the early 1980s, a group led by Iain Chalmers has provided critical appraisal of RCTs to establish confidence in certain practices, to raise doubt about others, and to define evidential lacunae for some surprisingly widespread interventions (see Enkin et al. 1989). As a result, perinatal medicine led the evidence-based medicine movement in what has become the Cochrane Collaboration. Perhaps this discipline accepted the challenge earlier than others for historical reasons: mortality statistics led Semmelweis to his insights; his successors have long held a certain respect for numbers.

The Feminist View: Criticism of Traditional Medical Ideas

So far, this history has tended to conform to the exponentially rising portrayal of Cianfranci. A similar perspective was endorsed by the

Toronto historian Edward Shorter in his lively book, *A History of Women's Bodies*. It tells how women could not contemplate liberation to vote and to seek outside employment until they were given control over their own biology. Shorter may be right about the timing, but feminists criticized his work on the grounds that women and society at large were also instrumental in these changes, and that medical practitioners often opposed women's education and work. Now we will slice this history from a different angle to illustrate the dichotomy in interpretations introduced at the beginning of this chapter.

The main actors in eighteenth-, nineteenth-, and twentieth-century obstetrics were men. But the proscriptions against women doctors may have been more severe in modern times than in the past. According to the sixth-century medical writer Aetius of Amida, a woman doctor practised in Athens in the fifth century B.C. – Aspasia, the mistress of Pericles. Female physicians also were known in Rome. In the great medieval school of Salerno, Trotula di Ruggerio (also called Dame Trot) was a well-respected professor, physician, and midwife, who is said to have been the author of an anonymous treatise on childbearing. With the advent of male midwifery in early modern times, women faded from medicine and obstetrical practice, especially in the cities. But in rural areas and in the New World, midwives were the primary accoucheurs.

Women have always wanted to study and practise medicine. Ironically, the nineteenth-century social values that thwarted their desires eventually provided an opening – through perceived inadequacies in the delivery of medical care for women. Man as midwife had frequently been the subject of mirth and ridicule. For example, in the eighteenth century, Mary Tofts staged herself giving birth to a litter of rabbits and convinced several prominent doctors of her claims, much to their later embarrassment. Victorian society in particular had difficulty reconciling the relationship between a woman and her male attendant, especially on matters involving her genitalia. To avoid offending sensibilities, doctors conducting an internal examination were taught not to look on a patient's nakedness but to gaze into her eyes or off into space.

In the early nineteenth century, women entered the professional workforce, first as teachers and later as nurses. At mid-century, driven by singular zeal and with few prior examples, Florence Nightingale improved the care given to soldiers in the Crimean War. Her action drew criticisms that were the corollary of the arguments both for and against women in medicine and men in midwifery: a lady should not be exposed to a nude male body; a gentleman should not attend a naked woman. But Nightingale built a profession on the 'womanly' virtues of cleanliness, patience, order, and service. Her legacy has been challenged by feminist historians, who decry the subservient, selfless position Nightingale's (always female) nurses were expected to adopt in deference to their (always male) superiors. From its inception, a Victorian sexism was embedded in nursing.

Women hid their sex in order to become doctors, but how many did so cannot be determined. Canada's first known woman physician was Dr James Miranda Barry, a British military officer and surgeon, who was appointed inspector of hospitals in 1857. A medical graduate of Edinburgh, her sex was not discovered until she was laid out for her funeral in 1865. She is said to have performed the first Cesarean section in the British Empire shortly after 1816, and because she travelled with the British army, she was the first woman to practise in other countries, including England and South Africa. Barry encountered Florence Nightingale in the Crimea. The Lady with the Lamp was furious because the doctor had kept her standing in the sun while 'he/she' chastised her from horseback. Nightingale's opinion of proper female delicacy of women is encapsulated in her account of their meeting.

Florence Nightingale on James Barry

(He) kept me standing in the midst of quite a crowd of soldiers, commissariat servants, camp followers etc. etc. every one of whom behaved like a gentleman, during the scolding I received, while (she) behaved like a brute. After (she) was dead, I was told that (he) was a woman. I should say (she) was the most hardened creature I ever met.

(cited in Hacker 1974, 10)

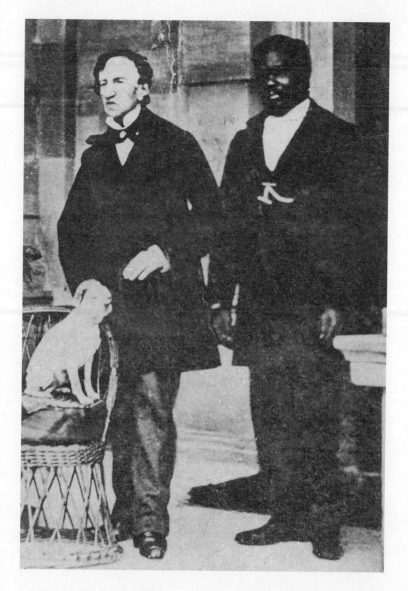

James Miranda Barry with her servant and dog in Jamaica, 1856. Widely thought to have been the first woman to practise Western medicine in Canada, Barry is said to have spent her life disguised as a man. Courtesy of RAMC Historical Museum, Aldershot, U.K.

In recognition of societal values, prominent women citizens, especially in the United States, began to insist that the best doctors for women and children ought to be other women. These same activists supported the temperance and suffrage movements. After 1850, medical schools slowly began to accept women students in response to this perceived need to provide care for their own. Nevertheless, as historian Thomas Bonner has said, to obtain the education that they desired, women were forced to travel 'to the ends of the earth.' In 1849 Elizabeth Blackwell became the first openly female person to graduate from a Western medical school in modern times; she had studied at Geneva College in rural New York State. Blackwell and Elizabeth Garrett Anderson, who had studied in Paris, were the only women known to practise in England before 1877. Two American women graduated from European schools in 1871 – Mary Putnam Jacobi at Paris and Susan Dimock at Zurich. But doors that had opened only a crack began to shut tightly, and segregated schools for women's training were founded in Philadelphia and in New York City. When the medical school of Johns Hopkins University opened in 1893, it was forced to offer 10 per cent of its places to women because of the unwelcome but intransigent condition of a key (lady) donor. Similar stories are now being told about the medical education of blacks, Jews, and other minorities.

Sometimes, medical training came with narrow expectations if not stipulations for subsequent practice. Emily Stowe, one of Canada's first woman physicians, was denied education in Toronto and did her training at a segregated medical college in New York City, graduating in 1867. But even after obtaining her formal credentials, she was refused (or did not seek) a licence to practice until 1880. In 1883, her daughter, Augusta Stowe-Gullen of Toronto, became the first women to graduate from a Canadian medical school. Gullen's alma mater and its successor, the University of Toronto, admitted no other women medical students for a quarter century more, referring all female applicants to segregated schools. Stowe-Gullen's achievement marked a watershed in higher education for women: a few years earlier, Mount Allison University had granted the first Canadian BSc (1875) and BA (1882) to women. Stowe and her daughter were outspoken advocates of temperance, education, and votes for females, and they confined their practices to women and children.

Kingston hosted Canada's earliest school for the professional education of women. Founded on 8 June 1883 after a failed attempt at integrating women students into Queen's University, the Women's Medical College opened that October, holding its classes in City Hall. The first three graduates were Elizabeth Smith-Shortt, Alice McGillivray, and Elizabeth Beatty. McGillivray became a professor of obstetrics and later devoted her career to improving the lot of women and children in Hamilton, Ontario. Beatty became a missionary, and Smith-Shortt was a prominent force in Kingston society. Approximately forty women graduated as doctors in the eleven years the college was in operation. A rival institution had scrambled to open in Toronto (also in October 1883), and the Women's Medical College closed because of the competition. It is no accident that the first woman physician to lead an academic medical department in Canada was an obstetrician: Elinor F.E. Black, who became professor and head of obstetrics the University of Manitoba in 1952. Until 1999, no woman had been chosen to serve as a medical dean in this country; in that year, both Dalhousie and the University of Western Ontario took the plunge.

Women physicians concentrated on women, babies, and birthing, but they also became important advocates of public health. Appalling conditions in hospitals were their special focus. Similarly, women doctors supported the legal attack on the patent drug industry, which promised to cure everything, although its nostrums consisted mostly of alcohol, opium, or water. Many unsuspecting clients became addicted to these useless products and avoided medical care. The advent of epidemiological methods, statistics, and public health made it possible for physicians to appreciate inequities in the quality of obstetrical care. Various campaigns were aimed at improving women's health, and frontier nurse-midwife facilities were founded.

Inability to control conception predicated female existence. Historian Judith Leavitt has used an American woman's diary to show how for the majority of her twenty-two years of married life, the diarist was either pregnant or nursing. In 1873 a Catholic theologian at Louvain had recommended sterile-cycle sex as a method of contraception; this 'rhythm method,' together with abstention and coitus interruptus, encompassed birth control. All other methods – including douching, sponges, condoms, caps, diaphragms, and abortion – were not only frowned upon; they were illegal. According to an 1892 Canadian law, disseminating information about contraception was obscene and carried a prison term of up to two years. Similar laws existed in Europe and the United States.

Women were instrumental in the birth-control movement. Science may have provided the mechanism for these techniques, but medical professionals – even women doctors – rarely helped to make them available. Some champions of this cause were jailed or prosecuted for their efforts: American nurse Margaret Sanger, English paleobotanist Marie Stopes, and Kitchener, Ontario, volunteer Dorothea Palmer. The latter had worked with A.R. Kaufman, a male philanthropist and manufacturer of rubber footwear who was never charged. She was acquitted on 17 March 1937 after a nineteen-day trial, which was the first Canadian case to use the defence issue of the 'public good.' The many witnesses for Palmer's defence included the Toronto psychiatrist Brock Chisholm, who later served as director general of the World Health Organization (see chapter 13).

Free centres for birth control information were set up in Vancouver (1923), Kitchener (1930), and Hamilton (1932). Two women doctors made the unusual choice of working toward birth control – Elizabeth Bagshaw and Helen MacMurchy. Graduating from the University of Toronto in 1900, MacMurchy was the first woman to intern at Toronto General Hospital and one of the first in Canada to hold a high-level bureaucratic post. Not only did she support birth-control education by authoring pamphlets on family planning, but she was concerned with infant mortality and mother-child welfare. Scrutiny of her methods, however, has revealed that MacMurchy's main targets were the poor and 'feeble minded,' and it has exposed her links to the now discredited eugenics movement (see chapter 13).

In 1969, through the efforts of international organization, a coalition of Protestant church representations, and citizen activists such as Barbara and George Cadbury, the 1892 Canadian birth control law was changed. In the same year, homosexual acts between two consenting persons over the age of twenty-one were decriminalized.

Abortion is another controversial issue. Physicians and volunteers working in abortion clinics in the United States and Canada have been shot and sometimes killed as part of the 'justifiable homicide' movement. The dead include Drs David Gunn in 1993 and John Britten in 1994, both of Pensacola, Florida, and in 1998 Barnett Stepian of Amherst, New York. In Canada, Drs Garson Romalis of Vancouver in 1994, Hugh Short of Hamilton in 1996, and Jack Fainman of Winnipeg in 1997 were shot and injured. In other societies, however, the procedure has not carried the stigma it bears in some sectors of North America today. Abortion (or at least a specific technique for abortion) was forbidden by the Hippocratic oath, but it was practised in other Greco-Roman circles. Amerindians used efficient methods involving natural dilators of the uterine cervix. Modern techniques have become increasingly safe, but the controversy is not about maternal safety. It revolves around the ethics of killing the fetus. Religious views of abortion as a sin inevitably influence the laws. In the last thirty years, the Canadian physician Henry Morgentaler has been prosecuted and acquitted many times for establishing abortion clinics in several provinces. Personal philosophy determines whether he is viewed as a criminal or a saint.

Control over female biology has indeed produced some changes: fertility rates have fallen, and women study, work, and vote. But the battle against sexism is not over. Women still make up less than half the workforce, and they are the lesser paid. In a world of five billion people in which thousands of children starve every year, some jurisdictions worry about the decline in their own birth rate. Fears that have a basis in xenophobia and nationalism are expressed as moral dilemmas. Women bear the brunt.

As the years passed, home delivery became less and less frequent. In 1989 some parts of Canada were reporting more than one in four deliveries done by Cesarean section, which made the country's rate among the highest in the world. Without rejecting the potential value of modern obstetrics, some historians question how much of it is needed. Does every birth need to be medicalized?

Hence the back-to-the-home-delivery movement in obstetrics, which began in the 1960s with 'innovative' methods that evoke a prehistoric past: the natural positions found in nonindustrialized

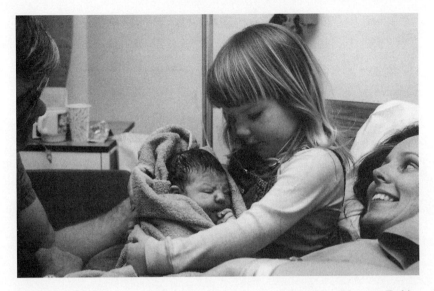

The happy results of a family-centred birth. Photograph by Eleanor Enkin, Hamilton

societies; the inclusion of family members in the delivery room (pioneered in Canada in the mid-1960s by Dr Murray Enkin of Hamilton); and special settings, like those endorsed by the French *accoucheurs* Frédéric Leboyer or Michel Odent, who aimed to mollify the trauma of birth with a dimly lit room, a warm-water bath, and music – private procedures that in France, at least, command high fees.

Proponents of family-centred, home delivery maintain that, in many cases, it is at least as safe as the hospital, because it avoids drug-resistant organisms and provides psychological benefits for mother-child bonding. Until recently, Canada was one of only eight World Health Organization member countries that did not regulate midwifery. Over the opposition of many obstetricians, several provinces have launched task forces to study the issue: Alberta (1988 and 1994), British Columbia (1993), Manitoba (1988 and 1993), Ontario (1987), and Saskatchewan (1996). In Ontario, midwifery training began in Sudbury, Hamilton, and Toronto in 1993, and the first cohort of students graduated in 1996. This change relies on public perception of the personal, psychological, and medical benefits of home delivery and is further prompted by the perceived economic advantages of shifting care to lesser-paid professionals. But whether we like it or not, state-funded birthing will continue to be medicalized to some extent. Governments wishing to avoid responsibility for disasters find solace in medical expertise.

Obstetrics and gynecology have indeed made remarkable progress. Childbearing is safer than it was a century ago, but the technological fix has not solved all the medical dilemmas. By creating a multiplicity of options, it has generated new ethical problems. Feminist historians, such as Veronica Strong-Boag and Deborah Gorham, find that women doctors abandoned the original purpose of their predecessors – to attend to the social and biological needs of women and children. The pioneer women in medicine were thoroughly sensitized and motivated by feminist issues. But women who choose medicine today are said to become plain ordinary doctors, undifferentiated from and just as conservative as their male peers. Women's medicine and medicine's women are now faced with the exciting challenge of integrating two historically rich traditions into a coherent and effective whole.

Suggestions for Further Reading

On Obstetrics and Gynecology and the Role of Women

Apple, Rima. *Women and Health in America: A Historical Handbook.* New York: Garland, 1990

Arney, William Ray. *Power and the Profession of Obstetrics.* Chicago: University of Chicago Press, 1982

Borst, Charlotte G. *Catching Babies: The Professionalization of Childbirth, 1870–1920.* Cambridge, Mass.: Harvard University Press, 1995

Cianfranci, Theodore. *A Short History of Obstetrics and Gynecology.* Springfield: Charles C. Thomas, 1960

Cohen, Estelle. ' "What the Women at All Times Would Laugh At": Redefining Equality and Difference, circa 1660–1760.' *Osiris* 12 (1997), 121–42

Daly, Mary. *Gyn/ecology: The Metaethics of Radical Feminism.* Boston: Beacon Press, 1978

Duden, Barbara. *The Woman beneath the Skin: A Doctor's Patients in Eighteenth-*

Century Germany. Trans. Thomas Dunlap. Cambridge, Mass.: Harvard University Press, 1991

Ehrenreich, Barbara, and Deirdre English. *For Her Own Good: 150 Years of Experts' Advice to Women*. Garden City: Anchor Books, 1989

Enkin, Murray, Marc Keirse, Iain Chalmers, and Eleanor Enkin. *A Guide to Effective Care in Pregnancy and Childbirth*. New York and Oxford: Oxford University Press, 1989

Farley, John. *Gametes and Spores: Ideas about Sexual Reproduction, 1750–1914*. Baltimore: Johns Hopkins University Press, 1982

Gallagher, Catherine, and Thomas Laqueur. *The Making of the Modern Body: Sexuality and Society in the Nineteenth Century*. Berkeley: University of California Press, 1987

Garrison, Fielding H. *An Introduction to the History of Medicine*. 3rd edn. Philadelphia: Saunders, 1922

Himes, Norman Edwin. *Medical History of Contraception*. 1936. Reprint, New York, Shocken Books, 1970

Jordanova, Ludmilla. *Sexual Visions: Images of Gender in Science and Medicine between the Eighteenth and Twentieth Centuries*. New York, London, Toronto, Sydney, and Tokyo: Harvester Wheatsheaf, 1989

Laget, Mireille. *Naissances: L'accouchement avant l'age de la clinique*. Paris: Editions du Seuil, 1982

Laqueur, Thomas Walter. *Making Sex: Body and Gender from the Greeks to Freud*. Cambridge, Mass.: Harvard University Press, 1990

Leavitt, Judith Walzer. *Brought to Bed: Birthing Women and their Physicians in America, 1750 to 1950*. New York: Oxford University Press, 1986

McLaren, Angus. *Birth Control in Nineteenth-Century England*. London: Croom Helm, 1978

– *A History of Contraception: From Antiquity to the Present Day*. Oxford, UK and Cambridge, Mass.: Blackwell, 1990

Martin, Emily, *The Woman in the Body: A Cultural Analysis of Reproduction*. Boston: Beacon Press, 1987

Merskey, Harold, and Paul Potter. 'The Womb Lay Still in Ancient Egypt.' *British Journal of Psychiatry* 154 (1989), 751–3

Merskey, Harold, and Susan J. Merskey. 'Hysteria, or Suffocation of the Mother.' *Canadian Medical Association Journal* 148 (1993), 399–405

Oakley, Ann. *The Captured Womb: A History of the Medical Care of Pregnant Women*. Oxford and New York: Blackwell, 1984

Pinto-Correira, Clara. *The Ovum of Eve: Egg and Sperm and Preformation*. Chicago: University of Chicago Press, 1997

Rose, June. *Marie Stopes and the Sexual Revolution*. London: Faber, 1992

Schiebinger, Londa. *Nature's Body: Gender in the Making of Modern Science.* Boston:
   Beacon Press, 1993
Semmelweis, I.F. *The Etiology, Concept, and Prophylaxis of Childbed Fever.* Trans.
   and ed. K. Codell Carter. Madison, Wis.: University of Wisconsin Press,
   1983
Shephard, David A.E. *John Snow: Anesthetist to a Queen and Epidemiologist to a
   Nation: A Biography.* Cornwall, P.E.I.: York Point Publishing, 1995
Shorter, Edward. *A History of Women's Bodies.* New York: Basic Books, 1982
Speert, Harold. *Obstetrics and Gynecology: A History and Iconography.* Rev. edn. San
   Francisco: Norman Pub., 1994
Thoms, Herbert. *Classical Contributions to Obstetrics and Gynecology.* Springfield,
   Ill.: Charles C. Thomas, 1935
Ulrich, Laurel T. *A Midwife's Tale: The Life of Martha Ballard, Based on Her Diary,
   1785–1812.* New York: Knopf, 1990
Wertz, Dorothy C., and Richard W. Wertz. *Lying In: A History of Childbirth in Amer-
   ica.* London: Macmillan, 1977
Wilson, Adrian, *The Making of Man-Midwifery: Childbirth in England 1660–1770.*
   London: University College London Press, 1995

On Women Doctors in the Western World

Bonner, Thomas N. *To the Ends of the Earth: Women's Search for Education in
   Medicine.* Cambridge, Mass.: Harvard University Press, 1992
Gorham, Deborah. 'No Longer an Invisible Minority: Women Physicians and
   Medical Practice in Late Twentieth-Century North America.' In *Caring and
   Curing,* ed. Dianne E. Dodd and Deborah Gorham, 183–211. Ottawa: Univer-
   sity of Ottawa Press, 1994
Hurd Mead, Kate. *A History of Women in Medicine from the Earliest Times to the Begin-
   ning of the Nineteenth Century.* Haddam, Conn.: Haddam Press, 1938
Lower, J. *Women Physicians: Career, Status, and Power.* New York and London:
   Tavistock, 1984
Marland, Hilary. '"Pioneer Work on All Sides": The First Generations of Women
   Physicians in The Netherlands, 1879–1930.' *Journal of the History of Medicine
   and Allied Sciences* 50 (1995), 441–77
Morantz-Sanchez, Regina Markell. *Sympathy and Science: Women Physicians in
   American Medicine.* New York: Oxford University Press, 1985
Rose, June. *The Perfect Gentleman: The Remarkable Life of Dr. James Miranda Barry.*
   London: Hutchinson, 1977
Walsh, Mary Roth. *'Doctors Wanted: No Women Need Apply': Sexual Barriers in the
   Medical Profession.* New Haven and London: Yale University Press, 1977

On Canadian Obstetrics, Gynecology, and Women

Collin, Johanne. *Changement d'ordonnance: Mutations professionelles, identité sociale et féminisation de la profession pharmaceutique au Québec, 1940–1980.* Montreal: Boréal, 1995

Dodd, Dianne. 'The Birth Control Movement on Trial, 1936–7.' *Histoire sociale/ Social History* 16 (1983), 411–28

Dodd, Dianne E., and Deborah Gorham, eds. *Caring and Curing: Historical Perspectives on Women and Healing in Canada.* Ottawa: University of Ottawa Press, 1994

Duffin, Jacalyn. 'The Death of Sarah Lovell and the Constrained Feminism of Emily Stowe.' *Canadian Medical Association Journal* 146 (1992), 881–8

Fryer, Mary Beacock. *Emily Stowe: Doctor and Suffragist.* Toronto: Dundurn Press and the Hannah Institute for the History of Medicine, 1990

Fuhrer, Charlotte. *The Mysteries of Montreal: Memoirs of a Midwife,* ed. W. Peter Ward. Vancouver: University of British Columbia Press, 1984

Hacker, Carlotta. *The Indomitable Lady Doctors.* Toronto: Clarke Irwin, 1974

Laforce, Hélène. *Histoire de la sage-femme dans la region de Québec.* Quebec: Institut québécois de recherche sur la culture, 1985

McLaren, Angus. *Our Own Master Race: Eugenics in Canada, 1885–1945.* Toronto: McClelland and Stewart, 1990

McLaren, Angus, and Arlene Tigar McLaren. *The Bedroom and the State: The Changing Practices and Politics of Contraception and Abortion in Canada, 1880–1997.* 2nd ed. Toronto: Oxford University Press, 1997

McPherson, Kathryn M. *Bedside Matters: The Transformation of Canadian Nursing, 1900–1990.* Toronto, New York, and Oxford: Oxford University Press, 1996

McPherson, Kathryn, and Meryn Stuart, guest eds. *Canadian Bulletin of Medical History.* Special issue on the history of nursing. 11 (1994)

Mitchinson, Wendy. *The Nature of Their Bodies: Women and Their Doctors in Victorian Canada.* Toronto: University of Toronto Press, 1991

Muzzin, L.J., G.P. Brown, and R.W. Hornosty. 'Consequences of Feminization of a Profession: The Case of Canadian Pharmacy.' *Women and Health.* 21, no. 2/3 (1994), 39–56

Skuy, Percy. 'Canadian Pioneers in Family Planning.' *Journal SOGC* 21 (1999), 377–84

Strong-Boag, Veronica. 'Canada's Women Doctors: Feminism Constrained.' In *A Not Unreasonable Claim,* ed. Linda Kealey, 109–29. Toronto: Women's Press, 1979

Vandervoort, Julie. *Tell the Driver: A Biography of Elinor F.E. Black, M.D.* Winnipeg: University of Manitoba Press, 1992

CHAPTER TWELVE

Wrestling with Demons: History of Psychiatry*

No one who, like me, conjures up the most evil of those half-tamed demons that inhabit the human breast, and seeks to wrestle with them, can expect to come through the struggle unscathed.

Sigmund Freud, *Dora*, 1905, in *Standard Edition*, vol. 7, 109

Mental illnesses are unique because they continue to be defined by the patient's symptoms or behaviours, rather than by physical, chemical, or anatomical tests. Many themes presented earlier come into play in this history of psychiatry: the long-standing importance of a life force in explaining the functions of living beings (see chapter 3); and the tension between two pairs of rival disease concepts: first, disease from the outside versus disease from within; and second, the disease of the individual versus disease of the group (see chapter 4).

The mind has often been equated with a vital spirit. Just as Galen's concept of a life force resonated for Christian theologians who saw it as the soul, vitalism has had explanatory power in psychological theories of illness. Vitalism is making a comeback in psychosomatic theories that link physical ailment to prior emotional suffering. As a result, psychiatric disturbances relate to physiological or holistic concepts (disease from within) when they are diagnosed by observation of the disturbed relationship between a body and its environment.

*Educational objectives for this chapter are found on pp. 398–9.

Ontological concepts can also be found in psychiatric explanations that implicate discrete changes inside the body caused by external agents, be they possession by demons or chemical derangements.

The word 'psychiatry,' derived from two Greek words meaning 'soul' (or 'mind') and 'healer,' was coined by the German physician Johann Christian Reil, and was first used in English less than a hundred and fifty years ago. The word 'psychiatry' implies that these conditions are of the *psyche*, not the *soma*. By definition, then, psychiatric disease is a disorder of the mind, not the body, with respect to its cause and manifestations. Mental disorders may be associated with alterations in the body, but they are not identified by them. Rather, they are distinguished by changes in behaviour, perception, thought, or affect. Yet throughout history, mental diseases were usually considered to be the product of unseen but physical causes, such as diet, poisonings, occult infections, or structural change.

Prior to the integration of anatomy with bedside medicine, the classification of all diseases, or nosology, was based on the study of patients' symptoms (see chapter 4). As physical pathology grew, some diseases of the mind were reclassified as diseases of the brain, the nerves, or the metabolism; examples include, epilepsy, tertiary syphilis, mental retardation, cretinism, and deafness. They appear in the psychiatric literature only because of associated symptoms, such as depression and anxiety. Psychiatric disorders are those ailments that are 'left over' because they cannot be, or have yet to be sorted into an anatomical or physiological realm.

Classification of disease in modern psychiatry remains in a state of subjective symptomatology akin to eighteenth-century nosology. Notwithstanding the discoveries of many scientists, no blood tests, biopsies, ultrasounds, scans, or electrodynamic studies can objectively confirm a psychiatric diagnosis.

Themes in the History of Psychiatry

First, the tension between the physical and psychological causes of mental disease has been apparent throughout the history of mental illness; the dichotomy pervades psychiatry today. Second, 'normal' behaviour is socially and culturally determined; therefore, behaviours that are labelled 'abnormal,' 'mad,' or 'insane' can also be socially determined. Actions that are considered normal in one culture may be unacceptable in another; examples include incest, cannibalism, killing, genital mutilation, and political dissent. As a result, the mental state that leads an individual to socially unacceptable actions can be viewed variously as criminal, sinful, or sick. Psychiatric diagnoses can and have been socially constructed; as a result, psychiatry is vulnerable to abuse. For example, the judiciary exploits the subjective nature of psychiatric diagnosis when expert witnesses are selected to contradict each other in court over questions of sanity.

Finally, mental illness has carried a stigma, deriving from the patient's apparent unreliability, unpredictability, and perceived responsibility for the illness. Unlike most bodily ailments, mental disorders can sometimes be feigned. Homer's Odysseus, the biblical King David, and other ancient heroes pretended to be mad to achieve specific ends. This common knowledge tends to imply that all persons who behave unacceptably may have consciously chosen behaviours that they could or should be able to control or prevent.

Historical Overview

Madness has been recognized since the earliest times, but it was not always a problem for doctors. In antiquity, it was identified by wide ranging symptoms, including convulsions, cries, screams, violence, emotional pain, and the inability to learn or remember. In Hellenic and Judeo-Christian traditions, people so afflicted were sometimes thought to be prophets; examples include the Trojan princess Cassandra and the Christian saint John the Baptist. A few ancient writers cited psychological or emotional causes to explain the behaviour, but most found physical explanations residing in naturalistic and material theories of the humours. For example, in the Hippocratic writings, epilepsy was the result of phlegm obstructed in the brain; depression was due to an accumulation of black bile – hence the term 'melancholia.' 'Hypochondria' referred to ailments originating in the upper abdomen below the ribs. Afflictions of women, both physical and mental, were attributed to a wandering womb – the origin of the term 'hysteria,' invented at a much later time (see chapter 11).

In the second century A.D., Aretaeus of Cappadocia, who vividly described diabetes and other physical ailments, defined 'mania' as delirium without fever, distinguishing it from 'phrenitis,' which was delirium with fever. He also recognized that periods of mania, or fury, could alternate with periods of depression (*Chronic Diseases I*, v, vi). Emphasizing the perceived physical causes for these conditions, treatments were also physical, including diets, baths, ointments, drugs, and rest. Greek and Roman societies created laws to protect families from dangers posed by the insane who were feared, shunned, prayed over, and mostly left alone.

The first institutions for the care of the insane were the ninth- and tenth-century *mauristans* in the Islamic cities of Baghdad, Cairo, Fez, and Damascus. Muslim societies believed that the insane were divinely inspired rather than demonically possessed; the words to describe them were either *majnoon* (veiled) or *majthoob* (pulled, by the grace of God). Because mad people were holy, emphasis was placed on giving them comfortable accommodation rather than treatment or confinement. *Mauristans* are said to have been luxurious, but restraints were used to control violent outbursts.

The first European mental institutions appeared in the parts of the continent that came under Islamic rule, especially fourteenth-century Spain at Granada, Valencia, Zaragoza, Seville, Barcelona, and Toledo. A Spanish merchant, who himself had suffered a psychotic episode, founded an order of hospitaliers, later called the Order of St John of God. Like their Middle Eastern predecessors, these institutions functioned as hospices for decent care, not for cure.

Citing literary sources, some scholars have suggested that the early Middle Ages conceived of emotional causes for mental disturbances and consequently sought emotional cures (Alexander and Selesnick 1966, 52). In the late Middle Ages and Renaissance, social control of deviance became a major preoccupation. Persons given to unusual behaviour were thought to have let down their moral guard and been possessed by demons. 'Treatments' were implemented, but in reality they resembled persecutions and included beating, whipping, expulsion, and execution. Care of the mentally disturbed was the responsibility of each community, and patients were lucky if they were simply neglected. Some communities in northern Europe are said to have hired sailors to remove the unruly – hence the origin of 'ship of fools,' a metaphor for the human condition in sixteenth-century Germany. Over a period of some three hundred years, unknown numbers of unconventional women were burned as witches by perpetrators who feared epidemics of madness – perpetrators who themselves have been portrayed, more recently, as victims of mass hysteria. Those whose distress did not interfere with their own survival or that of others, managed alone, doubting that help could be found in medicine.

> What physic, what chirurgery, what wealth, favour, authority can relieve, bear out, assuage or expel a troubled conscience? A quiet mind cureth all.
>
> Robert Burton, *Anatomy of Melancholy*, pt 3, 4.2.4, 1651

Hospitals founded to provide humane care gradually became horrifying places of incarceration. The Charité de Senlis, in France, run by the monastic order St John of God, forbade restraints and punitive therapies, but such lenience was the exception. Ostensibly to protect society, criminals, beggars, prostitutes, the poor, the chronically ill, and some mad people were held indefinitely in squalid, rat-infested places where they were subjected to punitive 'treatments,' designed to shock or humiliate them into behaving 'rationally.' The administrators of these so-called hospitals in France, Germany, and Britain enjoyed absolute power over the occupants and immunity from the courts and police.

By the eighteenth century, St Mary of Bethlehem Hospital in London, built in 1247, had become the fearful 'Bedlam.' In his series of engravings, *The Rake's Progress*, William Hogarth depicted Bedlam as the miserable and deserving end of a wanton *bon vivant*. Custodial rather than medical, these institutions employed few doctors and were little concerned with physical health. Their seemingly less than human occupants became objects of paid entertainment; however,

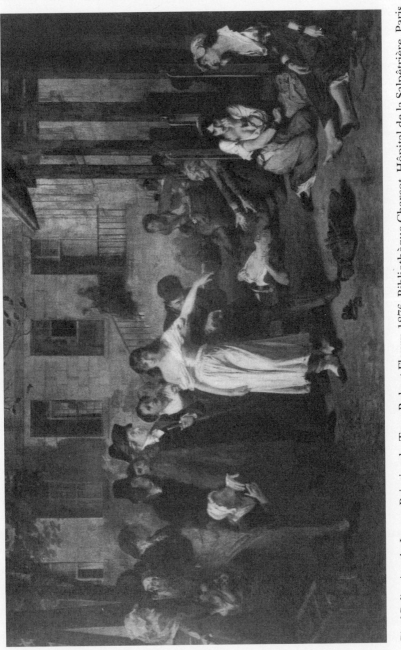

Pinel Delivering the Insane. Painting by Tony Robert-Fleury, 1876. Bibliothèque Charcot, Hôpital de la Salpêtrière, Paris

the oft-repeated claim that 96,000 annual spectators paid a penny apiece to stroll the wards of Bedlam is probably a gross exaggeration (Patricia Allderidge, in Bynum and Porter 1987, vol. 2).

Asylum reform spread over the Western world at the end of the eighteenth century. The 'asylum' was to be a safe place for seclusion, care, and restoration. The movement was fostered by Benjamin Rush in Philadelphia, William Tuke in England (who was a Quaker and not a physician), and Christian Reil in Germany. In France after the revolution, Philippe Pinel was appointed director of two Paris hospitals – the Bicêtre for men and the Salpêtrière for women, where he implemented a figurative 'unchaining' of the insane. Influenced by English writers, he argued that many patients were sick from emotional or 'moral' causes, and their treatment should be based on emotional or 'moral' principles. Unchaining is an appropriate metaphor for Pinel's work, and it has been portrayed many times in medical art, although the precise moment probably never took place in the literal sense. Controls were not abandoned. Patients continued to be confined, and violence was subdued by modified straitjackets or by other forms of coercion, such as hydrotherapy (baths).

Asylums gathered many people with like symptoms and gave physicians an opportunity is observe patterns of mental illness. Their goals were to protect and to 'console and classify.' In conjunction with the scientific *Zeitgeist*, classification of insanity (also called alienation, or vesania) became the cutting edge of research into mental disturbances. William Cullen of Edinburgh created the category called neurosis – a Latinization of the word for nervousness. He reasoned that functional conditions resulted from a highly sensitive reaction to outside stimuli mediated by the nerves. Within this physiological category of neurosis, he situated the older concepts of melancholia, hysteria, hypochondria, and sexual deviation. In France, Pinel and his student Jean-Etienne-Dominique Esquirol also devised classifications; they distinguished between mental retardation, cretinism, senility, melancholia, and a category called monomania, in which might be grouped the neuroses of today. These doctors were known as alienists – specialists in diseases that alienated patients from reality.

As explained in chapters 4 and 9, all disease concepts became

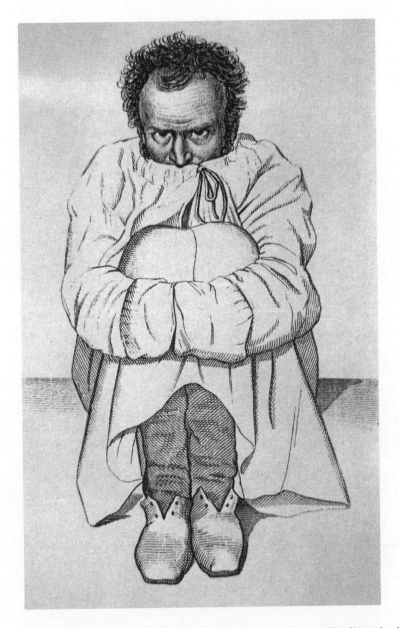

Mania Succeeded by Dementia. Engraving by Ambroise Tardieu, in J.E.D. Esquirol, *Les maladies mentales*, vol. 2, 1838

increasingly anatomical during the nineteenth century. In conjunction with the asylum movement, scientists were forging links between physical changes in the nervous system and certain behavioural disorders. Gradually, organic correlatives were found for conditions that could no longer be thought of as diseases of the mind: epilepsy, tertiary syphilis, vasculitis, allergy, and stroke. Neurology grew as a related but separate discipline, based on rigorous anatomical localization of specific changes in the nervous system. The anatomo-physiological explanations that had characterized Cullen's approach gave way to purely functional explanations. The category of neurosis persisted, but lack of physical findings led to its 'denervation.' 'Psychosis' became the mid-nineteenth-century term for serious alienation or complete disorientation. 'Neurosis,' or 'monomania,' was reserved for alienation in only one dimension.

Psychiatry dealt with what was 'left over' when the neurological disorders were removed. Reil's new word 'psychiatry' referred to 'healing' (of the soul) with pediatrics and podiatry and unlike most other medical designations, which end with the suffix '-ology' (= words or theory about). The etymological choice is telling: the newborn psychiatry of the early nineteenth century was confidently optimistic that it would not only care but cure.

Asylum architecture was designed to demonstrate the imposing stature, power, and authority of the new profession. Canada's first dedicated-use asylum was completed in 1850 at 999 Queen Street West, Toronto. It was quickly filled to capacity with over 500 patients. The address itself gradually became synonymous with madness and was changed, in the 1970s, to 1001 Queen Street West in an attempt to obliterate its gothic associations. Other Ontario institutions experienced rapid expansion. In Hamilton the 1875 asylum, built to house 200 patients, accommodated more than 1,300 by late 1914; in London during the same period, the asylum grew from 120 beds to 1,130. The superintendents, Joseph Workman at Toronto and Richard Maurice Bucke at London, became known for their practice based on the principles of moral restraint.

Historians are divided over whether or not the asylum keepers were heroes or villains. In the more traditional histories, they are portrayed as heroes because they attempted to improve conditions,

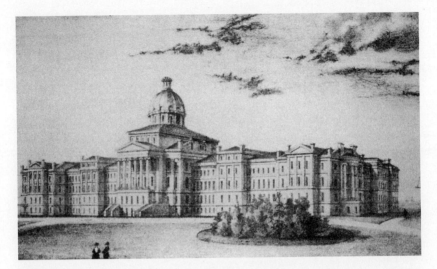

Design for the Provincial Lunatic Asylum, Toronto, ca. 1854. From Henry Hurd, *The Institutional Care of the Insane in the United States and Canada*, vol. 1, 1916

sought better understanding of psychiatric disturbances, adopted the ideals of moral cause and moral treatment, and tried to find cures. Despite the medical, verbal, and architectural trappings, however, asylums continued to be places of confinement, and diagnosis often incorporated prejudicial notions of class, gender, and race. Critics have shown that some new therapies were worse than useless, because they were harmful. Yet these therapies were not designed to hurt patients deliberately. Why did they once seem to be rational, justifiable, and effective? The answer lies in the generally accepted concepts of mental disease in the nineteenth and twentieth centuries and possibly also in the frequency of spontaneous remissions, now estimated to be 30 per cent.

By the late nineteenth century, psychiatry was losing professional credibility. Anesthesia, antisepsis, germ theory, and public health had fostered effective interventions for other human problems and had generated great optimism for surgeons, internists, obstetricians, and their patients. Psychiatrists, on the other hand, had yet to make equivalent discoveries – discoveries that could explain, predict, cure, or prevent. One Canadian scholar (Dowbiggin) cited this borderline professional despair as a reason why psychiatrists clung passionately and stubbornly to etiological theories of heredity, degeneracy, and self-abuse – hypotheses that tended to blame the patients, rather than medicine, for their incurability.

Notwithstanding the moral cause and moral treatment hypothesis, psychiatric disorders were increasingly perceived to be disorders of the brain, not of the 'soul.' If mental processes resided in the brain, then physical and physiological treatments seemed to be justified. Joannes B. Friedreich took a strongly somatist approach to mental disorders; Wilhelm Griesinger combined physical and emotional therapies. Jean-Martin Charcot, a French neurologist, studied hysteria and its modification through hypnotism, but some contemporaries and historians have demonstrated that his desire to find hysteria prompted his patients to reproduce it for him.

Sophisticated observation of the mentally ill continued with the longitudinal study of case histories and autopsies; modifications to the classification schemes were made. In 1899 Emil Kraeplin defined the two major psychoses as manic depression and dementia praecox, subdividing the latter into hebephrenia, catatonia, and paranoia. Two years later, dementia praecox was named schizophrenia by Paul Eugen Bleuler. With considerable modification, these categories are still in use.

Twentieth-Century Psychiatry

At the beginning of this century, psychiatric research expanded in three different directions, all of which continue: psychoanalysis, psychosomatics, and psychobiology.

Psychoanalysis

Psychoanalysis had precursors but did not receive medical approbation until the work of Sigmund Freud. A Viennese-born Jew, Freud began his career as a physician interested in physical and neurological disturbances. During 1885–6, he spent a few months in Paris with Charcot and Pierre Janet, where his interests turned from neuropathology to psychopathology. But as Freud himself later claimed, it was through the 'teachings' of his own patients, most of whom were wealthy and neurotic, that he was led to his theories of the unconscious.

The ideas expressed in Freud's extensive publications have become cultural icons: the interpretation of dreams, the unconscious, the ego and the id, the importance of childhood experience, sexual conflict, the hydraulic theory of neurotic defence mechanisms, repression, fixations (anal, oral, and genital), fantasy, wish-fulfillment, symbols (phallic and otherwise), catharsis, free association, analysis, and complexes named for mythic figures of antiquity. Critics claim that Freud's work applied only to himself or to the upper middle class in turn-of-the-century Europe, and that its ethnocentric and androcentric concepts, such as penis envy, made it irrelevant to others. Yet whether Freud is lauded or deplored, medicine, psychiatry, and Western culture in general were irreversibly altered. The rapid dissemination of his thought testified to a perceived need for the articulation of nonphysical etiologies.

Freud first began publishing in the 1890s. His ideas met with some opposition, but he and his collaborators, Carl Jung and Alfred Adler, found supporters almost immediately. His influential book, *The Interpretation of Dreams*, was published in 1900; the first international congress on psychoanalysis was held in Salzburg in 1908; and by 1911 the American Psychoanalytic Association had been founded. An important boost to psychoanalytic theories of disease came during both world wars, when psychiatrists interpreted the debility of soldiers exposed to the stress of war. Unlike other specialties and possibly due to the influence of Jung, psychoanalysis has accepted and sometimes welcomed the leadership of women: for example, Karen Horney, Anna Freud (daughter of Sigmund), Melanie Klein, and Canadian, Grace Baker. Because Canadian analysts participated in the American organizations, the Canadian Psychoanalytic Society was not formed until 1952.

Two of the eight founders of the American Psychoanalytic Association were from Toronto: Welsh-born Ernest Jones and Canadian-born John T. McCurdy. Jones first learned of Freud in 1903, and he brought analysis to Canada in 1908, when he began working for

Charles Kirk Clarke, Toronto's medical dean and first professor of psychiatry, after whom the prestigious psychiatric institute was named. Jones was charged with sexual misconduct several times, but he was never convicted. Perhaps the accusations were an occupational hazard of zealous application of the new psychoanalytic theory in a disbelieving society. Jones was one of Freud's many biographers, and his personal acquaintance with the master lent an authority to his opinions that has only recently been questioned.

Theoretical rifts in psychoanalysis developed. But Freud's ideas have been an important prototype, if not the basis of all psychotherapy – which is treatment by talking, without drugs or other physical modalities. Reflecting the biases of its creators, psychotherapy is generally thought to help the educated, middle- to upper-class neurotic and to be of little benefit to the uneducated, the poor, or the psychotic. Rifts among analysts are reflected in the medico-historical study of Freud, in which his life, his patients, and the evolution of his theories are debated with passion. Restrictions on access to his papers have led to media scandals (see Malcolm 1985; Gelfand and Kerr 1992).

Fortunately, analysis is not the only way to resolve inner conflicts. Life itself still remains a very effective therapist.

Karen Horney, *Our Inner Conflicts* (New York: Norton, 1945), 240

Psychosomatics

The second direction taken by psychiatric research is the psychosomatic approach, which began in the late nineteenth century and flourished in the 1930s with the founding of specialized journals. Challenging the historic and artificial distinctions between mind and body, research was conducted on the physical effects of strong emotions. The focus shifted from mental changes to the somatic damage caused by prolonged psychic stimulation. The Vienna-born Canadian, Hans Selye, studied the physical products of prolonged stress. Personality was classified into 'types,' following Jung, and was measured on newly devised scales, reflecting a spectrum of normal rather than pathology. Certain personality types were thought to favour certain diseases; for example, the psychic stressors associated with 'Type A personality' were correlated with ulcer and coronary heart disease. More recently, researchers have been turning to the effects of daylight, stress, burnout, and depression on the immune system and on other body functions to explain disorders such as chronic fatigue syndrome and seasonal affective disorder.

> As physicians, we cannot afford to lose sight of the physical aspects of mental states, if we would try to comprehend the nature of mental disease, and learn to treat it with success.
>
> Henry Maudsley, *Body and Mind* (New York: Appleton, 1870), 94

Psychobiology

The third direction taken by psychiatry early in this century was to embrace radical treatments of a physical nature. The discovery of the spirochete completed the anatomo-clinical definition of neuro-syphilis, and in 1917 a cause was found for viral encephalitis. The linking of these formerly 'mental' disorders to germs and organs raised expectations that physical links would eventually be found for the rest. Sometimes, treatments were developed in advance of a known cause. Historians have tried to explain this aspect of the psychiatric past by recalling the turn-of-the-century frustration felt by psychiatrists who cared for the mentally disabled but failed to find effective cures. The development of treatments now viewed with repugnance constitutes a fascinating but sobering collection of clinical vignettes and imaginative reasoning.

Ovariotomy, or the removal of ovaries, was one of the earliest gynecological operations, originating in the early nineteenth century before the advent of anesthesia (see chapter 11). By the end of the century, the removal of normal ovaries to produce a premature menopause had become a standard treatment for mental illness in North American women. Critics, including some physicians, warned of its dangers and deplored the apparent lack of positive results. Others justified the intervention, claiming that women's lives were unbearable when they were subject to menstruation, childbearing, and hormonal variation. Cultural justifications for the castration of women derived both from ancient disease concepts and from Victorian discomfort with expressions of female sexuality.

Mental diseases were also treated by deliberately invoking physical disease. Noticing that symptoms of syphilis remitted when patients were febrile, the Austrian psychiatrist Julius Wagner-Jauregg instigated malarial-fever treatment for patients with tertiary syphilis. His achievement was hailed as a model for the future of psychiatry – organic disease treated organically. In 1927 he was awarded the Nobel Prize and is the only psychiatrist to have been so honoured.

Insulin shock therapy was discovered in a similarly fortuitous manner. From 1927 to 1933, Polish-born Manfred Sakel worked at a Berlin hospital, where he treated narcotic addicts and noted that abstention led to overexcitation. He reasoned that the overexcitation arose from hyperactivity of adrenal and thyroid glands, the hormone products of which had only recently been discovered. His insight is said to have been inspired by a clinical experience with a famous German actress who was both diabetic and addicted to narcotics: an accidental insulin coma had reduced her craving for morphine. At first Sakel used insulin as addiction therapy, but when he treated an addict who was also psychotic, he saw a concomitant improvement in the mental disturbance. Between 1933 and 1935, Sakel wrote a series of papers, claiming to have found the first effective weapon against schizophrenia. Psychological and physiological explanations were developed (but never proven) to explain the regression in schizophrenic symptoms that followed insulin shock. The treatment was widely used for a short time and then abandoned in the 1940s, because of its dangers, cost, and displacement by safer ways of inducing shock.

Studies in epilepsy and psychosis led the Hungarian psychiatrist Ladislas Joseph von Meduna to the conclusion that epileptics were never psychotic (now proven wrong). He reasoned that convulsive agents might cure schizophrenia. Unaware of earlier reports, Meduna believed himself to be the first to have produced convulsions with camphor in 1933, and later with its less toxic derivative, metrazol. Reactions to these drugs were unpredictable and uncontrollable: convulsions followed at variable intervals after the adminstration, and seizures could be so powerful that bones were broken, tongues bitten, and teeth lost.

Electroconvulsive shock therapy (ECT) was developed by the Italians, Lucio Bini and Ugo Cerletti, who also had been studying epilepsy. By experimenting on hogs at a slaughterhouse, they established a safe dose of electricity and administered their first electroshock treatment to a human with schizophrenia in April 1938. By 1941, curare was being used to control the violent convulsions, and the more easily monitored ECT was considered safer and more effective than chemical shock therapies. ECT is still in use today for some psychotic disorders and for refractory endogenous depression. A typical dose might be 70 to 130 volts passed through the brain for 0.1 to 0.5 second, but much higher doses were used in the past. In 1948, L.E.M. Page and R.J. Russell developed intensive shock therapy using 150 volts for a full second, followed by five shocks of 100 volts during the convulsion; the process was repeated once or twice a day.

The first prefrontal lobotomies were performed in 1935 by Antonio de Egas Moniz and Pedro Manuel Almeida Lima. A Portuguese-born neurosurgeon, Egas Moniz had invented cerebral angiography in 1927; he also served for twenty years as a liberal politician. He and Lima reasoned that morbid thoughts cycled repeatedly through the brains of psychotics, and that interrupting the cycle might be beneficial. They had learned from American experiments on chimpanzees that after prefrontal lobotomy, animals were more manageable and less easily frustrated. By extrapolation, they predicted that obsessive persons who were refractory to shock treatment could be 'relieved' with surgery into a state of manageable indifference. Their initial report on lobotomy, published in 1936, dealt with twenty human patients: seven had been cured, they claimed, seven improved, and six showed no change.

Prefrontal lobotomy (removal of frontal lobe tissue) and its less invasive successor, the leucotomy (cutting tissue tracts), were widely practised in the 1930s and 1940s. A public outcry gradually caused the medical establishment to recognize that some patients so treated had become profoundly altered, tactless individuals, devoid of character – 'zombies.' Far from being a cure, the irreversible procedure was little more than a surgical straitjacket. What was obvious by the 1970s had been invisible two decades earlier. It is both humbling and instructive to notice how often doctor-written histories of psychiatry ignore the embarrassing fact that in 1949 Egas Moniz, like Wagner-Jauregg before him, was awarded the Nobel Prize.

Freud himself believed that mental processes would eventually find biophysical explanations, and some physical models of mental disease have found success, especially in genetics and psychopharmacology. In the latter half of this century, Alzheimer's disease moved out of the realm of psychiatry into neurology, genetics, and pharmacology. Studies of twins with schizophrenia examined the old theories of heredity in the light of modern genetics. Certain drugs have been found to be effective in the care of a variety of psychic conditions. Bromides were introduced as sedatives in the nineteenth century, and by 1928 they were so popular that they accounted for 20 per cent of all prescriptions (Alexander and Selesnick 1966, 287). But sedatives did little for persons with major psychotic disorders. In the mid-twentieth century, asylums were still full of people who could neither support nor care for themselves. This situation changed dramatically with the advent of effective psychoactive drugs.

The first major tranquillizers were derived from *Rauwolfia serpentina*, the snakeroot plant, long known in Asia for sedative properties; its products were also used for the treatment of hypertension, despite many unacceptable side effects. Phenothiazines were discovered as a side product of antihistamine research and introduced in the form of chlorpromazine in 1952 by the French psychiatrists Pierre G. Deniker and Jean Delay. Despite their many side effects – hepatitis, photosensitivity, tardive dyskinesia, and reduced seizure threshold – the phenothiazines did not cause as much drowsiness as earlier agents, while they calmed agitated patients, reduced the frequency of hallucination, and partially restored disordered thought patterns. They were brought to North America in 1954 by the Canadian Heinz Lehmann, who first used chlorpromazine at the Verdun Protestant Hospital in Montreal.

Other psychoactive drugs have contributed to our concepts of mental disease. Two types of mood elevators, first the monoamine oxidase (MAO) inhibitors and then the tricyclic antidepressants, were introduced in 1956–7 for the treatment of depression. Minor tranquillizers in the form of benzodiazepines, beginning with chlordiazepoxide (Librium) and then diazepam (Valium), were initially applied to depressive states. Now they are used to control anxiety, but in the 1960s they may have been overprescribed, especially to women.

More impressive was the effect of lithium on manic-depressive illness. In 1949 the Australian John F.J. Cade was looking for toxins in mania. His strange experiment studied the relative quantities of human urine needed to kill guinea pigs: manic urine from psychotic patients was more lethal than normal urine, but it became less lethal when mixed with lithium. After experimenting with the administration of lithium (without urine), first on guinea pigs, then on himself, he gave the drug to manic individuals with startling success. Lithium results in improvement so marked and so specific that it has been taken as proof of the organic nature of bipolar disorder.

The advent of phenothiazines and lithium resulted in a deinstitutionalization movement, or what historians call 'decarceration,' as the asylums emptied in the late 1960s and early 1970s. Public consternation was roused when group homes and outpatient facilities were created. Hallucinogenic drugs, such as LSD (a derivative of ergotamine and mescaline), seemed to mimic psychotic states and were employed in studies of psychosis. But in the midst of these pharmacologic successes, less felicitous outcomes tracked the use of other drugs, such as amphetamines and vitamin B_3.

Drugs are now used as a mainstay for psychosis and as adjuvants to psychotherapy for other problems. Some psychiatrists observe that they rely on biological methods, leaving psychic methods for psychologists. For fiscal and pharmacological reasons, most psychiatric patients are managed outside hospitals; but some relate the 1990s increase in homelessness to the inability of untreated and uncared-for psychotics to manage on their own.

Antipsychiatry Movement

Mental diseases still continue to be diagnosed 'eighteenth-century

---

The Great Canadian Schizophrenia Controversy

Beginning the mid-1950s, the team of Abram Hoffer and Humphry Osmond of Saskatchewan began to explore mega-doses of vitamins in the treatment of acute schizophrenia. Their experiment was prompted by concern over the side effects of the new psychoactive drugs and by biochemical understanding of the disease. Their popular claims to success were disputed and eventually rejected by the psychiatric establishment in Canada and the United States. In 1976 they marshalled the support of Nobel laureate Linus Pauling and responded with a blistering attack on the objectivity of their critics, the questionable methods of funding in psychiatry research, and the putative value of double-blind methodology in randomized controlled trials.

---

style' by observation of symptoms and behaviour. In open recognition of the subjectivity of such an approach, the American Psychiatric Association sponsored the production of the first *Diagnostic and Statistical Manual* (DSM-I, 1952). Like an annotated nosological tree, the DSM strives for standards in nomenclature and diagnosis by providing statistical analyses of many similar cases. Since 1952, and through four subsequent revisions at decreasing intervals (1968, 1980, 1987, 1994), new diseases are recognized, defined, and subdivided; others are eliminated. Decisions to establish or delete categories are taken by a panel of distinguished experts.

In parallel with this endeavour to standardize diagnosis and eliminate bias, an antipsychiatry movement emerged, motivated by abuses of the physical therapies and the failures and inaccessiblities of psychoanalysis. Some find it ironic that antipsychiatry grew during the period of psychopharmacologic achievements, the merits of which the movement refuses to acknowledge. Informed by the philosophies of social criticism, including feminism and Marxism, antipsychiatry strives to delineate and prevent abuses of power. Former patients are called 'survivors,' diagnosis is viewed with scepticism, and all treatments, including psychotherapy, are seen as methods of control, while psychiatry itself has become the enemy, if not the disease. The conflict between psychiatric power and self-determinism was vividly expressed in the acclaimed Hollywood film *One Flew Over the Cuckoo's Nest* (1975), loosely based on the novel by Ken Kesey. Like psychoanalysis, antipsychiatry has become an icon of popular culture.

Antipsychiatry garnered support from knowledgeable insiders such as Thomas Szasz, who claims that mental illness is a myth, because it does not fit the medical model. His stance exemplifies the extent to which organic-based diagnosis has permeated our world view; but it has a fundamental weakness. What, in Szasz's opinion, would happen to these 'nondiseases' if a physical basis for them were found? Would they become real diseases after all, like the many mental disorders that were quickly transmuted into neurological, metabolic, or chemical problems? For example, within a decade of EEG, epilepsy was distinguished from hysterical convulsions. Similarly, the efficacy of lithium argues for the chemical basis of bipolar disorders; and the advent of histamine-2-antagonists, Helicobacter pylori, and β-blockers closed prolix discussions of the personalities predisposing to ulcer disease and high blood pressure. Will the advent of technological diagnosis or an effective pharmaceutical invalidate the earlier psychic observations and correlations? Does it mean that they are wrong or nonexistent? Does 'pre-organic' suffering deserve to be ignored? Or, is psychiatric wisdom no longer relevant in a reductionist medical world?

An Ontario antipsychiatry periodical, *Phoenix Rising*, presented full-issue reports with dramatic titles: 'Death by Psychiatry,' 'A Close Up Look at the Enemy' (i.e., psychiatrists), 'Psychiatry Kills,' and 'Abolish Forced Psychiatric Treatment.' It inspired several spinoff publications, including David Reville's personal account of six months in Kingston Psychiatric Hospital, called *Don't Spyhole Me.* Support of *Phoenix Rising* was provided by the Ontario Arts Council until late 1988, when the folly of government-funded criticism of government-funded medical endeavour was exposed. The funds were withdrawn, sending *Phoenix Rising* into an irreversible death spiral.

Despite the fate of the phoenix, the antipsychiatry movement has come to pervade the field of medical history, where the debates within psychiatry itself are now championed by its historians. As described by the pro-biological-psychiatry historian Edward Shorter, 'zealot historians,' imbued with aberrant Freudian thought, peer at shameful episodes of the past through biased lenses. In contrast, historians, like Andrew Scull, remind us that Shorter's zealots strive only to use the language of the past in its context, especially since it is still early days to be claiming triumph over mental illness: 'chlorpromazine is no penicillin,' Scull wrote. Some episodes may be unpleasant to recall, but they should not be forgotten.

A Canadian example is the 'psychic driving' experiments conducted by Donald Ewen Cameron at the Allan Memorial Institute in Montreal in the mid-1950s. Born in Scotland and trained in the United States at Johns Hopkins University and in Switzerland, Cameron's first job was in Manitoba, where he organized a network of mental health clinics. In 1943 he was recruited to McGill by the Yale-trained neurosurgeon, Wilder Penfield. Two years later he was one of three North American psychiatrists invited to Nuremberg to assess the Nazi leader, Rudolf Hess. There he learned of the atrocities committed by Nazi doctors in the name of science. A medical historian, Werner Leibrandt, who was a witness for the prosecution at Nuremberg, suggested that Nazi doctors (45 per cent of all German doctors) laboured under an attitude called 'biological thought,' in which the patient had become simply an object for scientific study. Despite his trip to Nuremberg, Cameron would commit similar crimes.

In the postwar climate, Cameron and his colleagues feared the mind-control capacities of communist enemies. The aura of urgency and international importance led him to investigate ways of preventing mind control by creating it. In short, he experimented on mentally ill patients by administering so-called treatments that were not only unnecessary but damaging. Secret funding for his research came from the Canadian government and the U.S. Central Intelligence Agency.

Cameron had hoped that his institute at McGill would become the first successful centre for psychosomatic or biological psychiatry. In the mid-1950s, with his associate Hassan Azima, he developed 'psychic driving' by modifying a Russian technique of sleep treatment: patients were heavily sedated with the newly discovered tranquillizers, occasionally combined with hallucinogenic drugs. While asleep for hours, days, or weeks, they were forced to listen to repetitive, tape-recorded, personal messages that often dwelt on their faults. The theory used to justify such torture was that the regression so induced would disrupt resistance to psychotherapy.

In 1956 Cameron announced the success of his technique. But the real story, which emerged only thirty years later, is that many of his patients were irreparably damaged by the brainwashing – stripped of their personalities, their livelihood, and their families. Cameron's relationship with Penfield cooled, and he left Montreal in 1964 to direct a laboratory in Albany, New York. He died three years later with his reputation intact, having risen to the highest prominence in psychiatry, serving at various times as president of the Quebec Psychiatric Association, the Canadian Psychiatric Association, the American Psychiatric Association, the World Psychiatric Association, the American Psychopathological Association, and the Society for Biological Psychiatry. In 1992 the Canadian government compensated the victims of Cameron's psychic-driving experiments.

Ambivalent Status of Psychoanalysis

Important questions are raised by the definition of psychiatric diagnoses and by acceptance of therapies. Psychoanalysis is only partially reimbursed by Canadian health insurance and most patients must pay for this expensive treatment themselves. Payment of fees for outpatient psychotherapy is being reconsidered in Ontario, although recent assurances suggest it is secure for a few more years.

Yet why should psychotherapy be disallowed? Is it too expensive – or ineffective? Or inegalitarian in a society that demands equality for everyone in everything? Or is it because psychotherapy tends to downplay the importance of biological causes? And what will result from this change? Will it guarantee that only the wealthy will be able to afford psychotherapy and that the poor and middle classes will be increasingly obliged to accept drugs? Will it constitute a public pronouncement on the physicality of psychiatric illness?

Psychiatric diagnoses are made on the basis of observation, after the elimination of disorders with identifiable organic causes. A decision must be made about whether or not the behaviour, thought, and mood are appropriate or inappropriate, healthy or sick. Equating inappropriate behaviour with sickness leaves psychiatry open to the biases of culture, race, religion, politics, and class. In other words, in psychiatry more than in any other medical field, the definition of normal can be ethnocentric.

Historians have shown that biases contaminated psychiatry in the past. For example, asylums were used in the former Soviet Union to incarcerate political dissenters. In North America, hundreds of women were castrated because they could not conform to societal norms of comportment. Poor people and criminals have been kept in asylums in the absence of disease and sometimes over the protests of asylum keepers. Cultural beliefs, such as the evil eye and voodoo, also have been subjected to the psychiatric analysis of a different but dominant society. Certification has been used as a means of control, and mentally disturbed individuals have been stripped of their rights and inappropriately mutilated by experimentation. It would be naïve to suppose that our present system is devoid of prejudice.

With the rise in social criticism, some conditions previously thought of as sicknesses have become variations of normal; for example, homosexuality. In ancient Greece, homosexuality was tolerated. In Judeo-Christian cultures, it was a sin and, by extension, it also became a crime. In the late nineteenth century, it was retrieved from moral disapprobation (if not legal) and reconstituted as a disease by Richard von Krafft-Ebing and Henry Havelock Ellis. When I was at medical school in the early 1970s, homosexuality was still a disease, but physicians were uncomfortable with that label. As a disease, homosexuality theoretically required treatment, and if treatment was unavailable, then research should be undertaken. But homosexuality was not life threatening, it was rarely 'curable,' and few of its 'sufferers' wanted to be cured. Instead, homosexuals wished that society could be cured of its intolerance.

One way of dealing with an 'incurable' condition that does not kill is to decide that those who have it are not sick. In 1973 homosexuality was deleted from the DSM by a non-unanimous vote of mostly male, mostly white, mostly heterosexual psychiatrists. A heated debate followed over retaining an entry for homosexuals who were uncomfortable with their sexual orientation. Now, a quarter of a century later, homosexuality is recognized as a variation of normal. Changes in the cultural and sociopolitical climate have contributed to this decision.

Should the existence of diseases be decided by the votes of highly educated upper-middle-class professionals? Are physical diagnoses determined in this way, or is universal agreement implicit in their first definitions? How often were votes cast on the status of appendicitis? Diabetes? Leukemia? Epilepsy? Cancer? Arthritis? Should our recognition of psychiatry's special vulnerability and cultural subjectivity allow us to reject this method of diagnosis? My answer is no.

Psychiatry is a fascinating blend of sensitive humanitarian ideals with the latest in pharmacological and neurological research. Its goal is to help unhappy people move from chronic incapacity to contented living and self-sufficiency. Positive outcomes restore the well-being of patients and their contributions to communities. Perhaps the old ambition to effect radical cures for 'diseases' which had yet to be delineated has been softened to a more realistic yet worthy aim to help people adjust to themselves and their world. The successful practice of psychiatry is not hampered by acknowledging its vulnerability through an awareness of the triumphs and transgressions in its past. In history as in analysis, 'being entirely honest with oneself is a good exercise' (Freud, 15 Oct. 1897, in *Origins*, 1954, 223).

Suggestions for Further Reading

Alexander, Franz G., and Sheldon T. Selesnick. *The History of Psychiatry: An Evaluation of Psychiatric Thought and Practice from Prehistoric Times to the Present.* New York: Harper Row, 1966

Ayd, Frank J., and Barry Blackwell, eds. *Discoveries in Biological Psychiatry.* Philadelphia: Lippincott, 1970

Bayer, Ronald, and Robert L. Spitzer. 'Edited Correspondence on the Status of Homosexuality in DSM-III.' *Journal of the History of the Behavioral Sciences* 18 (1982), 32–52

Bonduelle, Michel, Toby Gelfand, and Christopher G. Goetz. *Charcot: Constructing Neurology.* New York: Oxford University Press, 1995

Braslow, Joel T. *Mental Ills and Bodily Cures: Psychiatric Treatment in the First Half of the Twentieth Century.* Berkeley: University of California Press, 1997

Bynum, W.F., and Roy Porter, eds. *The Anatomy of Madness: Essays in the History of Psychiatry.* 3 vols. London and New York: Tavistock, 1985–8

Dols, Michael W. *Majnun: The Madman in Medieval Islamic Society.* Ed. Diana E. Immisch. Oxford: Clarendon, 1992

Dowbiggin, Ian R. *Inheriting Madness: Professionalization and Psychiatric Knowledge in Nineteenth-Century France.* Berkeley, Calif.: University of California Press, 1991

Ellenberger, Henri F. *The Discovery of the Unconscious: The History and Evolution of Dynamic Psychiatry.* New York: Basic Books, 1970

Foucault, Michel. *Madness and Civilization: A History of Insanity in the Age of Reason.* Trans. Richard Howard. New York: Vintage Books, 1973

Freud, Sigmund. *The Origins of Psychoanalysis.* Ed. Marie Bonaparte, Anna Freud, and Ernst Kris. Trans. Eric Mosbacher and James Strachey. New York: Basic Books, 1954

Gelfand, Toby, and John Kerr, eds. *Freud and the History of Psychoanalysis.* Hillsdale, N.J.: Analytic Press, 1992

Goldstein, Jan. *Console and Classify: The French Psychiatric Profession in the Nineteenth Century.* Cambridge and New York: Cambridge University Press, 1987

Hansen, Bert. 'American Physicians' "Discovery" of Homosexuals, 1880–1900: A New Diagnosis in a Changing Society.' In *Framing Disease: Studies in Cultural History,* ed. Charles E. Rosenberg and Janet Golden, 104–33. New Brunswick, N.J.: Rutgers University Press, 1992

Jackson, Stanley W., *Melancholia and Depression: From Hippocratic Times to Modern Times.* New Haven: Yale University Press, 1986

MacDonald, Michael. *Mystical Bedlam: Madness, Anxiety, and Healing in Seventeenth-Century England.* Cambridge and New York: Cambridge University Press, 1981

Malcolm, Janet. *In the Freud Archives.* New York: Vintage Books, 1985

Micale, Mark S., and Roy Porter, eds. *Discovery of the History of Psychiatry.* Oxford: Oxford University Press, 1994

Pigeaud, Jackie. *Folie et cures de la folie chez les médecins de l'antiquité greco-romaine.* Paris: Belles lettres, 1987

Postel, Jacques, and Claude Quetel. *Nouvelle histoire de la psychiatrie.* 2nd edn. Paris: Dunod, 1994

Pressman, Jack D. *Last Resort: Psychosurgery and the Limits of Medicine.* Cambridge and New York: Cambridge University Press, 1998

Scull, Andrew T. *The Most Solitary of Afflictions: Madness and Society in Britain, 1700–1900.* New Haven and London: Yale University Press, 1993

– 'Chlorpromazine Is No Penicillin.' *Times Literary Supplement,* 16 May 1997, 8–10

Shorter, Edward. *From the Mind into the Body: The Cultural Origins of Psychosomatic Symptoms.* New York and Toronto: Free Press and Maxwell Macmillan, 1994

– *A History of Psychiatry: From the Era of the Asylum to the Age of Prozac.* New York: Wiley, 1997

Showalter, Elaine. *Hystories: Hysterical Epidemics and Modern Culture.* New York: Columbia University Press, 1997

Simon, Bennett. *Mind and Madness in Ancient Greece: The Classical Roots of Modern Psychiatry.* Ithaca, N.Y.: Cornell University Press, 1978

Szasz, Thomas Stephen. *The Myth of Mental Illness: Foundations of a Theory of Personal Conduct.* 2nd edn. New York: Harper and Row, 1974

Tomes, Nancy. *A Generous Confidence: Thomas Story Kirkbride and the Art of Asylum Keeping, 1840–1883.* Cambridge and New York: Cambridge University Press, 1984

Whyte, Lancelot Law. *The Unconscious before Freud.* New York: St Martin's Press, 1978

On Canada

Brown, Thomas E. 'Foucault Plus Twenty: On the Writing of Canadian Psychiatry in the 1980s.' *Canadian Bulletin of Medical History* 2 (1985), 23–50

Cellard, André. *Histoire de la folie au Québec de 1600 a 1850: Le désordre.* Montreal: Boreal, 1991

Collins, Anne. *In the Sleep Room: The Story of the CIA Brainwashing Experiments in Canada.* Toronto: Lester and Orpen Dennys, 1988

Dubé, Viateur, and André Paradis. *Essais pour une préhistoire de la psychiatrie au Canada, 1800–1885, suivi d'une anthologie de textes.* Trois-Rivières: Université du Québec à Trois-Rivières, Dep. de philosophie, no. 15, 1977

Edginton, Barry. 'Moral Treatment to Monolith: The Institutional Treatment of the Insane in Manitoba, 1871–1919.' *Canadian Bulletin of Medical History* 5 (1988), 167–88

'Half a Century of Stress Research: A Tribute to Hans Selye by His Students and Associates.' *Experientia* 41 (1985), 559–78

Hurd, Henry M. *The Institutional Care of the Insane in the United States and Canada.* 4 vols. Baltimore: Johns Hopkins University Press, 1916–17

Keating, Peter. *La science du mal: L'institution de la psychiatrie au Québec, 1800–1914*. Montreal: Boréal, 1993

Krasnick, Cheryl. '"In Charge of the Loons": A Portrait of the London Ontario Asylum for the Insane in the Nineteenth Century.' *Ontario History* 74 (1982), 138–84

Lowy, F.H., and R.O. Jones. 'The Canadian Certification Examination in Psychiatry. I. Historical Notes.' *Canadian Psychiatric Association Journal* 24 (1979), 275–84

Mitchinson, Wendy. 'Gynecological Operations on Insane Women, London Ontario, 1845–1901.' *Journal of Social History* 15 (1982), 467–84

Paradis, André, Hélène Naubert, and Clémence Bélanger. *Recension bibliographique: Les maladies infectieuses (2) transmissibles sexuellement (blennorragie, chancre mou, syphilis) et les maladies nerveuses et mentales dans les périodiques médicaux québécois du XIX siecle*. Trois-Rivières: Centre interuniversitaire d'études québecoises, Université du Québec à Trois-Rivières, 1995

Parkin, Alan. *A History of Psychoanalysis in Canada*. Toronto: Toronto Psychoanalytic Society, 1987

Reaume, Geoffrey. 'Accounts of Abuse of Patients at the Toronto Hospital for the Insane, 1883–1937.' *Canadian Bulletin of Medical History* 14 (1997), 65–106

Shortt, S.E.D. *Victorian Lunacy: Richard Maurice Bucke and the Practice of Late Nineteenth-Century Psychiatry*. Cambridge: Cambridge University Press, 1986

Simmons, Harvey G. *Unbalanced: Mental Health Policy in Ontario, 1930–1989*. Toronto: Wall and Thompson, 1990

Weinstein, Harvey. *A Father, a Son and the CIA*. Toronto: Lorimer, 1988

Yanacopoulo, Andrée. *Hans Selye, ou, La cathedrale du stress*. Montreal: Le Jour, 1992

CHAPTER THIRTEEN

No Baby, No Nation: History of Pediatrics*

Pediatrics does not deal with miniature men and women, *with reduced doses and the small class of diseases in smaller bodies, but ... has its own independent range and horizon, and gives as much to general medicine as it has received from it.*

Abraham Jacobi, 1889 (cited in P. English 1989, 254)

The wisdom that infants and children were subject to certain specific diseases and problems originated in antiquity. But medical – as opposed to parental – care for children emerged in the seventeenth and eighteenth centuries, together with a marked shift in social attitudes toward children. The specialty of pediatrics (from the Greek words for 'child' and 'healer') did not come into being until the nineteenth century. The history of this specialty cannot be separated from the history of concepts of childhood; in this chapter we will briefly examine both.

Pediatrics has focused on prevention of disease and disability, rather than on cure. To accomplish this goal, it was forced to wrestle with the social and economic determinants of health sooner and more effectively than all other medical endeavours.

*Educational objectives for this chapter are found on p. 399.

Have All Peoples Loved Their Babies?
History of Children and Childhood

With his influential book of 1960, Philippe Ariès claimed that childhood was culturally conditioned – a social construction (see chapters
4 and 7). He meant that care for growing children satisfied social
expectations. How often should a baby be fed? What should it eat?
How should it be dressed? At what games, where, and how often
should it play? What stories may it be told? When and where should
it sleep? And – the most important question for Ariès – should it be
educated? If so, how? Examining evidence from the Middle Ages to
the twentieth century, he found that the answers to these questions
varied widely and had evolved slowly through time. He concluded
that the notion of childhood as a time of innocence, play, and learning was entirely modern.

Several writers modified Ariès's arguments; some cited earlier
authors who had anticipated his ideas. Lloyd de Mause claimed
that child care was an indicator of human civilization as it moved
through six positivistic stages of improvement, beginning with
ancient brutality and ending with modern helping. Others simplified these rigid self-congratulatory categories to manifestations of
economic realities in time and place: were children perceived to
be 'financial assets,' born to increase family wealth and provide
for aging parents? Or were they 'financial liabilities,' whose
upbringing entailed investment and debts willingly incurred? The
extent to which societies embraced one or the other attitude
determined the extent to which children were granted a childhood.

Many scholars now reject the idea that brutality to children ever
formed part of any socially sanctioned tradition. They criticize it as
an unjustified presentist projection upon a scarcely knowable past;
and they point out that infanticide and abuse continue to be significant causes of child mortality in the seemingly civilized First World
of the twentieth century. Nevertheless, all historians who write about
children recognize that the length and nature of childhood has
varied.

Child Care and Health in Antiquity

In antiquity, pediatrics did not form a distinct body of medical knowledge. Several historians scoured extant ancient texts to dredge up references to children. The Hippocratic Corpus (of the fifth century B.C.) includes treatises on dentition and on premature infants, while the famous *Sacred Disease*, shows that astute observations on child patients were made.

On Childhood Epilepsy

Such as are habituated to their disease have a presentiment [aura] when an attack is imminent ... Young children at first fall anywhere, because they are unfamiliar with the disease; but when they have suffered several attacks, on having the presentiment they run to their mothers or to somebody they know very well, through fear and terror at what they are suffering.

Hippocrates, *Sacred Disease*, XV

References to children appear in the works of Celsus (first century A.D.), Soranus of Ephesus, Aretaeus, and Galen (all in the second century), and Oribasius (fourth century). Childhood diseases that are recognized in antiquity include *aphthae* (thought perhaps to be ulcers, thrush, or diphtheria), hydrocephalus, rickets, ophthalmia, rashes, 'epilepsy' (infantile convulsions), and *seiriasis* (possibly meningitis or dehydration). By their very scarcity, however, these citations indicate that the professional medicine of ancient Greece was generally not for kids. As if to endorse this conclusion, Mettler recalled that one of the most detailed ancient accounts of human birth is found in Aristotle's *History of Animals*. Children may have been the property of their fathers, as were their mothers and slaves; however, responsibility for their care resided with women – mothers, midwives, and wet-nurses – not with doctors.

What was baby care in antiquity? At birth, children were 'salted' with alkaline soda ash, avoiding the eyes, and then washed to remove the vernix. This practice probably arose in prehistory, and it persisted until approximately 1000 A.D. The Arabic authors preferred oil to soda ash, and later writers recommended dilute wine. Infants were 'swaddled' (bound tightly) to prevent movement, to keep them warm, and to ensure that they would grow straight. Sometimes they were hung on hooks to keep them out of the way. Breast milk was the food of choice. The obstetrical treatise of Soranus of Ephesus described the 'fingernail test' to assess the quality of mothers' milk: a drop should retain its form, being neither too runny nor too thick. This test was still being cited in the eighteenth-century work of William Smellie (see chapter 11). When a year old, the child would be offered gruel mixtures of honey, sprouts, barley porridge, and goat's or cow's milk. For irritability associated with teething and other ailments, infants were drugged with opium or wine.

Controversial evidence, both literary and demographic, from ancient Greece and Rome suggests that deformed infants and sometimes healthy females were left to die, but how many newborns perished in this way is unknown. Wealthy women used paid wet-nurses, and the practice eventually spread to all social classes, even slaves. Breast-feeding was known to be contraceptive; a slave was more 'useful' if her baby was sent away to be nursed, allowing the mother both to work and to breed another future slave. If a child fell ill, medicine would be given to the wet-nurse for transmission to her charge through her milk. If wet-nurses could not be found, artificial feeding preoccupied those who cared for orphaned or abandoned children. But effective compositions were elusive, and the mechanics of feeding small infants from sponges, spouts, boats, and spoons were complicated and risky. Until the twentieth century, artificial feeding usually meant disaster.

What we know of child care is derived not only from written sources but from artwork and from objects such as infant feeding vessels, catheters, cradles, clothing, shoes, amulets, and toys. Some congenital deformities, including dwarfism, club foot, and dislocated hip, can be recognized in ancient art. The Canadian pediatrician and nutritionist Theodore G.H. Drake amassed and researched an extensive collection of prints, books, and artifacts, including 250 feeding vessels, from antiquity to the present, now the property of the Canadian Museum of Health Care in Toronto (see Spaulding and Welch 1991).

Arabic, Medieval, and Renaissance Pediatrics

Arabic authors adopted the infant-care practices of their Greco-Roman precursors, but they also acknowledged society's responsibility for children. Perhaps because the prophet Mohammed had been an orphan, the Koran laid out provisions for children of divorced or deceased parents. It also condemned female infanticide and discrimination against women.

Again, evidence of 'pediatrics' in the Middle Ages is scant; most medical writings scarcely mention children. The tenth-century Persian, Rhazes (see chapter 4), distinguished smallpox from measles on the basis of symptoms and signs, recognizing their peculiarities in children; however, diseases thought to afflict children had changed little since antiquity. In his *Canon*, Ibn Sina (Avicenna) compiled views of his predecessors on infant ailments. Like them, he envisaged the wet-nurse as a therapeutic instrument; for example, a baby should not be bled, but the nurse might be bled or cupped on its behalf. Even female medical writers who might be expected to have had some existential familiarity with child care, including Dame Trot of Salerno and Hildegard of Bingen, refer to birthing, but say little about children.

The relative silence of medieval medics on the subject should not allow us to suppose that there was no tradition or theory in child care. This knowledge lay in oral traditions conveyed by wise (but illiterate) women to other women, beyond the sphere of learned men. The German historian Karl Sudhoff studied multiple manuscript copies of two treatises on the care of children, dating from the sixth to ninth century. The authors and their intended audience are unknown, but the treatises describe practices similar to those outlined in ancient and Arabic writings (see Ruhräh 1925, 22–6).

Another indicator that oral tradition played a role in child care is the special genre of pediatric poems. Shortly after the advent of

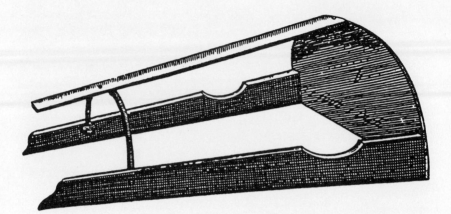

Arcutio, a device to prevent overlying. Inside the frame, a baby could not be accidently crushed by a parent who shared the bed. From *Philosophical Transactions* 422 (1732), opp. 223

printing, versified works on the care of babies and children appeared in the vernacular, rather than in Latin. The *Versehung des Leibs* (Proper Care of the Body) was composed by the monk Heinrich von Louffenburg and was printed in 1491 from a 1429 manuscript held in Munich. The inspiration is said to have been a much older and much-copied Latin manuscript, the *Regimen sanitatis* of Salerno (ca. 1000 A.D.). The appearance of these poems in the fifteenth century does not imply that they originated at that time. Like the songs of Homer, Norse sagas, nursery rhymes, and the Anglo-Saxon *Beowulf*, these poems may have been chanted for generations in easy-to-remember verse before being preserved in writing.

Christianity disapproved of infanticide, abortion, and contraception; the practices may have declined but did not disappear. Children continued to be sold or stolen into slavery; others were maimed to make them more effective beggars. A new cause of child death emerged during the Middle Ages – 'overlying' – and a special device, the *arcutio*, was invented to prevent the supposed fatal accident of an adult lying on a child who shared the same bed. Scholars now doubt the realistic probability of overlying, suggesting that this 'disease' may have been invented to conceal murder.

In contrast to the silence of previous writers, the earliest printed books on medicine were new works on diseases of children. Paolo Bagellardi published the first treatise devoted solely to childhood diseases – *De regimine infantiae* (On the life of children). It was printed in Padua in 1472. The following year, Bartholomaeus Metlinger of Augsburg produced a work in the German vernacular. A decade later, Cornelius Roelans did the same, but his book is so rare that only two copies are known to exist. Rösslin's much-reprinted midwifery treatise, *Rosengarten* (1513), also contained advice on child care (see chapter 11). The illustrated 1577 treatise of Omnibonus Ferrarius contained images of various ambitious gadgets, including a breast pump, a helmet to prevent head injury, a walker, and a toilet chair. Finally, Hieronymus Mercurialis of Padua prepared a compendium of children's diseases, which was liberally annotated with observations on parasitic worms and other topics. Artificial feeding continued to be an important preoccupation, and recipes were provided for broth, called 'panada,' and flour-based mixtures called 'pap.' Rather than presenting new discoveries, these books compiled the knowledge of the ancients and the Persians, finally bringing the child to the attention of medical practitioners.

Enlightenment: Diseases and the Discovery of Child Mortality

During the seventeenth and eighteenth centuries, two parallel processes emphasized the health status of children: first, nosology, or the definition of specific childhood diseases; second, the rise in medical statistics.

Nosology arose from a study of symptoms to classify and distinguish diseases as separate entities (see chapter 4). Most conditions had been recognized in antiquity, but a few new accounts of ailments peculiar to children distinguished them from other sufferers. Picking up where the tenth-century Rhazes had left off with his separation of measles and smallpox, several children's diseases were described in the seventeenth century (see table 13.1).

By 1689, Walter Harris of London had assembled many disease descriptions into a Latin treatise, which has been called the first modern textbook of acute pediatric diseases. The reputation of this

Table 13.1
'Classic' descriptions of childhood disease from the seventeenth century

---

Chicken pox (Chanael 1610)
Chorea (Sydenham 1686)
Cretinism (Plat[t]er 1625)
Diphtheria (Villareal 1611)
Neonatal syphilis (Guillemeau 1609)
Neonatal tetanus (Andreu 1678)
Rheumatism (Baillou 1640)
Rickets, or rachitism (Reusner 1582; Whistler 1645; Glisson 1650)
Scabies (Wurtz 1612)
Scarlet fever (Sennert 1641; Sydenham 1676),
Thrush (Wurtz 1612)
Thymic death (Plat[t]er 1614)
Whooping cough (Baillou 1640; Willis 1675)

---

book, one historian said, extended 'far beyond its merits'; yet he acknowledged the impact of the eighteen editions published over the next half century in English, French, German, and Latin (Still 1931, 291). Harris's treatise found an English successor in Michael Underwood's 1784 work, the last edition of which appeared nearly sixty years later. Extending the nosology of the preceding century, Underwood described neonatal icterus, poliomyelitis, and congenital heart disease. In the United States, Benjamin Rush gave a new account of the ancient cholera infantum, a form of diarrhea and vomiting that was called the 'summer complaint.' These descriptions of specific diseases invited a search for specific cures.

The second process to captivate the attention of would-be pediatricians was the shocking revelation of high mortality rates among children across Europe and North America. Because Islam and Christianity both condemned infanticide, formal provision was made for orphaned or abandoned infants. Beginning in 787 in Milan, asylums had operated throughout continental Europe, founded by bishops, priests, and other clerics, one of whom was St Vincent de Paul. But these dwellings were unlike the hospitals of today, although some, like Florence's Hospital of the Innocents, bore the name. Instead, they were warehouses rather than places of healing. Children were brought in the wagons of porters, who commanded fees for use of their regular circuits. To provide anonymity

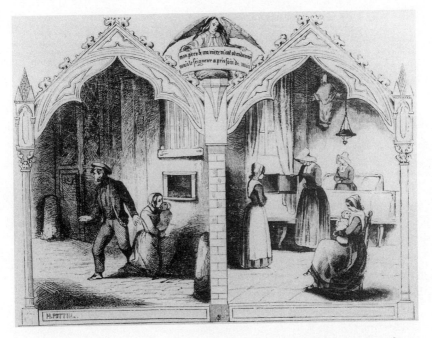

Enfants trouvés: Le tour, extérieur et intérieur. Engraving by Henri Pottin, after a seventeenth-century original. A foundling home. Outside, the parents leave their infant; inside, the nuns make ready to retrieve the babe. Drake Collection, Canadian Museum of Health and Medicine, Toronto

and to avoid exposure of infants awaiting discovery at the asylum door, the turnstile, called 'tour' (turn) in both English and French, was invented. Cities ran fostering systems for nurslings until they could feed themselves. Survivors were cared for, taught a trade, and eventually released, usually by the age of eight. Mothers of illegitimate infants were sometimes welcomed if they nursed their own children and one or more of the others.

The eighteenth-century discovery of the high mortality rates in these institutions seems to have come as a horrifying surprise. Furthermore, the rates were rising. Philip Gavitt demonstrated that foundling mortality in fifteenth-century Florence ranged from 12 to 60 per cent, and Joan Sherwood showed that in the Inclusa of Madrid three hundred years later, the annual death rates ranged between 53 and 87 per cent of admissions, with a rising trend. Economic and cultural factors meant that admissions increased, alms declined, and the price of wheat rose; more mouths to feed and fewer resources to pay for wet-nurses and provisions.

In Paris on the eve of the revolution, between five and six thousand children were abandoned annually. According to Dora Weiner, these numbers had been increasing steadily throughout the eighteenth century. Whether the foundlings were placed in the various city hospices or were fostered in the countryside, about 60 per cent succumbed in their first year; another 30 per cent died before the age of five. In London, a similar picture emerged. Bills of mortality from 1730 to 1750 reveal that 75 per cent of all infants did not live five years. The carnage did not respect class boundaries: Queen Anne bore seventeen or eighteen children, but none survived childhood. In any year, 40 per cent of all deaths were of children under five. The historian Daniel Teysseire, who analysed references to children in the *Encyclopédie* (1751–77) of Denis Diderot and Jean d'Alembert, concluded that to be a child in eighteenth-century France was to be sick. With the Industrial Revolution and the privations associated with poorly remunerated labour in factories and sweat shops, the health even of children who had not been abandoned or institutionalized began to deteriorate.

Malthus on Foundling Homes

The greatest part of this premature mortality is clearly to be attributed to these institutions, miscalled philanthropic ...

If a person wished to check population, and were not solicitous about the means, he could not propose a more effectual measure than the establishment of a sufficient number of foundling hospitals.

T.R. Malthus, *Essay on the Principle of Population*, bk 2, iii
(1803; reprint, Cambridge, 1989), 177–9

The fate of innocent children became a matter of national pride.

With a newly rising liberalism in social and political thought, and the ideas of philosophers like physician John Locke and Jean-Jacques Rousseau, the value of an extended period of youthful learning and play was endorsed. Combined with the appalling statistics, the new numerical methods in medicine also turned medical minds to prevention. The bleak outlook shamed reformers into action. But what exactly should or could be done to save the lives of children?

The Dawn of Child Welfare

Once they fell ill of the acute illnesses that tended to plague them, children rarely survived; it had to be admitted that medicine could not save them. On the other hand, most children were born healthy; the goal should be to keep them that way. Reformers moved on several levels at once: dispensaries and hospitals; policies to promote hygiene; advice literature; medical and surgical research; and legislation.

What Mothers Want and What They Need

La mère veut que son enfant soit heureux, qu'il le soit dès à présent, en cela elle a raison; quand elle se trompe sur les moyens, il faut l'éclairer.
(The mother wishes that her child be happy, as long as he is, she is right; when she is wrong in her methods, it is necessary to enlighten her.)

Jean-Jacques Rousseau, epigraph in Michael Underwood,
Traité sur les maladies des enfants (1784; trans., Québec:
Nouvelle Imprimerie, 1803)

Hygiene and Advice

Philanthropists tried to improve conditions in foundling homes, and they also created dispensaries for free care, in a process similar to the concurrent asylum movement for the mentally ill (see chapter

12). Unlike major cities in the rest of Europe, London had no children's hospice until after the realization of the high mortality rates. In response, the merchant Thomas Coram established London's Foundling Hospital in 1741; however, this gathering of healthy infants could not guarantee their survival. Coram and his reformers were immediately challenged on how to keep motherless children alive; once again, artificial feedings proved to be a failure. An advocate of artificial feeding ('dry-nursing'), George Armstrong opened a dispensary for the free care of the ailing 'infant poor' of London in 1767. Armstrong also wrote a description of pyloric stenosis. Three years later, a rival dispensary was inaugurated under the supervision of J.C. Lettsom, who launched vitriolic attacks on Armstrong. Philanthropy had become politically correct, and physicians vied for the spotlight. From 1730 to 1810, the London bills of mortality showed a steady decline in mortality before age five (from 75 to 40 per cent). Similarly, in postrevolutionary France, with the new provisions for cleanliness and accountability at child-care institutions, mortality of abandoned infants under five supposedly fell from 83 per cent in 1798 to 13.5 per cent in 1813.

The education of parents, especially the poor, became yet another arm of this multipronged attack on infant mortality. Medical experts took up the venerable practice of offering advice on how to rear healthy children. Guidelines for the London Foundling Hospital were based on the 1748 *Essay* of William Cadogan, who wrote (at first anonymously) against a tide of tradition by prescribing loose clothing (rather than swaddling), daily bathing, and maternal breast-feeding. In 1761 the Swiss hygienist Simon A. Tissot laid down rules for physical and mental health, through heating and aeration of homes, moderate diet, and exercise. Tissot was one of the first to describe the dangers of masturbation, which was much touted as a cause of somatic and moral degeneration until well into the twentieth century. Similar instructions emerged in Germany, where 'school hygiene' originated. In his 1780 treatise, Johann Peter Frank stipulated the state's obligations to care for and to educate children. Frank's work inspired the widely distributed and oft-translated *Catechism of Health* (1794) by Bernhard C. Faust. Inadvertently, or perhaps deliberately, however, the social hygiene movement tended to blame mothers and nurses for the suffering and loss of their children.

Communicating this wisdom to the often illiterate masses, especially to mothers, was not always easy. In some places, monetary rewards for the survival and number of children were established. Remnants of these programs survive today: France and Quebec maintain tax relief and price reductions for *familles nombreuses*, as part of an active pro-natalist policy. The rising literacy of women opened the door for advice literature for families – almanacs and self-help manuals – led by the multi-edition *Domestic Medicine* of William Buchan. Addressed to a rural elite, these 'family physician' books were novel in their emphasis on child care. Academic physicians also participated in the movement. In Germany, the distinguished liberal professor, Christoph W. Hufeland, published a vulgarization, *The Art of Prolonging Human Life*, just as he launched an early medical periodical. Similarly, the 1803 Quebec edition of Michael Underwood's treatise summarized his recommendations to mothers of ailing children. The practice continued with the work of Severin Lachapelle, professor of hygiene in Montreal, who wrote several advice manuals for the general public and translated the popular *Practical Home Physician* of the Chicago professor, Henry M. Lyman. Recommendations could vary widely, and some confident pronouncements on neonatal feeding now seem quite peculiar – for example, the early introduction of egg, or the withholding of banana. With modifications in specifics, this tradition continues into the present with the popular manual of Dr Spock (see below).

Medical and Surgical Advances

Anatomical research on childhood diseases led to surgical and medical solutions for long-standing problems. Even the fetus began to receive attention when in 1827 Hufeland wrote a treatise on diseases *in utero*. The life-saving method of tracheotomy for diphtheria, first suggested by several authors in the early seventeenth century, was promoted by Pierre Bretonneau in 1826. Chief among these impressive achievements was Jenner's discovery, published in 1798, that cowpox could protect people from smallpox (see chapter 7).

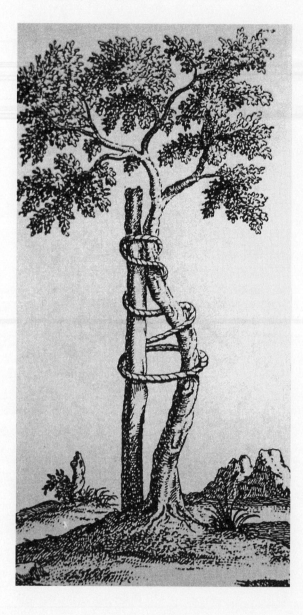

The tethered tree symbolizing the goals of orthopedics. From Nicolas Andry, *Orthopedia, or the Art of Correcting and Preventing Deformities in Children*, vol. 1, 1743, opp. 211

Chronic ailments also received attention. In 1741 Nicolas Andry introduced the word *orthopédie* (derived from the Greek for 'straight' and 'child'). His treatise described procedures for the correction of club foot and hip disorders, but not all his recommendations were surgical; he also prescribed for tics, chlorosis (anemia), rashes, nail problems, pimples, warts, lisping, and stuttering. Deaf children were taught to communicate through the efforts of T.H. Gallaudet in the United States and J.M.G. Itard in France.

Finally, medicine and surgery had something to offer sick or disabled children. Special hospitals were created for the specific treatment (as opposed to warehousing) of children suffering from specific diseases. Paris opened the world's first such children's hospital in April 1802. Infants with neonatal syphilis were transferred immediately to a special venereal hospital at Vaugirard, where they were 'treated,' in the ancient tradition – through wet-nurses taking mercury for their own syphilitic afflictions. Children's hospitals also appeared in Germany (1840s), London (1852), New York (1854), Philadelphia (1855), Edinburgh (1860), Chicago (1865), Boston (1869, after an 1846 precursor had closed), and Toronto (1875). Physicians hoped that these hospitals would provide treatment, as well as human resources for further research. Since most inpatients were poor and uneducated, reformers also envisaged the hospital as a locus of moral training.

Professionalization of Pediatrics

The following decades saw the professionalization of pediatrics as its own specialty, defined by professorships, associations, and journals. Many new periodicals devoted solely to child health were launched between the 1790s and 1920s (for a list, see Garrison and Abt 1965, 125–30). A chair in pediatrics was inaugurated in Paris in 1879, and in Berlin in 1894, while professional associations for pediatrics were founded in Germany (1883), Moscow (1885), and the United States (1888). The American specialty board was created in 1933; its Canadian equivalent in 1937, with certification being granted in 1942 by 'grandfathering' and in 1946 by examination.

Convinced that social solutions could be found for biological problems, many pediatricians maintained links to political liberal-

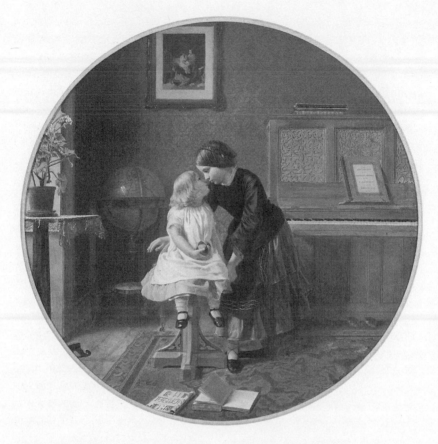

Enfance, by James Collinson, 1855. National Gallery of Canada

ism. The first president of the American Pediatric Society, Abraham Jacobi, had left his native Germany after the right-wing revolution of 1848. As the pediatrician and historian Peter C. English argues, Jacobi's vision of pediatrics was predicated on his concept of social intervention to disrupt the continuing high mortality in foundling homes (which was still 75 per cent or greater). Jacobi thought that the main killers of children, especially diarrhea and respiratory illness, could be eradicated only by attacking the underlying problems of poverty and housing.

The arrival of the new professional bodies followed hard upon Koch's 1882 discovery of the mycobacterium tuberculosis and the concomitant realization that the notorious killer, consumption, could be spread through milk. Pediatricians now were able to devise safer methods of artificial feeding through application of prior innovations in feeding and sterilization. The technology of the rubber nipple (U.S. patent, 1845) had been a boon to artificial feeding, while pasteurization, developed by Louis Pasteur in 1864, promised to improve its safety. At the end of the nineteenth century, keeping newborns healthy seemed to be an attainable goal.

At the turn of the century, public hygienists became increasingly preoccupied with childhood mortality. Dispensaries for advice and well-baby care were set up in all major cities, beginning with Paris (1892) and New York (1893). Similarly, milk depots were created to provide a steady affordable supply of clean milk. The municipal milk station that opened at Rochester, New York, in 1897 claimed to be the first on this continent. Success was measured by annual reviews of mortality. Montreal was reputed to have one of the highest rates of infant mortality in North America, and its *Gouttes de lait* clinics were opened in 1901 to offer safe milk services in French and English. The system quickly grew to twenty-eight depots by 1915. In cities and rural areas, public health nurses instructed mothers in the principles of hygiene and infant feeding. Between 1905 and 1911, international conferences on the provision of milk were held in Paris, Brussels, and Berlin, but discussion extended to all causes of infant death.

Due to improved hygiene, mortality rates began to fall; however, prior to antibiotics and vaccines against other childhood diseases, the life-saving power of hygiene alone was limited. In Canada, some decline in mortality may have been more apparent than real, as it coincided with increased reliability in recording of births. Early success may also have been due to a general willingness to let children live (see 'Social Pediatrics,' below).

Medicalizing Growth

In the early twentieth century, several exciting discoveries meant that what had once been the domain of wise women and entrepre-

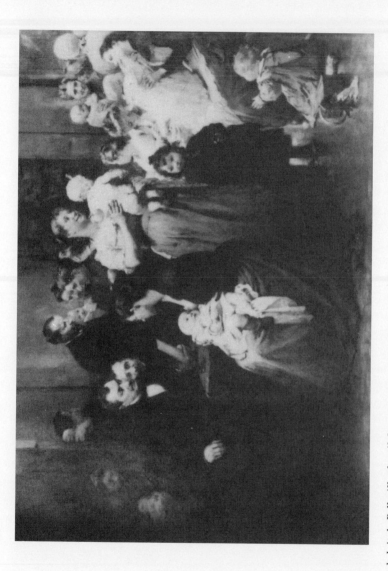

Goutte de lait de Belleville, detail from a triptych by Henri Geoffroy. At a clinic in a poor suburb of Paris, doctors dispense advice and milk to mothers who are eager to keep their babies healthy. Musée de l'Assistance Publique, Paris

neurs now became the purview of doctors, scientists, and industrial giants. These discoveries included germ theory, vaccines, diphtheria toxoid, hormones, genetics, vitamins, and antibiotics. One by one, the scourges of childhood were dramatically reduced – if not eliminated: measles, diphtheria, mumps, whooping cough, scarlatina, and rheumatic fever with its associated heart and kidney complications. An epidemic of poliomyelitis in the early 1950s was stemmed by the advent of Salk and Sabin vaccines; experts now predict the global eradication of this disease (see chapter 7). Even congenital abnormalities, including heart disease and hip displacement, which had once condemned children to chronic dependency if not early death, could now be repaired, allowing them to reach maturity as productive members of society. Several Canadians made important contributions to these surgical endeavours (see chapter 10).

Subspecialization

Pediatrics began to divide into various subspecialties, defined by child age. Neonatology arose out of specific achievements in the mid-1950s. New York anesthetist Virginia Apgar developed her simple score for rapidly assessing the status of the newborn (see chapter 11). In 1958 phototherapy was introduced for newborn jaundice, drastically reducing the sequelae of a very common problem. The role of surfactant in the respiratory distress syndrome of premature babies was discovered by Mary Ellen Avery and Jere Mead in 1959; it prompted the technological advances that have made it possible to save the lives of infants at only twenty-six weeks of gestation or less.

Keeping the emphasis on prevention, physicians soon became aware of the danger of maternal smoking, drinking, and drug use. By 1963, immunological prevention of erythroblastosis foetalis in children yet to be conceived could be accomplished by administration of rhesus antibodies to the Rh-negative mother. Pioneering work in this area was accomplished by Bruce Chown of Winnipeg, whose laboratory, founded in 1944, assessed and controlled the immune status of mothers throughout Manitoba.

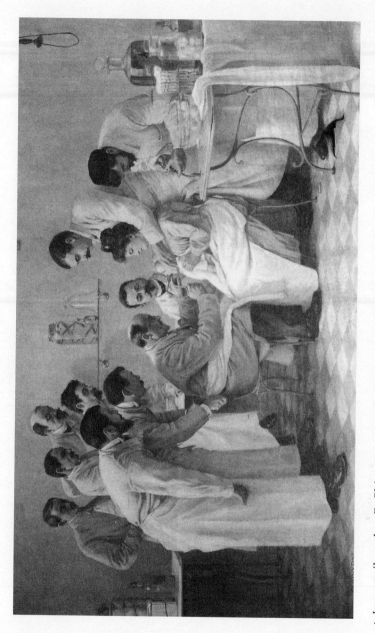

Le tubage, attributed to G. Chicotot, early twentieth century. Surrounded by concerned adults, a child with diphtheria is being intubated by a physician, who may be a partisan in the debate on intubation versus tracheotomy. Lines in the tableau converge on the infant's throat. Musée de l'Assistance Publique, Paris

Genetics and Eugenics

> No baby; no nation.
>
> Helen MacMurchy, *The Canadian Mothers' Book,*
> The Little Blue Book Mothers' series, no. 1
> (Ottawa: Dept of Health, 1927), 8

From its inception, the social hygiene movement was intimately connected to the aspirations of developed nations. Children were the future; their welfare reflected that of the state. The new possibilities for saving infant lives raised a deeper question: Should all lives be saved? Or, put differently, should all citizens become parents? The word 'eugenics' had been coined in 1883 by the British physiologist Francis Galton to signify 'ideal breeding.' On the one hand, science could identify and prevent inherited disorders; on the other, dominant races and ideologies could use this knowledge for political ends in defining 'superiority.' The philosophy of eugenics lent scientific approbation to that project.

In 1902 A.E. Garrod demonstrated that Mendelian laws governed the inheritance of alcaptonuria, making it the first human disorder to be identified as 'genetic.' Soon a succession of congenital abnormalities were linked to genetics (see chapter 4). Situating these complex problems in the structure of DNA informs genetic counselling and invites research into new biotechnologies to prevent or control them. In the past, however, states and physicians resorted to more drastic measures for producing 'ideal' genetics.

Nazi science was predicated on 'racial hygiene' and the notion of Aryan superiority. It pursued the 'final solution' of compulsory sterilization or genocide of Jews, gypsies, the mentally disabled, and people with physical deformities. A vast literature now tracks the role of physicians and scientists in unethical experimentation and the extermination of millions following the election of Adolf Hitler in 1933. After the war, a code of standards in medical research was established at Nuremberg, but scholars have found that it made little impact on American research.

Our confident disgust over the German Third Reich makes it all too easy to forget that eugenicist notions had currency in North America too. Critics of *in vitro* fertilization, for example, caution against complacency; they point to more subtle but disturbing examples from the past, including the sterilization policies of the so-called mentally retarded in Alberta. But Canadian eugenicists were neither 'monsters,' nor were they 'simple-minded reactionaries'; they 'saw themselves as progressives who were seeking to wed science, medicine, and social welfare' (McLaren 1990, 166). Enthusiastic bureaucrats and educators, like Helen MacMurchy, subscribed to a Canadian ideal that was white, middle class, and Protestant (see chapter 11). Their initiatives were packaged appealingly in the form of 'help' for the 'helpless,' and centred on issues of immigration, education, and sterilization of the 'feeble-minded.' The apparent reasonableness of these solutions in promoting what are now seen as offensive infringements of civil liberties is a sobering reminder of the difficulty in identifying all the subtle complexities of any process of intervention before it takes place.

Vitamins and Nutrition

Among the most intriguing of twentieth-century scientific achievements from a pediatric perspective is the discovery of vitamins. Since antiquity, manipulation of milk, food, and feeding practices had been the mainstay of therapy for children. With the concept of vitamins, a number of vague, apparently infectious illnesses were transformed into specific dietary deficiencies, which could now be identified and prevented by science.

Long before Vitamin C had been imagined, its deficiency disease, scurvy, was known to be the result of poor diet. In the sixteenth century, Jacques Cartier was shown how to prevent it by aboriginal people, who gave him a recipe for a tea (see chapter 5). In 1753 the English sea captain James Lind described the antiscorbutic properties of orange juice (though boiled). The practice of carrying citrus fruits is said to be the origin of the British epithet 'limey.' But many other diseases, now known to result from dietary deficiencies, could not be distinguished from infections. Like epidemics of influenza or measles, deficiencies occurred as 'outbreaks' in specific populations, localized by time and place. Following the advent of germ theory, avid researchers sought the bacterial causes of pellagra and rickets, and discovered instead that these 'epidemics' were nutritional rather than infectious.

In 1896 the Dutch physician Christiaan Eijkman noticed that pigeons fed on supposedly 'better quality' polished rice developed a paralytic disease resembling human beriberi, which resolved with a 'poor quality' whole-rice diet. In 1901 his colleague G. Grijns hypothesized that the rice hull contained an anti-beriberi substance. Similarly, Joseph Goldberger tried to transmit pellagra to himself and his associates by inoculation of secretions from human sufferers; his failure was taken as evidence of the non-infectious nature of the disease.

Chemical research on vitamins ultimately provided exquisitely specific causes and treatments for previously vague diseases with widespread effects. The word 'vitamin,' coined in 1912 by the Polish biochemist Kazimierz Funk, expressed the new theory of accessory foodstuffs. Frederick Gowland Hopkins also thought of vitamins as nutritional catalysts related to hormones. He studied synthetic diets and milk feeding in rats.

Over the next fifty years, individual vitamins were recognized, named, isolated, and synthesized. Once the biochemical concept was in place, the length of time from recognition to isolation or purification of each vitamin was greatly decreased. For example, in the case of thiamine (B_1), thirty years would elapse, but the time shrank to less than two years for riboflavin (B_2) and vitamin K (given its name by Henrik Dam for its role in 'Koagulation'). Reflecting the heady atmosphere created by this research, Nobel Prizes were awarded quickly: Hopkins and Eijkmann (1929); Whipple (shared, 1934); Szent-Györgyi (1937); Dam (1943).

The chemical reduction of infant food to component parts of vitamins, proteins, fats, and carbohydrates simply added to the rising authority of doctors. Now the composition of breast milk could be closely approximated with 'infant formula.' Emphasis on sterility and strict schedules prevailed, as medical experts explained how babies could be fed artificially in answer to the anxieties of mothers and the

Table 13.2
Milestones in vitamin history

	Named or postulated by	Year*	Purified or isolated by	Year*	Structure and/or synthesis year*
A	Bloch	1924	Karrer	1931-7	1937
B_1	Eijkman and Grijns	1896	Jansen	1926	1936
B_2	BMRC/Warburg	1927/1932	Kuhn	1933	1935
B_3	Goldberger/Voegtlin	1914–15	Funk/Subbarow	1914/1937	1867
B_6	Szent-Györgyi	1936	Keresztesy et al.	1938	1938
B_{12}	Whipple	1922	Rickes et al.	1948	1955
C	Funk	1911	Szent-Györgyi	1928	1933
D	Mellanby (chemistry)	1918	Pappenheimer	1921	
	Huldschinsky (light)	1919	Angus	1931	
E	Evans et al.	1922–3	Evans et al.	1936	1938
K	Dam	1934	Dam	1939	1939

Sources: *Goodman and Gilman's, Pharmacological Basis of Therapeutics* (New York: McGraw-Hill, 1996, and earlier editions); Roman J. Kutsky, *Handbook of Vitamins and Minerals and Hormones*, 2nd edn (New York: Van Nostrand Reinhold 1980).
* Years indicate date of either research or publication.

financial aspirations of industry. Motherless children were to benefit, but the impact of this achievement spread to the healthy infants of ordinary women, who trusted science to ensure that their babies would have enough good-quality milk. Ironically, the milk substitutes could never match the immunological value of breast milk; and the rubber nipple, once lauded for saving infants from choking and starving, is now the subject of toxicological investigations.

As historians Rima Apple and Katherine Arnup have shown, doctors continued to advocate maternal nursing, even as they provided more information on artificial feeding. But the bottles won. By the early 1970s, less than one-third of North American children were breast-fed. Worried about this trend, the La Leche League (founded in 1956) and health-care professionals actively promoted a return to natural methods; they feared that breast-feeding would continue to decline as women lost familiarity with it. Once again, a shift in cultural values, combined with increased scepticism over scientific expertise, helped the activists to reverse the trend and foster the late-

---

Breasts, Bovines, and Babies

Breast milk is for babies; cow's milk is for calves ... Breast milk is best because it doesn't have to be warmed, you can take it on picnics, the cat can't get at it, and it comes in such cute containers.

Alan Brown, physician at Toronto's Hospital for Sick Children
(cited in Arnup 1994, 97)

---

twentieth-century revival in breast-feeding. Nevertheless, industry is criticized for continuing to promote its more expensive and less effective formula feedings in the Third World.

Experts' Advice to Parents: Dr Blatz and Dr Spock

Behavioural and psychological research moved into the vacuum created by the First World's conquest of the biological killers. Child study and adolescent medicine became separate new fields with a special emphasis on behavioural and psychological well-being. The sociologist Sydney Halpern suggests that the trend to emphasize the psychological over the biological in academic pediatrics was influenced by government funding agencies.

As early as 1924, the physician-psychologist William Blatz headed a child-study centre at the University of Toronto, where he developed a relatively permissive approach to child rearing. Among many other activities, Blatz directed his controversial research on the Dionne quintuplets, whose nursery became a 'laboratory' for the analysis of nature versus nurture in child development. The project was terminated by the Ontario government in 1938 under pressure from the family. Nevertheless, the public had become aware of the promise of science in the rearing of healthy children.

The advice manual for parents written by the New York pediatrician Benjamin Spock became the world's third-largest-selling book, after editions of the Bible and Shakespeare. A Yale graduate, Spock held professorships at the Mayo Clinic and at Case Western Reserve

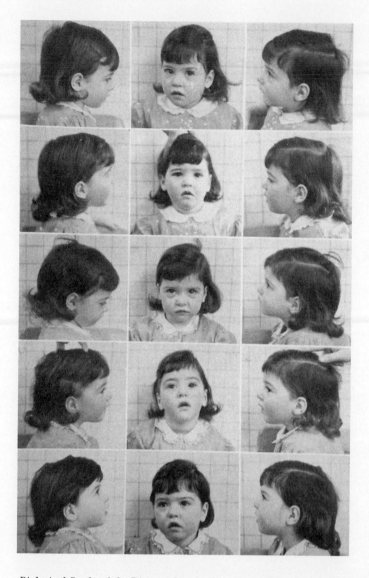

Biological Study of the Dionne Quintuplets. From J.W. MacArthur and Norma Ford, in Blatz et al., 1937, frontispiece. The composite image reflects the investigators' concerns in their study of nature versus nurture, but it also speaks eloquently of the now unacceptable 'scientific' incursions made into the lives of these five children and their family.

University. In simple words and short sentences, his *Baby and Child Care* brought Freudian theory to average Americans, by emphasizing the child's need for love and by relaxing the rigid standards for feeding, toilet training, clothing, and play that had prevailed in previous decades. Spock bolstered parents' confidence with understandable information; he appealed to common sense and reassured the innate parental desire to please children while guiding their physical, emotional, and moral growth. The first edition of 1946 sold more than half a million copies in ten months. Still a bestseller and translated into thirty-nine languages, total sales now exceed forty million copies a year.

In the mid-1960s, Spock was shocked by the Vietnam War and its wanton destruction of the very youth he had helped to raise. Becoming an outspoken advocate for disarmament and peace, he was arrested several times for participating in protests. In 1968 he was actually convicted for conspiracy to resist the draft and fined $5,000. Many Americans then turned against the aging pediatrician, angered by his adoption of an antigovernment stance seemingly in favour of communism. They claimed that his emphasis on love over discipline had caused an entire generation to be permissive and selfish; they also blamed Spock for the hippie movement, with its sexual, political, and social revolution.

Spock denied that his work had made such an extraordinary impact. He pointed to similar cultural turmoil in countries where his work was unknown, and he contrasted the upheaval in America with its absence in other nations where his book was equally successful. Scholars are reluctant to accept Spock's modest assessment of his own influence, even as they criticize dated aspects of his work. Never shy about publicity, the nonagenarian pediatrician participated in a September 1992 press conference to advocate breast-feeding and warn of the dangers of whole milk in early and later life. True to form, he succeeded in angering dairy farmers and business interests across North America.

Social Pediatrics

After the social hygiene movement, more infants survived to become adults, but the statistics still betray class-based and geographic imbalance. The realization that social provisions define child health did not come equally to all nations – even within each nation. As Preston and Haines have shown, American children of densely populated areas and those disadvantaged by poverty, race, or abandonment, did not enjoy the same life expectancy as their more privileged peers.

Child Labour and Child Experimentation

Laws against infanticide, like those against murder, have long been on the books of Western nations, but they were enforced only sporadically; convicted mothers rarely paid the full penalty, especially if they were single and poverty stricken. Legislation to protect children is vulnerable to interpretation through prevailing social attitudes about their value to society. Labour laws are similar.

In the early nineteenth century, young children were recruited into the labour force, where they encountered the dismal conditions so vividly portrayed in the novels of Charles Dickens. By the 1830s, Britain had enacted laws against child labour in factories. In North America, the economy was based on agricultural work, and industrialization came later; as a result, legislation to protect children in factories and mines on that continent was not passed until the 1870s and 1880s. But these laws did not apply equally to all children. London orphans, supposedly barred from work, grew more numerous and desperate. Thomas J. Barnardo founded homes across Britain, but in 1868 he began to export these children to families or labour situations in Canada. By 1883, the trickle had become a torrent, leading to the immigration of a total of 80,000 children – 30,000 of whom were 'Barnardo boys' or 'girls' – before the practice was abolished in 1925. Many destitute children may have been spared a short life on the London streets; but as Joy Parr has shown, most became workers rather than adoptees; at least one-third were not orphans; and as many as 10 per cent, usually from disadvantaged groups, were sent in a form of 'philanthropic abduction,' against the wishes or without the knowledge of their parents. Measures were taken to ensure the well-being of the children in care, and their wages were carefully collected; however, Barnardo's system also reduced the costs of caring for waifs in the home country, assuaging the financial interests of the banks and agencies directly involved. Special circumstances have always provided new justifications for keeping children at work rather than at school. Child labour continues to be a problem of global significance.

'Baby farms' also illustrate ambivalence in the application of laws to protect children. Homes for unwed mothers and their children served a 'black market' for adoption. Late-nineteenth-century legislation to curb the practice was not enforced, and many baby farms operated illegally under the guise of private hospitals. For example, the lax hygienic standards, cruelty, and high (but unreported) mortality rates of the Ideal Maternity Home in Nova Scotia were notorious among locals between 1925 and 1945; however, they did not receive wider attention until the 1988 report of investigative journalist Bette Cahill, entitled 'butterbox babies' – a grim allusion to the makeshift coffins remembered by former employees of the home.

Medicine, too, has witnessed an evolution in legislative attitudes surrounding children as experimental subjects. For several centuries, it strove to help children by investigating the diseases peculiar to them. Jenner's smallpox vaccine was tested on an eight-year-old boy, who was then challenged with active smallpox to prove the point. Other nineteenth-century trials – on measles prevention, for example – entailed inoculating blood from active cases into child subjects in the almshouses and orphanages of great cities. As Susan E. Lederer and her colleagues have shown, institutionalized children were similarly used in research on other vaccines, infections, and nutritional diseases – to their great good fortune, it was thought, when the experiments were a success. But not all experiments met with success; they could also cause pain and suffering. In 1970 public outrage greeted the discovery that, for fifteen years, children with severe mental retardation had been deliberately infected with 'inevitable' hepatitis at the Willowbrook State School of New York, supposedly with parental consent. The result was legislation to control biomedical research (U.S., 1974; Canada [MRC], 1978) and the subsequent laying down of guidelines and codes of conduct for the ethical use of all human subjects, especially children.

With control of infectious diseases and diarrhea, infant mortality rates in developed countries fell dramatically during the twentieth century, from roughly 150 deaths per 1,000 live births in 1900, to 26.6 in 1954 and to 13.1 in 1979 (Williams 1985, 29–34). Pediatricians gradually turned to the health of children elsewhere. For example, Jamaican-born and Oxford-trained physician Cicely Williams conducted research in Africa and Malaysia. In 1935 she published her classic description of kwashiorkor as a protein deficiency. The name, from a dialect of the African Gold Coast (now Ghana), literally means 'sickness of the deposed baby'; these peoples had long thought of the disease holistically, as a social problem created by a sibling birth. Working near Singapore in February 1942, Williams was captured – along with 70,000 Allied troops and thousands of Allied national citizens, including many other doctors – and was confined in a Japanese internment camp until August 1945. Following the war, she was invited to lead the Maternal and Child Health division of the World Health Organization (WHO). Overpopulation was a major concern, but Williams knew that women in developing countries would not be interested in birth control until child mortality had been staved.

The first director general of the WHO (1948–1953) was the Canadian physician G. Brock Chisholm. Having moved from general practice into psychiatry, he entered the Second World War as a private and rose through the ranks to head the medical services of the Canadian Army. Controversy surrounded Chisholm's views on child rearing, especially his agnostic stance on religion and his widely publicized opposition to the perpetuation of myths and superstitions, including Santa Claus. Repeated calls for his resignation from the Canadian bureaucracy were silenced only by his appointment to the WHO. Chisholm believed that war between nations would not be eliminated without conscious and enlightened efforts to develop tolerance and mutual understanding. An active promoter of Physicians for Social Responsibility, Chisholm also advocated birth control, acknowledging Williams's emphasis on the prior need for death control (see chapter 11). In concentrating on global health, Chisholm warned against the dangers of nuclear weapons, overpopulation, and pollution.

WHO statistics indicate that the problem of child mortality may have been lessened but is far from solved. Each year more than a million children die of malaria, while hundreds of thousands of others succumb to neonatal tetanus, diarrhea, and measles. Since the causes of these diseases are social as well as biological, effective control will inevitably entail delicate interference with cultural practices relating to gender, race, religion, and tradition. Solutions to these child killers will aggravate the problem of overpopulation, invoking the spectre of malnutrition and starvation. As a result, contraception continues to be an important issue. Birth-control methods have been developed as a lucrative product of industry – just like the infant formulas before them. But recent studies suggest that the limitation of birth rate is better correlated with the education of girls than with the provision of drugs or devices (see chapter 11).

The leadership of Chisholm, Williams, and others led pediatricians the world over to face a stark irony: efforts to save individual children from treatable, infectious illnesses pale when compared with the thousands who continue to die annually from starvation and filth, or the millions who stand to die from a war that might exterminate the entire species. Long schooled in prevention, pediatricians were aware that no medicine could help a nuclear disaster, and they supported the founding of the International Physicians for the Prevention of Nuclear War and similar organizations (see chapter 6).

Children without advocates – orphans and 'delinquents' – continue to be abused, especially those who are in 'havens' or are wards of the state. We realize with horror that money cannot begin to compensate the harm done, in the name of 'helping,' to native youth in residential schools. Even with loving care, children in poverty are disadvantaged physically, intellectually, and emotionally. As the figures for child poverty climb, the problems of global health hit closer to home. In 1997 the Canadian government promised to address the issue of rising child poverty, which remains a black mark on the country's otherwise stellar performance-rating by the United Nations.

Pediatricians continue to be experts in prevention, but there has always been a tension between reasonable intervention and unacceptable intrusion into other cultures and the private lives of individuals. Some methods, once touted as medical salvations, have been abandoned as shameful exploitations or regrettable mistakes, while others remain entrenched in law. In the midst of a process, it is sometimes impossible to discern the right way. With their focus on prevention and on the social (as well as biological) determinants of health, pediatricians have not only influenced the rest of medicine; they have created a model for enhancing survival of all life on the planet.

Suggestions for Further Reading

Apple, Rima D. *Mothers and Medicine: A Social History of Infant Feeding, 1890–1950.* Madison, Wis.: University of Wisconsin Press, 1987

Bel Geddes, Joan. *Small World: A History of Baby Care from the Stone Age to the Spock Age.* New York: Macmillan, 1964

Bloom, Lynn Z. *Doctor Spock: Biography of a Conservative Radical.* Indianapolis and New York: Bobbs-Merrill, 1972

Caulfield, Ernest. *The Infant Welfare Movement in the Eighteenth Century.* New York: P.B. Hoeber, 1931

Cone, Thomas E. *History of American Pediatrics.* Boston: Little, Brown, 1979

Cooter, Roger, ed. *In the Name of the Child: Health and Welfare, 1880–1940.* London and New York: Routledge, 1992

Craddock, Sally. *Retired Except on Demand: The Life of Dr. Cicely Williams.* Oxford: Green College, 1983

Cunningham, Hugh. *Children and Childhood in Western Society since 1500.* London and New York: Longman, 1995

English, Peter C. 'Not Miniature Men and Women: Abraham Jacobi's Vision of a New Medical Specialty a Century Ago.' In *Children and Health Care: Moral and Social Issues,* ed. Loretta M. Kopelman and John C. Moskop, 247–73. Dordrecht and Boston: Kluwer Academic Publishers, 1989

Fellman, Anita Clair, and Michael Fellman. *Making Sense of Self: Medical Advice Literature in Late Nineteenth-Century America.* Philadelphia: University of Pennsylvania Press, 1981

Fissell, Mary E. *Patients, Power, and the Poor in Eighteenth-Century Bristol.* Cambridge and New York: Cambridge University Press, 1991

Garrison, Fielding H., and Arthur F. Abt. *Abt-Garrison History of Paediatrics, with New Chapters on the History of Paediatrics in Recent Times.* Philadelphia and London: W.B. Saunders, 1965

Gavitt, Philip. *Charity and Children in Renaissance Florence: The Ospedale degli Innocenti, 1410–1536.* Ann Arbor: University of Michigan Press, 1990

Grodin, Michael A., and Leonard H. Glantz, eds. *Children as Research Subjects: Science, Ethics, and Law.* New York and Oxford: Oxford University Press, 1994 (esp. 3–25)

Hawes, Joseph M., and N. Ray Hiner, eds. *Children in Historical and Comparative Perspective: An International Handbook and Research Guide.* New York: Greenwood Press, 1991

Kamminga, H., and M.W. Weatherall, 'The Making of a Biochemist' [on Frederick Gowland Hopkins]. *Medical History* 40(1996), 269–92 and 415–36

Lawrence, Christopher J. 'William Buchan: Medicine Laid Open.' *Medical History* 19 (1975), 20–35

Lederer, Susan E. *Subjected to Science: Human Experimentation in America before the Second World War.* Baltimore: Johns Hopkins University Press, 1995

Lifton, Robert Jay. *The Nazi Doctors: Medical Killing and the Psychology of Genocide.* New York: Basic Books, 1986

Markel, Howard. 'Orphanages Revisited: Some Historical Perspectives on Dependent, Abandoned, and Orphaned Children in America.' *Archives of Pediatrics and Adolescent Medicine* 149 (1995), 609–10

– 'Academic Pediatrics: The View of New York City a Century Ago.' *Academic Medicine* 71 (Feb. 1996), 146–51

– 'Henry Koplik, MD, the Good Samaritan Dispensary of New York City, and the Description of Koplik's Spots.' *Archives of Pediatrics and Adolescent Medicine* 150 (May 1996), 535–9

Preston, S.H., and Michael R. Haines. *Fatal Years: Child Mortality in Late-Nineteenth-Century America.* Princeton, N.J.: Princeton University Press, 1991

Proctor, Robert. *Racial Hygiene: Medicine under the Nazis.* Cambridge, Mass.: Harvard University Press, 1988

Rosenberg, Charles E. 'Medical Text and Social Context: Explaining William Buchan's *Domestic Medicine.*' *Bulletin of the History of Medicine* 57 (1983), 22–42

– 'Catechisms of Health: The Body in the Pre-Bellum Classroom.' *Bulletin of the History of Medicine* 69 (1995), 175–97

Ruhräh, John, ed. *Pediatrics of the Past: An Anthology.* New York: P.B. Hoeber, 1925

Sherwood, Joan. *Poverty in Eighteenth-Century Spain: The Women and Children of the Inclusa.* Toronto: University of Toronto Press, 1988

Spaulding, Mary, and Penny Welch. *Nurturing Yesterday's Child: A Portrayal of the Drake Collection of Paediatric History.* Philadelphia: B.C. Decker, 1991

Still, George Frederic. *The History of Paediatrics: The Progress of the Study of Diseases of Children up to the End of the Eighteenth Century.* London: Oxford University Press, 1931

Teysseire, Daniel. *Pédiatrie des lumieres: Maladies et soins des enfants dans l'Encyclopédie et le Dictionnaire de Trévoux.* Paris: Vrin, 1982

Weiner, Dora B. *The Citizen-Patient in Revolutionary and Imperial Paris.* Baltimore and London: Johns Hopkins University Press, 1993

Williams, Cicely D. *Mother and Child: Delivering the Services.* 2nd edn. London and New York: Oxford University Press, 1985

On Canada

Arnup, Katherine. *Education for Motherhood: Child-Rearing Advice for Canadian Mothers.* Toronto: University of Toronto Press, 1994

Baillargeon, Denyse. 'Care of Mothers and Infants between the Wars in Montreal: The Visiting Nurses of Metropolitan Life, Les Gouttes de Lait, and Assistance Maternelle.' In *Caring and Curing,* ed. Dianne E. Dodd and Deborah Gorham, 163–81. Ottawa: University of Ottawa Press, 1994

Brown, Alan. *The Hospital for Sick Children.* Toronto: Hospital for Sick Children, 1984

Cahill, Bette L. *Butterbox Babies.* Toronto: Seal, 1992

Corbett, Gail H. *Barnardo Children in Canada.* Peterborough, Ont.: Woodland, 1981

Dodd, Dianne E. 'Advice to Parents: The Blue Books, Helen MacMurchy, M.D., and the Federal Department of Health.' *Canadian Bulletin of Medical History* 8 (1991), 203–30

McLaren, Angus. *Our Own Master Race: Eugenics in Canada, 1885–1945.* Toronto: McClelland and Stewart, 1990

Milloy, John Sheridan. *To Kill the Indian in the Child: A History of the Aboriginal School System.* Rev. edn. Winnipeg: University of Manitoba Press, 1998

Parr, Joy. *Labouring Children: British Immigrant Apprentices to Canada, 1869–1924.* Montreal: McGill-Queen's University Press, 1980

Raymond, Jocelyn Motyer. *The Nursery World of Dr Blatz.* Toronto: University of Toronto Press, 1991

Smandych, Russell Charles, Gordon Dodds, and Alvin A.J. Esau, eds. *Dimensions of Childhood: Essays on the History of Children and Youth in Canada.* Winnipeg: Legal Research Institute of the University of Manitoba, 1991

Stuart, Meryn. 'Ideology and Experience: Public Health Nursing and the Ontario Rural Child Welfare Project, 1920–1925.' *Canadian Bulletin of Medical History* 6 (1989), 111–31

Sutherland, Neil. *Children in English-Canadian Society: Framing the Twentieth-Century Consensus.* Toronto: University of Toronto Press, 1976

CHAPTER FOURTEEN

A Many-Faceted Gem: Decline and Rebirth of Family Medicine*

Never could I see myself listening all day with a stethoscope to chest sounds, or looking down throats or up rectums ... General practice [is] one of the most difficult fields of medicine because a competent general practitioner must be one of the most expert diagnosticians. He not only must know when he can help, but what is just as important, he must be quick to recognize a situation that is beyond him and refer such a seriously ill patient to more expert care than he can give.

W. Victor Johnston, *Before the Age of Miracles*, 1972, 8–9

Historians of family medicine often begin by commenting with surprise on how little has been written on their subject. After all, they contend, general practice is the oldest medical activity, predating the formation of any specialty; by rights, then, it should have the longest tradition of documentation. But two good reasons account for this apparent neglect.

First, general or family practice is *not* ancient; it is the newest of specialties. As medical and surgical specialties developed in the early twentieth century, doctors who did everything – the *omnipracticiens*, as they are tellingly called in French – began to fade into nostalgia, becoming the stuff of legend or backwardness. The rise of family medicine was a post-war phenomenon.

---

*Educational objectives for this chapter are found on p. 399.

Second, history of medicine – indeed all history – underwent a shift in focus after 1950. Historians used to be preoccupied with medical elites, academic issues, and the vast intellectual and technological transformations of science. General practitioners did not qualify for their attention. Only in the middle of the twentieth century did historians turn to 'everyday life.' Rather than fixing their sights on pivotal moments with lasting effects, they began to explore the context of continuity – history of the *longue durée*. Given this double caveat – that family medicine is new and that historians tended to ignore the ordinary and the continuous – it is scarcely surprising that the history of family medicine is yet to be written.

In this chapter, we will briefly examine the prehistory of family medicine – what is known of the life and work of ordinary doctors of the past. Then we will explore the social, political, economic, and intellectual forces underlying the professionalization of family medicine. Finally, we will examine the influence of this discipline on other specialties.

Prehistory of General Practice

After the advent of man-midwifery in the seventeenth and eighteenth centuries and the conceptual melding of surgery and medicine in the early nineteenth, there followed a century during which most doctors were 'general' practitioners (see chapters 10 and 11). Only professors and researchers could claim to be specialists, but some resented the label. The rules governing practice were dictated by legislation in each country and reflected societal expectations. In Canada, for example, from the late eighteenth century on, doctors were licensed by credentials and/or examination in the triple disciplines of medicine, surgery, and midwifery.

Our knowledge of general practitioners (GPs) has increased with the shift in historical focus from the exceptional to the ordinary and with the advent of computer technology. In projects covering a long period and numerous interactions, volumes of data must be assimilated and manipulated to produce reliable statements about practice, its stability, and its gradual change. Recent scholarship has unveiled the more distant past of general practice in a variety of ways.

A Doctor Remembers

My first introduction to the tragedy of diseases ... A long line of teams came slowly down that road. Driving the lead team ... was my father ... In the bed of the farm wagon were three oblong boxes ... As days wore on I learned that the wagon had borne the coffins containing the bodies of three of my playmates. Five more followed in quick succession. Eight of the nine children in that one family died of diphtheria in ten days. There remained only a baby of nine months. The mother took to carrying this child constantly even while she did the farm housework. Clutched to her mother's breast, this child seemed inordinately wide-eyed as though affected by the silent grief which surrounded her ...

Prayers for protection literally filled the air in those days of doom. There was no appeal to the science of medicine because there was none.

Arthur Hertzler, *The Horse and Buggy Doctor*
(New York and London: Harper, 1938), 1–2

One approach involves the examination of community records pertaining to health, illness, birth, and mortality in specific places and times. Using records of dispensaries, hospitals, and religious and philanthropic organizations, historian Hilary Marland traced the medical facilities in two contrasting towns in nineteenth-century England. She found a variety of practices, ranging from pluralistic 'self-help' to 'institutional' care. Similarly, Estes and Goodman, who set out to commemorate the centennial of a hospital in Portsmouth, New Hampshire, discovered a wealth of sources pertaining to the town, and they extended their research to cover three and a half centuries of births, diseases, mortality, and practitioners – both 'regular' and 'irregular.' Their achievement serves to represent an ordinary American town, since few municipalities have preserved equally rich sources. Future studies on regions and climates will undoubt-

edly reveal patterns of disease and practice that differ from those of
Portsmouth.

Another approach has been to analyse groups of practitioners in a
specific period or place. Fine studies of this type exist for both Britain and France. The historian Irvine Loudon examined the nature
of medical practice in Britain between 1750 and 1850, attending to
its relationship with pharmacy, surgery, and obstetrics. His sources
included parliamentary papers, medical periodicals, the professional archives, and the personal records of individual practitioners.
He found that the status of general practice rose following the
Apothecaries Act of 1815 – which, despite its name, had little to do
with pharmacy; it was a preliminary attempt to create national standards for practice and for regional licensing bodies. The Apothecaries Act resulted in a conscious movement to organize general
practice, but GPs had to wait another century before they acquired
full autonomy over accreditation.

Using a similar approach for his work on perirevolutionary
France, the historian Matthew Ramsey scoured the archives in scores
of *départements*, medical faculties, and professional bodies for records
pertaining to health and medicine in order to construct a complex
picture of diverse practitioners. He showed that in 1770 the boundaries of practice were diffuse: 'officially' trained doctors worked
beside, and in competition with a wide range of folk healers, moun-
tebanks, empirics, druggists, and 'witches.' By 1830, legislation and
custom had considerably altered the scene; a single profession of
certified practitioners had come to the fore, clearly distinguished
from their competitors and theoretically capable of all types of medical work. Similar studies of later periods have been conducted by
Gelfand, Léonard, and Weisz. Weisz's comparison of specialization
in Britain, France, and the United States will provide an interesting
corollary – statistics on general practice. For Canada, historians
Bernier, Connor, Gidney, Millar, Romano, and Tunis studied groups
of regular doctors and their alternative competitors, and they uncovered patterns in identity, work, and income.

The extent to which practice was regulated through legislation
indicates the extent to which the general public was willing to grant
autonomy to formally trained physicians. In the United States, the

medical profession was impressively successful in retaining control over licensing and practice. The American Medical Association was formed in 1846 as a monopolistic lobby against homeopathists and other 'irregulars.' By contrast, European countries and Canada were relatively more tolerant of alternative health care – not, it should be recognized, because physicians welcomed it, but because they failed to convince their governments to ban the competition. For example, a homeopathic representative sat on the council of the Ontario College of Physicians until 1967.

A variation on the doctor-based approach to the history of general medicine is the study of individual practitioners. Some doctors actually wrote their own histories, diaries, or autobiographies. These documents provided diverting reading for generations of physicians, but they were ignored or at least mistrusted by historians, because of the potential distortions embedded in any subjective writing. Now, however, scholars understand that these classic and antiquarian tales reveal issues that were significant for doctor and patient, even if they seem to be of little consequence to their successors. A number of these first-hand records have recently been published, opening fascinating vistas on medical life of the past (see table 14.1). Memoirs by Canadian practitioners were analysed by S.E.D. Shortt, who found that the triad of medicine, surgery, and midwifery typified their work, while the gap between the theoretical training of medical school and the realities of practice was a common complaint.

Ordinary medical practice can also be explored through medical daybooks and hospital records. Here, especially, microcomputers help to exploit the historical potential in the records that chart doctors' daily lives. To analyse the practice of the Ontario physician James Miles Langstaff, I transcribed information contained in forty years of daybooks and accounts into a database program to build a profile of his patients, their diseases, his diagnostic and therapeutic methods, the journals he read, and the money he earned. The results showed how his practice changed through time.

The average medical practice of the late nineteenth and early twentieth centuries was challenging and diverse. Most patients were seen on house calls, although doctors also kept offices in their homes. As Hertzler so vividly reminds us, infectious diseases, includ-

---

General Practice in Fiction

A list similar to table 14.1 could be made from the stirring fiction of several physician-writers who drew on their own experience. They include John Brown (Scottish), Anton Chekhov (Russian), Oliver Wendell Holmes (American), Tobias Smollett (English), and William Carlos Williams (American).

Nonphysician writers also created memorable vignettes of general practice. Among the most celebrated are the doctor stories in George Eliot's *Middlemarch* and Gustave Flaubert's *Madame Bovary.*

For more examples, consult the printed *Online Database of Literature and Medicine* or its website, http://endeavor.med.nyu.edu/lit-med/lit-med-db/topview.html

---

ing diphtheria, chest problems, diarrhea, postpartum fever, and scarlet fever, dominated the diagnostic spectrum. Doctors were also called to deliveries, often using forceps at the request of women attendants. They performed small operations, such as extracting teeth, lancing abscesses, suturing wounds, and reducing fractures and dislocations. On rare occasions, they undertook major operations, including amputations, mastectomies, and repair of congenital abnormalities such as club foot and hare lip. Operating on a kitchen table in Fergus, Ontario, in 1883, the intrepid Abraham Groves is said to have been the first in North America to remove an appendix (see chapter 10). Groves had already performed a vaginal hysterectomy, an ovariotomy, and a small transfusion. Of his long travels to make house calls, he wrote, 'One had time when driving alone to go over every aspect of the case, and I found the time so spent far from wasted' (1934, 5).

Work on billing records suggests that nineteenth-century doctors rarely expected to be paid in full. When Haddy and colleagues compared the finances of a mid-1930s physician with those of a general practice sixty years later, they found that the number of surgical pro-

Table 14.1
Some first-hand accounts of general practice

Period	Place	Author*
1832–42	British Columbia	Tolmie
1871–1930	Ontario	Groves
1893	Labrador	Curwen
1894–1930s	Kansas	Hertzler
1885–1965	SW Quebec	Geggie
1907–12	Saskatchewan	MacLean
1929–31	N. Alberta	Jackson
1930s	SW Newfoundland	Rusted
1933–47	Yukon	Duncan
1935	Aklavik	Urquhart
1924–54	Ontario	Johnston

*For full references, see 'Suggestions for Further Reading.'

cedures had declined and the most common diagnoses of the 1930s had almost disappeared because of vaccines and antibiotics. This change through time is apparent even within individual practices. Langstaff's prescribing habits altered more slowly but in concert with the changes described for major centres. Country doctors also adopted the new technologies for diagnosis and treatment, such as anesthesia, antisepsis, thermometers, and electrical machines. In the 1880s Langstaff's surgical practice seemed to wane, perhaps in competition with (or through relieved recognition of) specialists in nearby Toronto.

Despite rarely having time off work and, even less often, enjoying full payment, rural doctors usually managed to live quite comfortably and with the respect of their communities. By the turn of the century, however, doubts about competence had tarnished the image of the kindly GP and respect began to wane.

'I'm Just a GP': The Threat to General Practice

The threat to general practice was manifested first by declining numbers in specific geographic regions and by criticisms of incompetence. At the end of the nineteenth century, specialists were increasingly numerous in urban areas. General practice became the

---

Specialists versus Generalists

The rapid increase of knowledge has made concentration in work a necessity; specialism is here, and here to stay ... The desire for expert knowledge is ... now so great that there is a grave danger lest the family doctor should become ... a relic of the past.

William Osler, *Boston Medical and Surgical Journal* 126 (1892), 457–9, esp. 457

---

equivalent of rural practice and was characterized by culture-based assumptions about the 'modern city' and the 'backward country.' Ambient optimism about science meant that specialists were thought to be more effective than their humble rural colleagues because they were perceived to be more 'scientific.' Before the telephone, the automobile, highways, and air transportation, availability preserved a role for GPs – people in isolated areas had to be satisfied with one doctor for all their needs. But with shrinking distances and more trainees, some GPs began to predict the eventual demise of their metier with 'doleful misgivings' upon 'looking into the gloom' (Hattie, *Canadian Med. Ass. Journal* 22 [1930], 548).

In the more populated centres of the United States, France, and Great Britain, the proportion of general practitioners began to decline. Sociologist William G. Rothstein showed that from 1930 to 1962, the number of GPs in the United States fell in both absolute and relative terms from 90 to 37 per 100,000 population, or from 71 per cent of all doctors to only 27 per cent. In Canada and Australia, with their huge distances and vast areas of low population, specialty practice was both impractical and unprofitable; specialists there concentrated in cities, but the overall numbers of GPs remained proportionately higher. Nevertheless, by 1948, more than two-thirds of Toronto graduates planned to seek specialty training, although at least three-quarters eventually found themselves in general practice. That outcome was perceived to be a second choice for (presumably) second-rate doctors.

A Vignette from Vancouver Island

When [the city of] Victoria was young ...you did not have a special doctor for each part. Dr. Helmcken attended to all our ailments ... You began to get better the moment you heard [him] coming up the stairs. He did have the most horrible medicines ... Once I knelt on a needle which broke into my knee ... The Doctor cut slits in my knee and wiggled his fingers around inside it for three hours hunting for the pieces of the needle ... [He] said, 'Yell, lassie, yell! It will let the pain out.' I did yell, but the pain stayed in.

Emily Carr, *The Book of Small* (London and Oxford: Oxford University Press, 1942), 199–200

By the mid-1940s, general practice was experiencing a massive identity crisis, which constituted yet another threat. With few mechanisms for maintaining and guaranteeing standards, competence could be questioned. The public and the profession alike were aware that some doctors were more conscientious than others. Made to feel like second-class citizens, many GPs seemed almost resigned to the inevitable disappearance of their way of life. But the more optimistic formed professional associations, touting the undeniable merits of their enterprise: hard work, diagnostic challenge, diversity, continuity, and comprehensive care. Calls for the recognition of general practice as a specialty in its own right became more insistent and frequent.

In delineating the early-twentieth-century competition between obstetricians and GPs, Charlotte Borst observed a fundamental irony: GPs, who had once been the very doctors arguing for physician-assisted births 'would, in the end, find themselves eliminated from the birthing room' by their specialist competitors (1995, 130). Historian David Adams found a similar development in the 1945 attempt of a hospital in Cincinnati, Ohio, to limit privileges for tonsillectomy to Ear, Nose, and Throat (ENT) specialists. Increasing in numbers, the ENT specialists knew that the incidence of medically

Table 14.2
Some milestones in general/family practice

	Professional association	Specialty training	'Family' medicine
United States	1947	1969	1969
Great Britain	1952	1965	
Canada	1954	1966	1967
Australia	1958	1973	

unmanageable tonsillitis was stable or was likely to decline with the promise of antibiotics: more doctors; fewer procedures. They perceived the operating GP as a financial threat, but they cloaked their opposition in the morally superior issue of patient safety. The posturing failed. The GPs formed their own association, and the resultant uproar caused the hospital to rescind its decision. The organizational momentum of these GPs spilled well beyond the borders of the city to both the state and the nation. By 1947 the American Academy of General Practice had been formed. As postwar incursions on the scope and profitability of their work grew ever more hostile, GPs became angry, and they mobilized.

Professionalization of General Practice

As the diamond with its many facets is the finest of gems, so ... the family physician with his multiple viewpoints should be inferior to no other.

W. Victor Johnston, 1948 (cited in Woods 1979, 28)

The newly formed professional associations immediately went to work on several fronts. They countered the charge of incompetence in two ways: first, through workshops for the training and continuing education of their colleagues; second, by demanding the right to certify their own trainees. They also sought recognition within hospitals and medical schools. As they reminded their critics, ambulatory

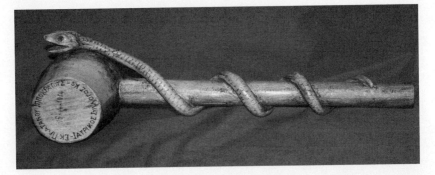

Gavel representing the snake and the staff of Asklepios, made of wood from the tree under which Hippocrates supposedly taught. Presented to the Canadian College of Family Physicians by the physicians of Cos

care comprised the bulk of practice after graduation (even for specialists); medical education should somehow reflect that fact. The initiative immediately raised the morale of the much-maligned GPs, who seemed to revel in their annual (and soon to be tax deductible) meetings. But achieving their goals took some time.

The Canadian College of General Practitioners (CCGP) was inaugurated in 1954 at a salmon luncheon in Vancouver; its permanent home would be Toronto. W. Victor Johnston, a GP from Lucknow, Ontario, was appointed the first executive director, a post he occupied for a decade. To mark the occasion, the Hippocratic society of physicians on the Greek island of Cos presented the new college with a gavel, entwined with the serpent of Asklepios and carved in wood taken 'from the plane tree under which Hippocrates taught.' The CCGP immediately sought advice and support from its slightly older siblings in the United States and Great Britain; in turn, it mentored similar groups in other countries. This national body emerged within the age of jet travel, easily linking it to events elsewhere in the world. In 1964 Montreal was selected to host the first international conference of general practice. This meeting was the first gathering of what in 1972 came to be called the World Organization of National Colleges, Academies, and Academic Associations of General Practitioners/Family Physicians (WONCA). It has held triennial meetings since 1980.

Opposition from specialists was a major obstacle to CCGP goals. Early organizers recall a frosty reception by the executive of the Royal College of Physicians and Surgeons of Canada (RCPSC), which had been founded in 1929 to certify specialists. The two bodies held a joint meeting in 1960 in an attempt to melt the ice, but friction persisted for some time. Specialists, who dominated undergraduate medical education, were loathe to yield structural or curricular space. Hospitals were slightly more receptive, and GPs continued to find admitting and practice privileges through departments of obstetrics, pediatrics, and psychiatry, where they performed routine tasks for lower fees than the specialists. The federal government sponsored pilot projects to develop GP training in Calgary, Alberta, and in London, Ontario. By 1960 thirty-three Canadian hospitals offered postgraduate work in general practice, although certification and academic departments had yet to be established.

Political differences, either actual or perceived, no doubt played a role. Specialists, who were well trained, older, and better paid, tended to be conservative, while the young physicians, medical students, and interns more commonly leaned to the left. During the war, younger medics had been intrigued by the decentralized community health-care initiatives and *feldsher* system of their Russian ally, and they willingly contemplated similar arrangements for the Canadian scene. These idealistic doctors, who worried less about money or prestige and more about public welfare, joined with the tired, rural practitioners to promote general practice issues. They also supported the simultaneous struggle for universal healthcare (see chapter 6) and called for collaboration with nurse-practitioners, social workers, rehabilitationists, and other health care providers. But in the Cold War of the following decades, their zeal was characterized as naive, amateurish, and dangerous. This multiplicity of political perspectives within the Canadian medical profession constitutes a striking difference between it and its neighbour to the south.

Once the specialist group finally became resigned to the tenacity of the generalists, it tried to 'hug them to death' by promoting certification in general medicine as a branch of the RCPSC. The GPs firmly resisted this new threat, viewing the right to certify their own as a necessary prerequisite for autonomy. Further impediments arose in 1963 with the formation of the Fédération des médecins omnipracticiens du Québec (FMOQ), which promoted the political and economic interests of Quebec GPs but opposed certification. When the residencies began in 1966, the CCFP viewed the achievement as a major victory; certificates of examination were first awarded in 1969. Thirty years later, these three professional bodies seem to have forgotten the initial mistrust; they maintain cordial relations and reciprocate on many levels.

Having solved the residency problem, the GPs moved on to tackle the medical schools. Some universities had already nodded in the direction of general medicine. For example, nonspecialists were employed in specialty programs; students received credit for preceptorships in private offices; and general practice units were created in existing departments of epidemiology and public health. Canada was a North American leader in academic family medicine – the residency at McMaster University was the first educational program launched by the fledgling medical school in 1967. The following year, the University of Western Ontario lured the general practice guru Ian R. McWhinney from Britain to be the first professor. Other universities soon followed suit, and by 1979 all sixteen medical schools in Canada could boast departments of family medicine. The United States moved at a slightly slower pace. In 1976 its federal government launched a project of grants designed to raise the percentage of medical schools with general practice departments above the 67 per cent level reached in that year.

The presence of an academic department did not guarantee the visibility of general practice in the undergraduate curriculum, which was still dominated by specialists. In 1983, according to Rothstein, only 56 per cent of American and Canadian schools required family practice rotations in the final year of training. Its presence was even less frequent in the more junior years, and it continues to pose a challenge in many schools. Nevertheless, what came to be called 'family medicine' is the residency choice for approximately 40 per cent of graduates in Canada. During the process, the name itself gained great significance.

The Advent of 'Family Medicine'

What's in a Name?

The American founders of the Board of Family Medicine have found it necessary to repudiate the name 'general practice' because of its associations with a type of practice which is deplored in academic circles ... 'Family medicine' as a name for our discipline and 'family physicians' for its members are both descriptive and dignified. Most of us, however, would recoil from a formal change of name and would be content, I think, to let evolution take its course.

Ian R. McWhinney, *Lancet* 1 (1966), 419

Irvine Loudon traced the use of the words 'general practice' back to 1809, but he warned that seeking the expression in the more distant past is hopelessly anachronistic. When used in the eighteenth and nineteenth centuries, 'general practice' referred not to the work of the family doctor or the *omnipracticien*, but to the usual or customary course of medical action. The older usage resurfaced in the late twentieth century, when 'general internal medicine' and the 'general internist' came along to threaten GPs on the issue of primary care. In contrast, the term 'family physician' rarely appeared in nineteenth-century medical literature. Instead, it was used in the titles of 'self-help' medical encyclopedias and other forms of advice literature for people who wished either to demystify or to avoid their doctor. In her study of the popular literature of France, historian Martha Hildreth found that the new sciences of disease meant that an emphasis on 'family' could act as an antidote to the fear that medical practice was becoming overly scientific.

Names are symbolic. The conscious and almost universal renaming of 'general practice' as 'family practice' in English-speaking North America was a political as well as an etymological act, with both economic and cultural implications. It can be narrowly located in the late 1960s and is intimately connected to another threatened issue – primary care.

In 1966 Canada enacted a health-care system that was to provide universal access to free or affordable services. Doctors would be paid for all their services, but anonymous taxpayers rather than individual patients would be obligated for medical fees. Confident in the status of their scientific training, pediatricians, obstetricians, and general internists knew that the relative differences in their fees would no longer inhibit patients desirous of their attentions. Surely, demands on their services would and should increase. What more pleasant way to supplement coffers than by looking after people who are not very sick? Already, well-off people in the United States relied on specialists for primary care – pediatricians for children, gynecologists for women, and internists for adults and the aged. The specialist as a primary caregiver became a new and intriguing possibility, occupying increasing space in medical literature.

Canadian GPs helped to nip this process in the bud in two interesting ways. First, GP-versus-specialist became a matter of fiscal responsibility within the new fee schedules. Taxpayers should not be on the hook for unnecessary services. To see a specialist, patients would normally need the referral of another physician; without a referral, the specialist would have to accept a lower fee. In Ontario, for example, these restrictions are stated in 'Terms and Definitions' of fee schedules and follow sections on the 'Principles of Ethical Billing.' Suddenly, primary care seemed somewhat less attractive to the specialists in this country, although it is still hotly debated in the United States.

Second, GPs redefined their enterprise as 'family medicine.' The word 'family' implied all-inclusive practice in a positive way that evoked comfortable images of hearth and home. 'Family' also eliminated – or 'repudiated,' to use Ian McWhinney's term – the negative connotations of that vague word 'general,' which had always seemed to invite the charge of incompetence. How could any doctor be an expert in everything? Unlike 'general,' the word 'family' was not apologetic and needed no justification. It implied that one doctor could serve each person well without forgetting the significant context of the others. Children, women, the elderly – all could trust a family doctor to provide primary care.

The renaming of the CCGP as the CCFP formally took place in 1967 just as the residencies were launched. A similar change soon took place in the United States and in this instance again, Canada – with its new health-care system – seems to have led the way. In 1968 Malcolm Hill and colleagues conducted a survey in Hamilton, Ontario, to assess the validity of the term 'family doctor': 86 per cent of respondents representing 600 families in the care of four different doctors reported that one physician looked after the whole family. 'Is family doctor a valid term?' The answer, they concluded, was yes. For our purposes, the date of the survey and the fact that the question needed to be asked at all exemplify a fascinating shift.

McWhinney predicted that British GPs would resist the trend, but in 1984 when Oxford University launched its new journal, the title was *Family Practice.*

Research in Family Medicine: Oxymoron, Phoenix, or Sop?

The Collings Condemnation

My observations have led me to write what is indeed a condemnation of general practice in its present form, but they have also led me to recognize the importance of general practice and the dangers of continuing to pretend it is something which it is not.

Joseph S. Collings, *Lancet* 1 (1950), 555

Having secured its place in both undergraduate and postgraduate education, family medicine began to consolidate its position by claiming to provide exceptional research opportunities. The thought of GPs conducting research was ridiculed by many medical professionals. GPs themselves were divided on the issue. Some feared that research would be self-defeating by detracting from the central clinical purpose of holistic, comprehensive, and continuing care. Research seemed to be an unnecessary concession to the new and hard-won academic status – a concession that would inevitably turn family doctors into specialists by making them experts on the tiny topics that lent themselves to scientific investigation. Having successfully resisted the specialists on certification, they saw no reason to offer this sop to the old specialist-dominated structure of academe.

Others, like American leader John P. Geyman, saw tremendous research potential in the very nature of family practice, with its emphasis on continuity and comprehensive care. They argued that consortiums of GPs could use epidemiological methods on their practice records to answer those burning questions that left specialists bored. In Britain, classic works were reprinted on general practice research, describing it as the 'most alluring of occupations.'

One of the earliest general practice research projects was a British epidemiological investigation, published in 1956, which demonstrated that penicillin was of no value in measles. More recently, international committees of WONCA collaborated to create classification systems for assessing functional capacity that can be applied to research into common biological problems. In some places, however, population-based research – especially when it involved patterns of morbidity and mortality – seemed to encroach on the realm of public health experts, who doubted the conceptual and statistical sophistication of their family medicine colleagues. At the 1992 WONCA meeting in Vancouver, the four thousand delegates were exhorted to preserve global health by promoting peace and protecting the environment.

GPs also turned their research on themselves and their work, or they invited sociologists to do so on their behalf. What assumptions influenced the individuals and services that made up family practice? How could activities be made more efficient? Was solo work better than working in a group? Could a well-equipped office eliminate the need for house calls? Prompted by the famous Collings Report (1950), several British studies made recommendations for changes. In 1963 Kenneth Clute analysed Canadian general practice by comparing two provinces. He identified problems in physician distribution and work-related stress, including lack of time for professional renewal, patients, family, and friends. He predicted that the impending changes in health-care provision would be detrimental. A decade later, Wolfe and Badgley took up the same theme. Studies of the quality and quantity of life and work still constitute a major research issue within the discipline.

Next, family medicine research shifted from epidemiological investigations to behaviourist and psychotherapeutic issues. Disillusionment with statistics may have been one reason for the change. According to Thomas Osborne, GPs perceived limitations in population-based research and were uncomfortable with remote collective surveys. 'Sensitive to singularity,' he said, GPs were trained to focus on individuals and were attuned to a person-centred model. As a result, 'a subjectivizing surveillance of self was substituted for an objectivizing surveillance of morbid populations.' Research came to be motivated by what Osborne called a 'salvationist ideology,' centred on doctor-patient relations, communication, accountability, and introspection.

Thirty years later, research is still a contentious issue in family medicine. GPs have not rushed into scientific investigation, although the university systems of promotion and tenure urge them to do so with tangible rewards. The early 1990s witnessed the advent of 'evidence-based medicine' for validity of practice issues as described by epidemiologists and internists, especially at McMaster University in Hamilton, Ontario. Family practitioners seem to be eyeing the new trend with both scepticism and interest.

Impact of Family Medicine on the Specialties

Vive la différence!

Academic family medicine has made considerable progress in the last 20 years, yet we still do not fit comfortably into the academic milieu. To gain acceptance, it is said, family medicine must become less pragmatic, more theoretical, and more productive in quantitative research.

I believe that family medicine is marginal because it differs in some fundamental ways from the academic mainstream and that our main value to medicine lies in the differences. Eventually I think the academic mainstream will become more like us than vice versa.

Ian R. McWhinney, *Canadian Family Physician* 43 (1997), 193

Family medicine has influenced all medical practice in a wide variety of ways, the most obvious being the importance of Continuing Medical Education (CME) and the need for ongoing evaluation. From its very inception, the CCGP required members to seek a minimum of one hundred hours of postgraduate study every two years. In other words, the historically informed recognition that medicine will continue to change is embedded in the structure of the organization. Patients are assured that a CCFP-certified doctor has met the recognized standard of practice, not once but repeatedly. With its commitment to lifelong learning and public accountability, family medicine has helped to generate a market for the rising industry of CME and has stimulated research in original forms of pedagogic communication. As public mistrust of physicians grew, the enterprise rubbed off on specialist groups concerned about accountability. Thirty years after the founding of the CCGP, the Royal College implemented 'maintenance of competence' programs for Canadian specialists, and similar programs are being considered by specialist groups elsewhere in the world. By 1999, family doctors were deans in several medical faculties.

In trying to promote itself to the well-established schools as an academic discipline, organized family medicine also embarked on the philosophic task of self-definition. Not only did it establish the boundaries for its own identity and pedagogy, but it set criteria that could eventually be applied to the recognition of other newcomers. Having done so, it invited scholars from several nations to develop parameters of evaluation for training programs, for CME, and for evaluation of the evaluations themselves.

The 'miracles' of technology and subspecialization provide yet another justification for the integrative capacity of family medicine. The family practitioner permits the subspecialist to function in a restricted space. Conversely, the chronic problems of an aging population, polypharmacy, iatrogenic illness, and the impersonal face of a medical establishment centred on hospitals have combined to create a continuing role for the family physician. The doctor who actually knows and remembers the patient and her family is essential. Researcher or not, the family doctor *selects, coordinates,* and above all *explains* the specific expertise that will help to diagnose or treat a patient. And with the long-established features of continuity and context, only family medicine can provide the holistic care that an increasingly sceptical public now demands.

Suggestions for Further Reading

Ackerman, Evelyn Bernette. 'The Activities of a Country Doctor in New York State: Dr. Elias Cornelius of Somers, 1794–1803.' *Historical Reflections/Réflexions historiques* 9 (1982), 181–93

Adams, David P. 'Community and Professionalization: General Practitioners and Ear, Nose, and Throat Specialists in Cincinnati, 1945–1947.' *Bulletin of the History of Medicine* 68 (1994), 664–84

Borst, Charlotte G. *Catching Babies: The Professionalization of Childbirth, 1870–1920*. Cambridge, Mass.: Harvard University Press, 1995

Collings, Joseph S. 'General Practice in England Today.' *Lancet* 1 (1950), 555–85

Coulter, Harris L. *Divided Legacy: The Conflict between Homeopathy and the American Medical Association*. Richmond, Calif.: North Atlantic Books, 1973

Cule, John. *A Doctor for All the People: Two Thousand Years of General Practice in Britain*. London: Update Books, 1980

Day, Patricia. 'The State, the NHS, and General Practice.' *Journal of Public Health Policy* 13 (1992), 165–79

Doherty, William J., Charles E. Christianson, and Marvin B. Sussman, eds. *Family Medicine: The Maturing of a Discipline*. New York: Haworth Press, 1987

Estes, J. Worth, and David M. Goodman. *The Changing Humours of Portsmouth: The Medical Biography of an American Town, 1623–1983*. Boston: Francis Countway Library of Medicine, 1986

Freidson, Eliot. *Profession of Medicine: A Study of the Sociology of Applied Knowledge*. New York: Harper and Row, 1970

Gelfand, Toby. 'The Decline of the Ordinary Practitioner and the Rise of the Modern Medical Profession.' In *Doctors, Patients, and Society: Power and Authority in Medical Care*, ed. Martin Staum and Donald E. Larsen, 105–29. Waterloo, Ont.: Wilfrid Laurier University Press, 1981

Geyman, John P. 'Family Practice in Evolution: Progress, Problems, and Projections.' *New England Journal of Medicine* 298 (1978), 593–601

Gray, Denis Pereira. 'History of the Royal College of General Practitioners: The First Forty Years.' *British Journal of General Practice* 42 (1992), 29–35

Haddy, R.I., et al. 'A Comparison of Rural Family Practice in the 1930s and Today.' *Journal of Family Practice* 36 (Jan. 1993), 65–9

Haggerty, Robert J. 'The University and Primary Medical Care.' *New England Journal of Medicine* 281 (1969), 416–22

Hertzler, Arthur E. *The Horse and Buggy Doctor.* New York and London: Harper, 1938

Hildreth, Martha L. 'Doctors and Families in France, 1880–1930: The Cultural Reconstruction of Medicine.' In *French Medical Culture in the Nineteenth Century,* ed. Ann La Berge and Mordechai Feingold. Amsterdam, and Atlanta, Ga: Rodopi Press; and *Clio Medica* 25 (1994), 189–209

Lawrence, Christopher. *Medicine in the Making of Modern Britain.* London and New York: Routledge, 1994

Leavitt, Judith Walzer. 'Fielding H. Garrison Lecture. "A Worrying Profession": The Domestic Environment of Medical Practice in Mid-Nineteenth-Century America.' *Bulletin of the History of Medicine* 69 (1995), 1–29

Léonard, Jacques. *La France médicale: Médecins et malades au XIXe siècle.* Paris: Gallimard, 1978

Loudon, Irvine. *Medical Care and the General Practitioner, 1750–1850.* Oxford: Clarendon Press, 1986

McDonell, Katherine Mandusic. *The Journals of William A. Lindsay: An Ordinary Nineteenth-Century Physician's Surgical Cases.* Indianapolis: Indiana Historical Society, 1989

McWhinney, Ian. 'General Practice as an Academic Discipline: Reflections after a Visit to the United States.' *Lancet* 1 (1966), 419–23. See also *Lancet* 1 (1967), 91–6

– 'William Pickles Lecture (1996): The Importance of Being Different.' *British Journal of General Practice* 46 (1996), 433–6

Marland, Hilary. *Medicine in Wakefield and Huddersfield, 1780–1870.* Cambridge: Cambridge University Press, 1987

Osborne, Thomas. 'Epidemiology as an Investigative Paradigm: The College of General Practitioners in the 1950s.' *Social Science and Medicine* 38 (1994), 317–26

Ramsey, Matthew. *Professional and Popular Medicine in France, 1770–1830: The Social World of Medical Practice.* Cambridge: Cambridge University Press, 1988

Reiser, Stanley J. 'The Coming Resurgence of the Generalist in Medicine: Its Technological and Conceptual Basis.' *Pharos* 58 (1995), 8–11

Rothstein, William G. *American Medical Schools and the Practice of Medicine.* New York and Oxford: Oxford University Press, 1987

Stephens, G. Gayle. *Basis of Family Practice.* Tuscon, Ariz.: Winter Publishing, 1982

Stone, M.C. 'James Mackenzie Lecture: The Most Alluring of Occupations.' *Practitioner* 216 (1976), 77–89

Truman, Stanley R. *The History of the Founding of the American Academy of General Practice.* St Louis, Mo.: Warren H. Green and American Academy of General Practice, 1969

Weisz, George. 'Medical Directories and Medical Specialization in France, Britain, and the United States.' *Bulletin of the History of Medicine* 71 (1997), 23–68

On Canada

Bernier, Jacques. *La médecine au Québec: Naissance et évolution d'une profession.* Québec: Presses de l'Université Laval, 1989

Campbell, C.M. 'The Maintenance of Competence Programme of the Royal College of Physicians and Surgeons of Canada (MOCOMP).' *Postgraduate Medical Journal* 72, suppl. 1 (1996), S41–2

Clute, Kenneth F. *The General Practitioner: A Study of Medical Education and Practice in Ontario and Nova Scotia.* Toronto: University of Toronto Press, 1963

Connor, J.T.H. '"A Sort of Felo-De-Se": Eclecticism, Related Medical Sects, and Their Decline in Victorian Ontario.' *Bulletin of the History of Medicine* 65 (1991), 503–27

Curwen, Eliot. *Labrador Odyssey: The Journal and Photographs of Eliot Curwen on the Second Voyage of Wilfred Grenfell, 1893*, ed. Ronald Rompkey. Montreal and Kingston: McGill-Queen's University Press, 1996

Duffin, Jacalyn. *Langstaff: A Nineteenth-Century Medical Life.* Toronto: University of Toronto Press, 1993

Duncan, Allan. *Medicine, Madams, and Mounties: Stories of a Yukon Doctor, 1933–1947.* Vancouver: Raincoast Books, 1989

Geggie, H.J.G. *The Extra Mile: Medicine in Rural Quebec, 1885–1965*, ed. Norma and Stuart Geggie. Wakefield, Que., 1987

Gidney, R.D., and W.P.J. Millar. 'The Origins of Organized Medicine in Ontario, 1850–1869.' In *Health, Disease, and Medicine: Essays in Canadian History*, ed. Charles G. Roland, 65–95. Toronto: Hannah Institute for the History of Medicine, 1982

– *Professional Gentlemen; The Professions in Nineteenth-Century Ontario.* Toronto: University of Toronto Press, 1994

Groves, Abraham. *All in a Day's Work: Leaves from a Doctor's Casebook.* Toronto: Macmillan, 1934

Hill, Malcolm, R.G. McAuley, W.B. Spaulding, and Margaret Wilson. 'Validity of the Term "Family Doctor": A Limited Study in Hamilton, Ontario.' *Canadian Medical Association Journal* 98 (1968), 734–8

Jack, Donald. *Rogues, Rebels, and Geniuses: The Story of Canadian Medicine.* Toronto and Garden City, NY: Doubleday, 1981

Jackson, Mary Percy. *Suitable for the Wilds: Letters from Northern Alberta, 1929–1931.* Ed. Janice Dickin McGinnis. Toronto: University of Toronto Press, 1995

Johnston, William Victor. *Before the Age of Miracles: Memoirs of a Country Doctor.* Toronto: Fitzhenry and Whiteside, 1972

MacLean, Hugh. 'Recollections and Reminiscences: A Pioneer Prairie Doctor.' *Saskatchewan History* 15 (1962), 58–66

MacNab, Elizabeth. *A Legal History of the Health Professions in Ontario.* Toronto: Queen's Printer, 1970

McWhinney, Ian R. 'General Practice in Canada.' *International Journal of Health Services* 2 (May 1972), 229–37

Norris, John. 'The Country Doctor in British Columbia.' *B.C. Studies* 49 (1981–2), 15–39

Roland, Charles G. 'The Diary of a Canadian Country Physician: Jonathan Woolverton (1881–1883).' *Medical History* 14 (1971), 168–80

Roland, Charles G., and Bohodar Rubashewsky. 'The Economic Status of the Practice of Dr. Harmaunus Smith in Wentworth County, Ontario, 1826–1867.' *Canadian Bulletin of Medicial History* 5 (1988), 29–49

Romano, Terrie. 'Professional Identity and the Nineteenth-Century Ontario Medical Profession.' *Histoire Sociale/Social History* 23 (1995), 77–98

Rusted, Nigel. *Its Devil Deep Down There.* St John's, Nfld: Creative Publishers, 1987

Shephard, David A.E. *The Royal College of Physicians and Surgeons of Canada: The Pursuit of Unity.* Ottawa: RCPSC, 1985

Shortt, S.E.D. '"Before the Age of Miracles": The Rise, Fall, and Rebirth of General Practice in Canada, 1890–1940.' In *Health Disease and Medicine: Essays in Canadian History*, ed. Charles G. Roland, 123–52. Toronto: Hannah Institute for the History of Medicine, 1984

Tolmie, W.F. *The Journals of William Fraser Tolmie: Physician and Fur Trader.* Vancouver: Mitchell Press, 1963

Tunis, Barbara Logan. 'The Medical Profession in Lower Canada: Its Evolution as a Social Group, 1788–1838.' BA thesis, Carleton University, 1979

Urquhart, J.A. 'The Most Northerly Practice in Canada.' 1935. Reprinted *Canadian Medical Association Journal* 147 (1992), 1760–1

Wolfe, Samuel, and Robin F. Badgley. *The Family Doctor: Has He Disappeared? Can We Get Him Back?* Toronto: Macmillan, 1973

Woods, David. *Strength in Study: An Informal History of the College of Family Physicians of Canada.* Toronto: College of Family Physicians of Canada, 1979

CHAPTER FIFTEEN

Sleuthing and Science: How to Research a Question in Medical History*

History as a simple recitation of names and dates is dusty, boring stuff. But questions about why we do what we do or think what we think are compelling. Similarly, it can be equally compelling to seek answers to questions about why people used to think or do certain things, especially if those thoughts or deeds are now considered wrong. Historians can enjoy all the excitement and intrigue of detective work with a much lower risk of getting shot.

Bad medical history gives the entire enterprise an undeservedly poor reputation; it may explain why books about teaching history to health-care students seem obliged to begin with self-justification. Anatomy, physiology, and pharmacology do not apologize for their presence in the curriculum. Yet good history is also directly relevant to health-care education. It revolves around a fundamental truth: things change at different rates in different times and places, and for different reasons. Exploring the dimensions of that statement with respect to any aspect of health-care provision, in any culture, is history. Historical investigation relates to the goals of lifelong learning and evidence-based choice, which are essential for competent practice. Furthermore, good historical research resembles the scientific enterprise in many ways; it is about questions and answers.

This chapter contains my advice for conducting historical research. It is a subjective product of personal trial and error. I make no claims for originality. A history project can be approached

*Educational objectives for this chapter are found on p. 399.

in countless other ways. My method was and still is being shaped by my professors in medicine and history, and by colleagues, writers, editors, and especially my students. Since I am unable to perceive its weaknesses and biases, I advise you to use these ideas with care.

Framing a Clear Question

> The question is like the hypothesis in a scientific experiment.

The would-be investigator of history must understand exactly what is being sought and why she or he is seeking it. Presenting rounds, writing a report or an after-dinner speech, contemplating a change in practice, developing a policy, or simple curiosity are some of the many reasons that lead a student or practitioner to ask an historical question. The question will inevitably be refined by the available sources of information, by the results, and by the individual conducting the investigation. The final form of the question may bear little resemblance to the original.

At all times, the investigator should have in mind an honest and concise statement of the current question. Sophisticated questions take into account theoretical explanations that have usually been generated by other scholars for application to similar problems; however, simple questions are not intrinsically boring, nor does anything preclude creating a new theory.

Thoughout the process, the historian must acknowledge his or her role as a participant in the project – in matters of taste pertaining to the selection of subject, in the choice of research avenues that appeal, and in the neglect of pathways that seem less promising.

Identifying Sources

> Sources are like the materials in a scientific experiment.

The evidence for statements about the past are the sources. In general, sources are of two types – primary and secondary – but they may overlap. Sometimes it is simpler to begin with the secondary sources, where you may quickly find an answer to your question. Appendix B, on resources and research tools, introduces general secondary sources on various subjects. But answers derived from secondary sources should be handled with care. The best evidence comes from primary sources.

Primary Sources

Primary sources are documents produced during the period under investigation or produced by the subject of the study. Sometimes – for example, in the case of a newly discovered manuscript – they become the question, because their origin and purpose are unknown. If the project focuses on a person, the primary sources encompass that individual's publications and manuscript papers, including diplomas, practice records, laboratory notebooks, diaries, letters written and received, and scrapbooks. Primary sources also include other collections of manuscripts, contemporary books, journals, and newspapers. If the subject is a disease, a treatment, or a technology, the primary sources could include original descriptions, subsequent modifications, commentary, and possibly extant artifacts. If the subject is an institution, a period, or a place, the primary materials are found in anything emerging from that institution, period, or place. To learn about the health of populations, government documents, census statistics, and agency surveys are invaluable.

In defining primary sources, context is important. A historian must strive to situate the topic in time and place. No medical subject – be it a person, a practice, an institution, a technology, or an idea – can be fully explored without also studying its political, social, economic, and cultural environment. Sometimes, the environmental conditions are revealed by contrasting them with those elsewhere. For example, revolution or famine in one country will influence its medicine, while the medicine of another country, which may be enjoying peace and prosperity, will not be so affected.

History – itself made up of writing – has traditionally placed a special value on the written word as the ultimate form of evidence.

But this practice can obscure or skew the past by excluding the testimony of those who were not able to publish or write – women, children, patients, and illiterate or disadvantaged peoples. Moreover, just because something had been written does not make it accurate. Historical documents are powerful witnesses, but they have certain problems: quantities are variable; they reflect the authors' priorities; and their contents may be flawed. In recent decades, historical emphasis shifted away from great men, great discoveries, and great nations. Consequently, primary sources have become more eclectic and include 'oral histories' (the result of interviews), pictures, films, novels, art, music, and objects.

In the search for printed primary sources, the historian must rely on libraries – the bigger the better – and on bibliographies and indexes. For example, when dealing with a subject from antiquity, claims and quotations found in a secondary source must be verified with scholarly editions (e.g., the Loeb Classical Library or the Corpus Medicorum Grecorum). With electronic resources, it is possible to stay at home and browse the catalogues of great institutions such as McGill's Osler Library and the National Library of Medicine. Printed (and online) catalogues of the national libraries of France (Bibliothèque Nationale), Britain (British Library), and the United States (National Union Catalogue) are available in most university libraries and provide a wealth of bibliographic information.

Most health sciences libraries hold the early series of the *Index Catalogue of the Library of the Surgeon General's Office*. From 1880, it listed the holdings of what is now the U.S. National Library of Medicine, including references to a host of medical books and journal articles dating back several centuries. Early editions of the *Index Medicus* also are useful, but they must be examined year by year. For recent topics, both Medline and periodical literature indexes, including newspapers (such as *The New York Times Index*, *The Times Index*, and *Canadian Periodical Index*) provide a start, but they have limitations (see below). Morton's *Bibliography* is an attempt to list the most significant contributions to Western medical literature. (See also Appendix B2.)

Tracing unpublished primary sources is usually more complicated. Historians are rarely confident that they have examined every scrap of paper that could be seen. Archives exist in a surprising variety of forms and places. National and institutional archives are good places to begin. Published catalogues of holdings are helpful; specific collections are often indexed in unpublished guides called 'Finding Aids.' Archivists will usually respond to questions by mail or e-mail. But the scholar must know (or imagine) that an archive exists in order to find it. Again, archivists can be of assistance.

In a perfect world, all important papers would be kept in archives. Government and institutional documents are ordered by law to be preserved. Every country, every province or state, many cities, all universities, and most hospitals, organizations, and associations maintain records. In reality, however, complete preservation is rare. Even when a scholar is confident that the papers must reside in a particular archive, locating them there through a baffling classification system can be daunting. Having found the 'official' government records, scholars must remember that they are precisely that – official. They tell a version of the story chosen by a bureaucrat. Unknown quantities of papers may have been lost or deliberately destroyed. Indeed, the most salacious, controversial, and intriguing aspects in the life of an individual or institution can be forever excised in this way. Some papers may belong to friends, relatives, or descendants who refuse to open them to historians. Still others are withdrawn from scholarship, having become the property of private dealers and investors. Occasionally, an obituary or an entry in a biographical or national dictionary will indicate where the papers of an individual are kept. Finding papers is time-consuming and frustrating, but it is also deeply rewarding. For this kind of discovery – a piece of evidence to support an idea – the historian shouts, 'Eureka!'

Secondary Sources

Secondary sources are produced by fellow historians, be they living or dead. They include all attempts to explore the same or similar questions. The authors may be other practitioners, historians, sociologists, or philosophers, but they may also be contemporaries of the subject, such as colleagues, eulogists, and descendants. Sometimes, the secondary source will provide an immediate and satisfying answer to your question; however, before accepting such information at face value, it is wise to contemplate the nine caveats described below.

On Secondary Sources: Beware!

1 Assume someone else has already asked (and answered) your question.
2 Find out who, when, and where.
3 If you find no predecessors, be creative and search in tangential fields.
4 Exploit others' references for additional primary and secondary sources.
5 Be aware that you are not obliged to agree with your predecessors.
6 Find reviews of the sources on which you rely heavily. Is your opinion shared by experts? Is your confidence well placed?
7 Do not trust history without references, a.k.a. 'scholarly apparatus.'
8 Believe nothing you read if it does not refer to primary sources.
9 Believe nothing you read if you cannot understand why it was written.

When asked for help with a research question, I begin with the accessible *Bibliographies of the History of Medicine,* prepared by the National Library of Medicine since 1964. These five-year cumulative indices of the historical publishing recorded in the *Index Medicus* are cross-referenced by subject, author, and period. Individual diseases appear under the main heading of 'Disease.' Medline is also an excellent guide to secondary sources (as well as primary sources for late-twentieth-century topics). Separate entries on the history of a MeSH subject can be located by adding a '/hi' subheading (e.g., 'nursing/hi'). MeSH subject headings for history are organized by century only; to narrow a search, a strategic combination with key words must be made. Do not rely on Medline alone. It includes only some of the scholarly journals that have an interest in history; it does not always assign historical subject headings or key words to articles with historical information; it contains nothing published prior to 1966; and it ignores books and edited volumes (unless they happen to have enjoyed essay reviews). Other print tools, such as the *Index Medicus* and the *Science Citation Index*, cover the years prior to 1966 and include books.

A thorough search should extend beyond health-care literature. Relevant information may have appeared in periodicals devoted to philosophy, anthropology, history, sociology, economics, geography, political studies, and public administration. Database and print tools are available for the scholarly literature in the humanities and social sciences, and for newspapers and other periodicals. Ask a reference librarian for help.

The distinction between primary and secondary sources can blur in several situations. For example, an obituary can be both a primary and a secondary source. Similarly, a history written at the time of the subject of study can be a primary as well as a secondary source. A survey of several volumes of a journal counting the frequency of articles on a certain topic, will turn a primary source into a secondary source; or vice versa, as the numerical results raise new questions. Analysis of what other historians have said about a topic transforms secondary sources into primary sources, as part of the fascinating enterprise of historiography. Historiography examines trends, problems, methods, gaps, and interpretive styles. It can help to orient confused enthusiasts (see the suggestions below).

Method and Interpretation

> For figures in the past, including other historians, the most important question is this: How did writers come to know what (they thought) they knew? In other words, how did they justify their beliefs?
>
> Mirko Grmek, physician and historian

Analysis of the sources reveals the evidence, or 'argument,' to support the answer to your question. Historical methods are the direct cognate of methods in scientific experiments. Reading may be its basis, but this work also entails selection, interpretation, and manipulation – actions strongly influenced by current standards of historical practice and by the taste and imagination of the investigator.

In gathering evidence, examination of all relevant primary and secondary sources is ideal. Sometimes, however, an overwhelming abundance of information – for example, in the case of hospital records – can be dealt with only by devising a sampling system. Microcomputers have revolutionized historical research and enhanced the potential of voluminous collections, but this technology demands selection. Decisions to rely on some data and reject others must be made with care, confronting any biases that the historian may introduce.

Secondary sources must be analysed too. Like a review of the literature in scientific writing, this analysis locates your research – questions and answers – in the context defined by predecessors. Being human, historians like to see their work cited – but citation is much more than a placebo to vanity or a homage to reputation. It distinguishes good history from bad. Here's how it works:

Good historical product is not only information about the past; it situates data and ideas within the domain described by predecessors. It may support existing ideas with new data, or, even better, it may introduce original ideas to explain the past. Exciting new theories about why and how things came to be, or to change, can be applied and tested in future projects. In other words – and still drawing parallels to science – a thorough history project may conclude with questions to guide future research.

The political and philosophical biases of an investigator enter into the interpretation of data, just as they enter into framing the research question. Marxists, capitalists, socialists, feminists, chauvinists, racists, creationists, scientists, Baptists, atheists, deconstructionists, midwives, nurses, physicians, surgeons, and patients will find radically different explanations to account for the same past (see for example, Chapter 11). The laudable, positivistic aim of controlling all subjective variables, which dominates laboratory work, is simply not attainable in history, nor may it be in science. Unlike scientists, however, historians admit it – although, for a short time earlier in the twentieth century, they too strove for elusive objectivity. Instead, historians deal with interpretive bias by recognizing it and by bolstering their arguments with convincing evidence comprised of a swathe of sources chosen by complete and/or systematic sampling in a openly reproducible fashion. An eclectic array of evidence, selected simply because it tends to support an investigator's hypothesis, does not inspire confidence. A project that ignores mainstream historical thought may be entertaining, stimulating, plausible, and well written, but it is not history; it is journalism or editorializing. These principles are reflected in the writing process.

Writing It Up

> Acknowledge your biases, but do not judge the past by the standards of the present.

Even if publication is not your goal, recording your findings in a summary or bibliography is a good idea. Names and dates are easily forgotten or confused; sources are tricky to recall; and ideas – even brilliant ones – prove evanescent. Retracing one's steps in historical research should be unnecessary, but all too often historians come to check their references and find holes or mistakes. A passage, which seemed trivial on first reading, can suddenly loom crucially large after further research sparks a related idea. Finding it again can be daunting. Even if your work was only for an introduction to case rounds, keep your notes, overheads, and slides; you have become an expert, but you are no good without your evidence.

For health-care professionals, writing history is inhibiting. Like scientific reporting, however, the best composition is not a solid, seamless block of narrative – it needs a structure. The steps included on these pages outline the process I generally use, its sequence, and the reasons for it. Many other procedures exist, but starting at the beginning and writing to the end is perhaps the least popular approach.

Steps for Writing History

1 Start in the middle with the results of your research, i.e., the evidence and argument, a description of primary sources, method, and interpretation.

2 Next, draft the conclusion. With the argument set down in step 1, conclusions (hopefully) become obvious. The conclusion contains the answer to the question used to guide the work.

3 Next, write the introduction. In it, review the secondary literature and present the final version of your question. In other words, (re)compose your question *after* you have decided on its answer. Sometimes, the most intriguing version of the question will not have been discovered until after the research is done and the answer (conclusion) found.

4 You may then return to the conclusion, modifying it with commentary on how your question and your findings differ from those of your secondary-source predecessors. Historians are often excited by the unanticipated discovery that their research on a tiny topic challenges existing ideas about the past on a much broader scale. Another historiographic 'Eureka!' is possible here too.

5 Leave traceable references for everything you write.

Publication of historical research, just like that of scientific research, demands originality. A rehash of other work is not usually very interesting. Again as in science, there is vast scope for originality in topics, questions, sources, methods, analysis, and conclusions. New topics are constantly being discovered. For example, the rise of feminism brought women practitioners and patients to the fore; shifts in political views revealed gaps in knowledge about alternative medicines and the experience of patients. Even well-studied topics merit re-examination in the light of new sources, histories, methods, theories, and questions. Because questions about the past emerge from the present, it is often said that all history needs to be rewritten in each generation.

Historical writing is distinguished from scientific writing by the relative permissibility of the first person and the active voice. By convention, scientific reports use the passive voice and the third person to reflect the positivistic ideals of experimentation: 'The blood was let, then it was boiled.' In clinical reports, patients become 'cases' who do not take pills but are passively 'treated.' Rarely, and usually only in the conclusion, does the first person 'I' or 'we' appear.

Here, history is different from science. Modesty and style may dictate sparing use of the first person and the active voice, but their relative acceptability reminds authors of their own creative role at each step of the project. This acknowledged subjectivity is the open recognition that history is not limited to information about the past: history is also made up of the writing that expresses it, thereby marking it as a humanities discipline akin to art, music, and literature.

Pitfalls of Crossing Boundaries

The meetings of the national and international societies for the history of medicine are sometimes dominated by two artificial solitudes: doctors (generally older and often male) congregating in one room, historians (generally younger and more often female), in another. Sometimes plenary sessions will force one group to listen to the other, and much mutual grumbling will follow. Editorials proclaim who should be doing history and how. This particular dichotomy – a woeful intellectual apartheid – is not the only controversy in a fractious field, but it is perhaps the most counterproductive. It derives, I believe, from intolerance and a failure to communicate. If I could bequeath one contribution to my discipline, I would chose to heal this rift. Neither group functions well without the other.

Doctors complain that historians are boring, abstract, divorced from clinical reality, absorbed with minutiae, and too frequently hostile to the medical profession. They know that medicine is not perfect, but they respect it, and like generations of their predecessors, they strive to do no harm. They resent history being used for political purposes; for them, history is a collection of 'facts' or 'truths.' They do not salivate over effete references to obscure historians. At the mention of Foucault – or, worse, his cognate adjective, Foucauldian – their eyes glaze over.

Historians are not boring to each other; theory turns them on. They celebrate the creativity of humanities writing, thinking, and speaking. They love convincing arguments and imaginative yet well-reasoned interpretations anchored in detailed examinations of sources, inevitably constrained by time and space. For them, 'facts' do not exist and 'truth' is relative. They are suspicious of a medical preoccupation with what has survived, misinterpreting it either as unwillingness to face up to past mistakes or as a desire to glorify present practice. Trained through and by 'the word,' historians are baffled by doctors' love of images, which they find distracting, especially when the 'pictures' are made up entirely of words. For them, images trivialize communication, turning history into entertainment, a slide show, a travelogue. And if historians do not mention Foucault, some clever listener, reader, or editor will punish them by archly pointing out the omission. The trick is to refer to important theorists first – nod in the direction of common ground – and carry on. Some historians dislike the medical profession – a few may even be motivated by hatred for it – but editors try to assess quality by evidence and argument, not by opinion.

Historians complain that doctors who attempt history are bumbling amateurs or devout antiquarians, dabbling in a professional discipline that they neither respect nor understand. They invoke an obvious analogy – that retired historians do not take up brain surgery. How dare these rich interlopers think that age and experience alone can turn them into historians?

On either side of this useless debate, the criticisms are both valid and unjust. Beyond jealousy and intolerance, there is a happy mean. From practitioners, historians could learn how to challenge their assumptions and communicate their findings. Here, however, I will concentrate on the problems of health-care providers who want to write history. How do you convince an anonymous, sceptical, academic historian that your work is worth publishing?

Common Problems and How to Avoid Them

With pressures stemming from the 'publish or perish' mentality, editors of quality medical journals turn increasingly to professional historians for advice on submissions. Rejection letters can be baffling as well as disappointing. The criticisms cite 'problems' that appear to be inconsequential or mysterious to clinicians. Yet these faults are rarely insurmountable. To overcome them, the first step is to understand them. The second step, accepting them, is often more difficult, but it helps to set aside the readers' reports for a few weeks before responding. Whether or not you agree with the comments, it is foolish to ignore them. If you hope to carry on with this editor (or another), you are obliged to reframe your work in a manner that addresses the criticisms with respect. The most common faults of doctor-written history are summarized below.

1 Failure to ask a question. An assemblage of names, dates, and events set out in chronological, thick description is not history. The editor will wonder, 'Why should I or the readers care?' Enthusiastic historians who have done their research well should have no difficulty supplying a question, but they must remember to write it. Sometimes, a statement of why you yourself are interested in the topic now, or of why others ought to share that interest, is sufficient to remedy this problem. More attractive questions will feature the originality of your work.

2 Failure to use primary sources or to reveal the method used to exploit them – a serious flaw in much of the history once published in medical journals. One variation of this ubiquitous problem is the exclusive use of translations, something many of us are obliged to do when it comes to using ancient, medieval, or Asian sources. It may be unavoidable, but it should be acknowledged with humility. Translations inevitably contain interpretations.

3 Failure to contextualize a subject in time or place. Research that ignores social factors is often called 'internalist.' The topic is examined from within – inside the boundaries of medical knowledge – a process that is inappropriately equated with history of ideas (intellectual history). As a result 'external' issues, which may be of equal importance, are overlooked, leading the author into anachronistic assumptions. The reverse criticism, 'externalist,' could be applied to some social history writing, although critical doctors do not resort to that word. Instead, they deride it as 'medical history without the medicine.' Just as doctors and historians

need each other, historical accounts either of an idea or of a social phenomenon are incomplete without the context provided by the other.

4 Failure to cite relevant secondary literature. This failing has two vast dimensions. The first relates to the nature of history; situating the work within the body of ideas defined by fellow historical writers is an important part of the process. The second is common sense; the reader who is invited to assess your work will most likely be a person who has already published on the same topic or a related one. How would you react if you were asked to evaluate an essay by some young upstart (or old codger) who proposed to publish in your area of expertise without having read your brilliant book?

5. Overreliance on secondary literature. Why should any article be printed if it merely rehashes what has already been published elsewhere? Explicitly state the originality of your work. Be honest. If it is not original, why do you think it deserves to be published? It may be difficult, though not impossible, to justify its publication. For example, perhaps you are the first to bring two bodies of secondary literature together; or maybe you can enhance your research by going back to primary sources to test the claims of the secondary sources that you used. Sometimes such an exercise may surprise you by showing errors made by the other historians on whom you relied. It may also provide you with a new question. Do not allow yourself to perpetuate the mistakes of others. Expert readers will notice and trace the genealogy of your research to a certain second-rate history rather than to a credible primary source.

6 Presentism and whiggism (see below).

Presentism and Whiggism

We are not obliged to forget what we know, if we use it with care.

Presentism and whiggism are serious flaws from a historical perspective – they could even be called sins or crimes. Presentism is the tendency to judge the past by the standards of the present. It is unfair and anachronistic to blame predecessors for not saying, seeing, or knowing what could not yet be said, seen, or known. It is better history (and more interesting) to understand why they saw things as they did. 'Whiggism,' a term directly related to the progressive political philosophy of the British Liberal Party, is similar; it portrays the past as a series of events progressing to a better present. The assumption is that things change by improving and that progress has brought us to where we are now.

Historians are wary of 'progress.' The very word sets off mental alarms and shrieking whistles. Are things really getting better? Many technologies and treatments have been touted as miracle cures only to be rejected because of unforeseen side effects. The most ingenious discovery may have negative ecological considerations when the passage of centuries is taken into account. Not only is it premature to judge our own practices, but it is simplistic to reduce the past to a mere preparation for the future (a.k.a. our own glorious present). For postmodern scholars, progress, like facts, may no longer exist. Progress, in the sense of desirable improvement, is certainly problematic when those doing the labelling are also its proponents. We can be curious about the present without believing in its immutable superiority.

What to do? Never use the word 'progress.' If you feel an urge to do so, ask yourself why you think it is necessary and what you might really be avoiding. Take a deep breath, and if that doesn't work, take a Valium.

For health-care professionals, presentism and whiggism are the most difficult problems to avoid, since our questions emerge from a present anchored in practice. We cannot suppress our awareness of current medicine, and we lapse into 'medicalese' as a vehicle for our ideas. Pretending that we do not know what we do know is dishonest posturing. To that extent, Marxists, feminists, deconstructionists, and a host of other theoreticians also use questions, interpretations, and language that emerge from their present. Indeed, their works are presentist too. But somehow they manage to avoid the charge. I think the key is language. Medical verbiage should be kept to a minimum. For nonpractitioners, it is exclusionary jargon, a red flag; and even for practitioners, it can mask a superficial understanding of the past.

An Example: Hypothetical Histories of Bloodletting

All authors have carefully researched how and when bleeding was done when it worked, failed, or appeared to work in situations that we might now think of disastrous. But individual writers produce different histories.

The presentist history suggests that some applications were more 'rational' than others, since bleeding 'works' or is still used in a few cognate conditions of the present (e.g., polycythemia, hemochromatosis, or heart failure), none of which were diagnosed in the period under study.

The whiggish account of bloodletting is governed by the assumption that less bleeding is better. It extols a noble (but nonexistent) crusade marching into the present, intent on eradicating phlebotomy.

Here's where it gets tricky. A medically trained historian might explain the popularity of bleeding by appealing to neurovascular responses to depletion – a red-faced, hot individual turns pale, cool, and clammy – thus providing immediate positive feedback for the practice. Such use of modern concepts is neither presentist nor whiggish, but it makes some nonmedical reviewers nervous.

Sometimes accusations of presentism are unjust. They are inspired by the ideas we use or the way we write. If you must resort to current medical ideas or terminology, provide a footnote to explain why, and deal directly with the potential criticism of presentism or whiggism. Make it clear that you understand the flaw and explain why you think it does not apply in your case. Show that you know what you are doing.

The Last Word

Have fun. Remember that these ideas are far from infallible. I have a drawer full of unpublished papers. If you know an editor who might like to see them, please let me know.

Suggestions for Further Reading

Barry, Jon. 'Problems and Methods in the History of Medicine.' *English Historical Review* 105 (1990), 482–3

Benison, Saul. 'Oral History: New Technique in Medical Historiography.' *Ohio State Medical Journal* 68 (1972), 770–3

Brandt, A.M. 'Emerging Themes in the History of Medicine.' *Milbank Quarterly* 69 (1991), 199–214

Burnham, John C. 'The Past of the Future of Medicine.' *Bulletin of the History of Medicine* 67 (1993), 1–27

Church, O.M. 'Historiography in Nursing Research.' *Western Journal of Nursing Research* 9 (1987), 275–9

Clarke, Edwin, ed. *Modern Methods in the History of Medicine.* London: Athlone Press, 1971

Connor, J.T.H. 'Bigger than a Bread Box: Medical Buildings as Museum Artifacts.' *Caduceus* 9 (1993), 119–30

Cook, H.J. Correspondence. *Journal of the History of Medicine and Allied Sciences* 45 (1990), 99

Gelfand, Toby. 'The *Annales* and Medical Historiography: *Bilan et perspective.*' In *Problems and Methods in the History of Medicine*, ed. Roy Porter and Andrew Wear, 15–39. London: Croom Helm, 1987

Grmek, Mirko D. 'Introduction.' In *Histoire de la pensée médicale en occident*, ed. Grmek, 1:7–24. 4 vols. Paris: Seuil, 1995

Hannaway, Caroline. 'Historiographical Trends in the History of Medicine: An Editor's Perspective.' In *New Perspectives in the History of Medicine: First National Conference of the Australian Society of the History of Medicine, 1989*, ed. H. Attwood, R. Gillespie and M. Lewis, 75–84. Melbourne: University of Melbourne, 1990

Jarcho, Saul. 'Some Observations and Opinions on the Present State of American Medical Historiography.' *Journal of the History of Medicine and Allied Sciences* 44 (1989), 288–90

– Correspondence. *Journal of the History of Medicine and Allied Sciences* 45 (1990), 99–100

Jordanova, Ludmilla. 'Has the Social History of Medicine Come of Age?' *Historical Journal* 36 (1993), 437–49

Joy, Robert J.T. 'Occupying the Visual Cortex: Using Slides to Teach the History of Medicine.' In *Teaching the History of Medicine at a Medical Center*, ed. J.J. Bylebyl, 103–14. Baltimore and London: Johns Hopkins University Press, 1982

King, C.R. 'The Historiography of Medical History: From Great Men to Archaeology.' *Bulletin of the New York Academy of Medicine* 67 (1991), 405–26

Laudan, Larry. *Progress and Its Problems: Towards a Theory of Scientific Growth.*
   Berkeley: University of Calfornia Press, 1977
Leavitt, Judith. 'Medicine in Context: Review Essay of the History of Medicine.'
   American Historical Review 95 (1990), 1471–84
Ludmerer, Kenneth M. 'Writing the History of Hospitals.' *Bulletin of the History of
   Medicine* 56 (1982), 106–9
Micale, Michael S. 'Paradigm and Ideology in Psychiatric History Writing:
   The Case of Psychoanalysis.' *Journal of Nervous and Mental Disease* 184 (1996),
   146–52
Miller, Genevieve. 'The Fielding H. Garrison Lecture. In Praise of Amateurs:
   Medical History in America before Garrison.' *Bulletin of the History of Medicine*
   47 (1973), 586–615
Nuland, Sherwin B. 'Doctors and Historians.' *Journal of the History of Medicine
   and Allied Sciences* 43 (1988), 137–40
Porter, Roy. 'The Patient's View: Doing Medical History from Below.' *Theory and
   Society* 14 (1985), 175–98
Porter, Roy, and Andrew Wear, eds. *Problems and Methods in the History of Medicine.*
   London: Croom Helm, 1987
Prioreschi, P. 'Physicians, Historians, and the History of Medicine.' *Medical
   Hypotheses* 38 (1992), 97–101
Risse, Guenter B., and John Harley Warner. 'Reconstructing Clinical Activities:
   Patient Records in Medical History.' *Social History of Medicine* 5 (1992),
   183–205
Shortland, Michael. 'Bodies of History: Some Problems and Perspectives.'
   History of Science 24 (1986), 303–26
Teigen, Philip M. 'An Apology for Commemorative History: An Essay Review.'
   Journal of the History of Medicine and Allied Sciences 50 (1995), 79–85
Tomes, Nancy. 'Oral History in the History of Medicine.' *Journal of American
   History* 78 (1991), 607–17
Wilson, Leonard G. 'Medical History without Medicine.' *Journal of the History of
   Medicine and Allied Sciences* 35 (1980), 5–7

On the History and Historiography of Medicine in Canada

Bernier, Jacques. 'La place de l'histoire de la médecine.' *Health and Canadian
   Society/Santé et Société Canadienne* 1 (1993), 19–49
Crowley, Terry, ed. *Clio's Craft: A Primer of Historical Methods.* Toronto: Copp-
   Clark Pitman, 1988
Laver, A.B. 'The Historiography of Psychology in Canada.' *Journal of the History of
   the Behavioral Sciences* 13 (1977), 243–51

Mitchinson, Wendy. 'Medical Historiography in English Canada.' *Health and Canadian Society/Santé et Société Canadienne* 1 (1993), 205–27

Roland, Charles G. *Harold Nathan Segall: Cardiologist and Historian.* Toronto: Hannah Institute and Dundurn Press, 1995

Shortt, S.E.D. 'Antiquarians and Amateurs: Reflections on the Writing of Medical History in Canada.' In *Medicine in Canadian Society: Historical Perspectives,* ed. Shortt, 1–17. Montreal: McGill-Queen's University Press, 1981

Spaulding, W.B. 'How Can University Presses Publish Canadian Medical History?' *Canadian Bulletin of Medical History* 7 (1990), 5–7. See also reactions to this essay in Correspondence, *Canadian Bulletin of Medical History* 7 (1990), 121–30

Teigen, Philip M. *Books, Manuscripts, and the History of Medicine: Essays on the Fiftieth Anniversary of the Osler Library.* New York: Science History Publications, 1982

The Nobel Prize in Physiology or Medicine, 1901–1998

1901	Emil von Behring	serum therapy, diphtheria and tetanus
1902	Ronald Ross	anopheles mosquito and malaria
1903	Niels Finsen	light therapy for lupus
1904	Ivan Pavlov	digestive physiology – conditioned reflex
1905	H.H. Robert Koch	discovery of tubercle bacillus
1906	C. Golgi	neural structure
	S. Ramón y Cajal	"
1907	Charles Laveran	malarial parasite
1908	Paul Ehrlich	immune function – side chain theory
	Elie Metchnikoff	immune function – phagocytosis
1909	E.T. Kocher	thyroid physiology, pathology, and surgery
1910	A. Kossel	biochemistry of cell nucleus; amino acids
1911	A. Gullstrand	dioptrics of the eye
1912	Alexis Carrel	vascular anastomosis and organ grafts
1913	C.R. Richet	anaphylaxis, passive immunity
1914	R. Bárány	vestibular apparatus of ear and equilibrium
1915–18	No award	
1919	Jules Bordet	immune lysis, antibody complement
1920	S.A.S. Krogh	regulation of microcirculation
1921	No award	
1922	O. Meyerhoff	bioenergetics of muscle physiology
	A. Hill	"

1923	Frederick Banting	insulin (shared with C.H. Best)
	J.J.R. Macleod	insulin (shared with J.B. Collip)
1924	Willem Einthoven	electrocardiography
1925	No award	
1926	J.A.G. Fibiger	bacterial cause of cancer
1927	J. Wagner-Jauregg	malaria therapy for syphilis
1928	C.J.H. Nicolle	role of lice in typhus transmission
1929	C. Eijkmann	vitamins in nutrition (thiamine)
	F.G. Hopkins	"
1930	Karl Landsteiner	human blood groups
1931	Otto Warburg	cellular respiration enzymes (cyto-chrome a)
1932	E. Adrian	neurophysiology
	C. Sherrington	"
1933	T.H. Morgan	genetics, chromosomes in heredity
1934	George Minot	liver therapy for pernicious anemia
	William Murphy	"
	George Whipple	hemoglobin metabolism (liver, iron)
1935	Hans Spemann	experimental embryology
1936	H. Dale	acetylcholine
	O. Loewi	"
1937	Albert Szent-Györgyi	vitamin C (metabolism of)
1938	C.J.F. Heymans	aortic and carotid chemoreceptors
1939	Gerhard Domagk	Prontosil (prototype of sulfa drugs)
1940–2	No award	
1943	Henrik Dam	vitamin K discovery
	Edward Doisy	vitamin K structure
1944	J. Erlanger	nerve conduction
	H.S. Gasser	"
1945	Ernst B. Chain	penicillin
	Alexander Fleming	"
	Howard W. Florey	"
1946	H.J. Muller	X-Ray induced gene mutations
1947	C.F. Cori	catalytic conversion of glycogen
	G.T. Cori	"
	B.A. Houssay	pituitary hormones in sugar metabolism
1948	P.H. Müller	DDT as an insecticide
1949	W.R. Hess	brain mapping, neurophysiological methods

	A.A.C. Egas Moniz	frontal leucotomy and cerebral angiography
1950	P.S. Hench	adrenocortical hormones
	E.C. Kendall	"
	T. Reichstein	"
1951	Max Theiler	yellow fever virus and vaccine
1952	S. Waksman	streptomycin
1953	H.A. Krebs	citric acid cycle acetyl-coenzyme A
	F.A. Lipman	"
1954	John F. Enders	culturing of poliomyelitis virus
	Frederick Chapman Robbins	"
	Thomas Huckle Weller	"
1955	Axel H.T. Theorell	oxidation enzymes
1956	A. Cournand	cardiac catheterization, circulatory pathology
	W. Forssmann	"
	D.W. Richards, Jr	"
1957	Daniel Bovet	acetylcholine, epinephrine, histamine
1958	G.W. Beadle	one-gene one-enzyme theory
	E.L. Tatum	"
	J. Lederberg	genetic properties of bacteria
1959	A. Kornberg	DNA and RNA synthesis
	S. Ochoa	"
1960	F. Macfarlane Burnet	immune tolerance
	Peter Medawar	"
1961	G. von Békésy	mechanism of cochlear stimulation
1962	F. Crick	structure of DNA
	J.D. Watson	"
	M.H.F. Wilkins	"
1963	J. C. Eccles	membrane potential of nerves
	A. Hodgkin	"
	A. Huxley	"
1964	K. Bloch	cholesterol and fatty acid metabolism
	F. Lynen	"
1965	F. Jacob	operon theory of genetic control
	A.M. Lwoff	"
	J. L. Monod	"
1966	C.B. Huggins	hormonal treatment of prostate cancer
	F.P. Rous	tumor viruses
1967	R.A. Granit	physiology of retina and vitamin A

	H.K. Hartline	physiology of retina and vitamin A
	G. Wald	"
1968	R.W. Holley	genetic code in protein synthesis (RNA)
	H.G. Khorana	"
	M.W. Nirenberg	"
1969	M. Delbrück	molecular structure of viral genes (phage)
	A.D. Hershey	"
	S.E. Luria	"
1970	J. Axelrod	neurotransmitters, catecholamines
	B. Katz	"
	U. von Euler	"
1971	E. W. Sutherland, Jr	hormone action (cyclic AMP)
1972	G.M. Edelman	chemical structure of antibodies
	R.R. Porter	"
1973	Konrad Lorenz	ethology: animal behaviour
	Nikolaas Tinbergen	"
	Karl von Frisch	ethology: communication in bees
1974	A. Claude	microstructure of the cell
	C.R. de Duvé	"
	G.E. Palade	"
1975	D. Baltimore	tumor viruses and host genetics
	R. Dulbecco	"
	H.M. Temin	"
1976	B.S. Blumberg	Australian Ag, hepatitis B vaccine
	D. Carelton Gajdusek	slow virus infections (kuru)
1977	R.C.L. Guillemin	hypothalamic hormones (brain peptides)
	A.V. Schally	"
	Rosalyn Yalow	hypothalamic hormones (radio-immunoassay)
1978	W. Arber	molecular genetics: host-virus interaction
	D. Nathans	restriction enzymes (DNA cleavage)
	H.O. Smith	"
1979	Allan Cormack	computer axial tomography
	G.N. Hounsfield	"
1980	Baruj Benacerraf	HLA antigens (gene control of)
	Jean Dausset	HLA antigens (recognition of)
	G.D. Snell	"

1981	D.H. Hubel	neurophysiology of vision
	T.N. Wiesel	"
	R.W. Sperry	'split-brain' hemispheric neuro-physiology
1982	S.K. Bergström	prostaglandins
	B.I. Samuelsson	"
	J.R. Vane	"
1983	Barbara McClintock	chromosome crossover, gene transposition
1984	N. Jerne	immune theory: anti-antibody
	G.J.F. Köhler	immune technology: hybridoma
	C. Milstein	"
1985	Michael Stuart Brown	hypercholesterolemia and cell metabolism
	Joseph Leonard Goldstein	"
1986	S. Cohen	cell (epidermal) growth factors
	R. Levi-Montalcini	"
1987	S. Tonegawa	model of antibody production
1988	James W. Black	rational derivatives (histamine-, β-blockers)
	Gertrude B. Elion	rational derivatives (anti-DNA drugs)
	G.H. Hitchings	"
1989	J. Michael Bishop	genetic causes of cancer
	Harold E. Varmus	"
1990	E. Donnell Thomas	bone marrow transplant
	Joseph E. Murray	kidney transplantation
1991	E. Neher	cellular ion channels
	B. Sakmann	"
1992	Edwin Krebs	protein phosphorylation
	Edmond Fisher	"
1993	Philip Sharp	eukaryotic (split) genes
	Richard Roberts	"
1994	Martin Rodbell	G-protein cell signal transmission
	Alfred Gilman	"
1995	Edward B. Lewis	studies on drosophila
	Christianne Nusslein-Vohard	"
	Eric Wieschaus	"
1996	Rolf Zinkernagel	cellular immune recognition
	Peter Doherty	"
1997	Stanley B. Prusiner	prion hypothesis

1998	Robert F. Furchgott	nitric oxide as cardiovascular signal
	Louis J. Ignarro	"
	Ferid Murad	"
1999*	Günter Blobel	protein signals in cells

For profiles on some Nobel laureates, see Tonse N.K. Raju's Series 'Nobel Chronicles' in *Lancet*, 1998–1999.

* To keep up with Nobel prizes, visit the Karolinska Institute website at http://info.ki.se/ or the Nobel Foundation at http://www.nobel.se/.

Resources and Research Tools for the History of Medicine

1 Important Library Catalogues

Bibliotheca Osleriana: A Catalogue of Books Illustrating the History of Medicine and Science ... Montreal: McGill-Queen's University Press, 1969

The British Library General Catalogue. London

Catalogue général des livres imprimés de la Bibliothèque Nationale. Paris

Index Catalogue of the Library of the Surgeon General's Office. Washington: 1st series, 1880–95; 2nd series, 1896–1916; 3rd series, 1918–32, 4th series, 1926–55, fifth series, 1959–61

National Library of Canada (see 'Some Online Resources' below)

The National Union Catalogue. Washington (covers hundreds of U.S. libraries)

Wellcome Institute Library (see 'Some Online Resources' below)

2 Print Tools: Bibliographic Guides to the History of Medicine

(i) General

Bibliography of the History of Medicine. Bethesda, Md.: U.S. Public Health Service. Issued by the National Library of Medicine, 1965–97, annually and cumulated every five years

Connor, J.T.H. *The Artifacts and Technology of the Health Sciences: A Bibliographic Guide to Historical Sources.* London, Ont.: University Hospital Medical Museum Monograph, no. 1, 1987

Corsia, Pietro, and Paul Weindling. *Information Sources in the History of Science and Medicine.* London: Butterworth Scientific, 1983

Craig, Barbara L. 'A Guide to Historical Records in Hospitals in London,

England and Ontario, Canada, c 1800–1950.' [Two parts] *Canadian Bulletin of Medical History / Bulletin canadien d'histoire de la médecine* 8 (1991), 263–388, and 9 (1992), 71–142

Current Work in the History of Medicine: An International Bibliography of Reference

ISIS Current [also Critical] Bibliographies (annual since 1912) and *Isis Cumulative Bibliography: a Bibliography of the History of Science formed from ISIS Critical Bibliographies*; available online from 1975

Kelly, Howard A., and Walter L. Burrage. *Dictionary of American Medical Biography: Lives of Eminent Physicians of the United States and Canada, from the Earliest Times.* New York: Appleton, 1928

Miller, Genevieve. *Bibliography of the History of Medicine of the United States and Canada, 1939–1960.* 2d edn. Baltimore: Johns Hopkins Press, 1964

Morton, L.T. *A Bibliography of Medical – Biomedical Biography.* Brookfield, Vt: Scolar Press, 1989

Morton, L.T., and Jeremy M. Norman. *Morton's Medical Bibliography: An Annotated Check-list of Texts Illustrating the History of Medicine (Garrison and Morton).* 5th edn. Aldershot: Scolar Press, 1991

Norman, Haskell F., and Hope Mayo, eds. *One Hundred Books Famous in Medicine.* New York: Grolier Club, 1995

Pengelly, Eric T., and Daphne M. Pengelly. *A Traveler's Guide to the History of Biology and Medicine.* Davis, Calif.: Trevor Hill Press, 1986

(ii) On Canada

Connor, J.T.H., and Jennifer J. Connor. 'Medical and Related Museums, Historic Sites, and Exhibits in Ontario: An Annotated Guide and Review.' *Canadian Bulletin of Medical History / Bulletin canadien d'histoire de la médecine* 8 (1991), 101–20

Dunn, M. Margaret. *A Directory of Medical Archives in Ontario.* Toronto: Hannah Institute for the History of Medicine, 1983

Goulet, Denis, and André Paradis. *Trois siècles d'histoire médicale au Québec: Chronologie des institutions et des pratiques (1639–1939).* Montréal: VLB Editeur, 1992

Hunter, Isabel, and Shelagh Wotherspoon. *A Bibliography of Health Care in Newfoundland.* St John's: Faculty of Medicine Memorial University, 1986

Mychajlunow, Lorraine, and Sharon Richardson. *Directory of Nursing Archival Resources in Alberta.* Edmonton: University of Alberta Press, 1996

Paradis, André, and Hélène Naubert, with Denis Goulet. *Recension bibliographique: Les maladies infectieuses dans les periodiques médicaux québécois du XIXe siècle (I).* Trois-Rivières: Centre de recherche en études québécoises et Université du Québec à Trois-Rivières, 1988

Roland, Charles G. *Secondary Sources in the History of Canadian Medicine: A Bibliography*. Toronto: Hannah Institute for the History of Medicine, 1984. 2nd edn. J. Bernier and C.G. Roland, eds. Waterloo: Wilfrid Laurier University Press, 1999

Roland, Charles G., and Paul Potter. *An Annotated Bibliography of Canadian Medical Periodicals*. Toronto: Hannah Institute for the History of Medicine, 1979

3 Specific Periods in Western Medicine (See also pp. 9 and 10)

(i) Ancient, Islamic, and Judaic Medicine

Connor, J.T.H. 'An English Language Bibliography of Classical Greek Medicine.' *Canadian Bulletin of Medical History / Bulletin canadien d'histoire de la médecine* 3 (1986), 225–46

Estes, J. Worth. *The Medical Skills of Ancient Egypt*. Canton, Mass.: Science History Publications U.S.A., 1989

Friedenwald, Harry. *Jewish Luminaries in Medical History*. 1946. Reprint, New York Ktav Pub. House, 1967

Kottek, S.S., Leibowitz, J.O., and Richler, B. 'A Hebrew Paraphrase of the Hippocratic Oath.' *Medical History* 22 (1978), 438–45

Maloney, Gilles. *Cinq cents ans de bibliographie hippocratique, 1473–1982*. St-Jean-Crysostome, Quebec: Editions du Sphinx, 1982

Potter, Paul. *A Short Handbook of Hippocratic Medicine*. Quebec: Sphinx, 1988

– 'Some Principles of Hippocratic Nosology.' In *La maladie et les maladies dans la Collection Hippocratique: 6e Colloque international hippocratique, 1987*, ed. Paul Potter, Gilles Maloney, and Jacques Desautels, 237–53. Quebec: Sphinx, 1990

Rosner, Fred. *Medicine in the Bible and the Talmud: Selections from Classical Jewish Sources*. Augm. ed. Hoboken, N.J.: KTAV Pub. House; and New York: Yeshiva University Press, 1995

Savage-Smith, Emilie. 'Gleanings from an Arabist's Workshop: Current Trends in the Study of Islamic Science and Medicine.' *Isis* 79 (1988), 246–66

Scarborough, J. 'Ancient Medicine: Some Recent Books.' *Clio Medica* 16 (1981), 141–49

Sigerist, Henry E. *A History of Medicine*. Vol. 1, *Primitive and Archaic Medicine*. Vol. 2, *Early Greek, Hindu and Persian Medicine*. New York and Oxford: Oxford University Press, 1951

Smith, Wesley D. 'Notes on Ancient Medical Historiography.' *Bulletin of the History of Medicine* 63 (1989), 73–109

Society for Ancient Medicine Newsletters and *Reviews* since 1976 contain bibliographies of recent publications.

(ii) Medieval and Early Modern Medicine

French, Roger, and Andrew Wear, eds. *The Medical Revolution of the Seventeenth Century*. Cambridge: Cambridge University Press, 1989

King, Lester S. *The Road to Medical Enlightenment, 1650–1695*. London: Mac-Donald, 1970

McVaugh, Michael R. *Medicine before the Plague: Practitioners and Their Patients in the Crown of Aragon, 1285–1345*. Cambridge and New York: Cambridge University Press, 1993

McVaugh, Michael R., and Nancy G. Siraisi, eds. *Renaissance Medical Learning: Evolution of a Tradition*. Philadelphia: History of Science Society, *Osiris*, 2nd ser., 6 (1990)

Schatzmiller, Joseph. *Jews, Medicine, and Medieval Society*. Berkeley and Los Angeles: University of California Press, 1994

Siraisi, Nancy G. 'Some Current Trends in the Study of Renaissance Medicine.' *Renaissance Quarterly* 37 (1984), 585–600

– *Medieval and Early Renaissance Medicine: An Introduction to Knowledge and Practice*. Chicago: University of Chicago Press, 1990

Wear, Andrew, R.K. French, and I.M. Lonie, eds. *The Medical Renaissance of the Sixteenth Century*. Cambridge: Cambridge University Press, 1985

(iii) Modern Medicine, from the Eighteenth Century

Bynum, W.F. *Science and the Practice of Medicine in the Nineteenth Century*. Cambridge: Cambridge University Press, 1994

Bynum, W.F., and Roy Porter, eds. *William Hunter and the Eighteenth-Century Medical World*. Cambridge: Cambridge University Press, 1985

Cunningham, Andrew, and Roger French, eds. *The Medical Enlightenment of the Eighteenth Century*. Cambridge: Cambridge University Press, 1990

Fox, Daniel M., Marcia Meldrum, and Ira Rezak, eds. *Nobel Laureates in Physiology or Medicine: A Biographical Dictionary*. New York: Garland Publishing, 1990

King, Lester S. *The Medical World of the Eighteenth Century*. Chicago: University of Chicago Press, 1958

Lessard, Renald. *Health Care in Canada during the Seventeenth and Eighteenth Centuries*. Hull, Quebec: Canadian Museum of Civilization, 1991

Lindemann, Mary. *Health and Healing in Eighteenth-Century Germany*. Baltimore: Johns Hopkins University Press, 1996

Shryock, Richard Harrison. *The Development of Modern Medicine: An Interpretation of the Social and Scientific Factors Involved*. Madison: University of Wisconsin Press, 1974

4 Non-Western and Alternative Medicines and Their Interfaces

(i) Chinese Medicine

Bates, Don, ed. *Knowledge and Scholarly Medical Traditions.* Cambridge: Cambridge University Press, 1995, esp. 175–276

Hoizey, Dominique, and Marie-Joseph Hoizey. *A History of Chinese Medicine.* Trans. Paul Bailey. Vancouver: University of British Columbia Press, 1993 [also in French, Paris: Payot, 1988]

Huard, Pierre, and Ming Wong. *Chinese Medicine.* Trans. Bernard Fielding. New York: McGraw-Hill, 1968

Minden, Karen. *Bamboo Stone: The Evolution of a Chinese Medical Elite.* Toronto: University of Toronto Press, 1994

Unschuld, Paul U. 'The Chinese Reception of Indian Medicine in the First Millennium A.D.' *Bulletin of the History of Medicine* 53 (1979), 329–45

– ed. *Approaches to Traditional Chinese Medical Literature.* Dordrecht, Boston, and London: Kluwer, 1986

Van Alphen, and Anthony Aris, eds. *Oriental Medicine: An Illustrated Guide to the Asian Arts of Healing.* Boston: Shambhala, 1996

Wang, Chi-min, and Wu Lien-Teh. *History of Chinese Medicine: Being a Chronicle of Medical Happenings in China from Ancient Times to the Present Period.* 2d edn. Tientsin, China: Tientsin Press, 1932. Reprinted from Ann Arbor, Mich.: Xerox University Microfilms, 1975

Zimmermann, Francis. 'From Classic Texts to Learned Practice: Methodological Remarks on the Study of Indian Medicine.' *Social Science and Medicine* 12 (1978), 97–106

(ii) Ayurvedic, Hindu, Indian Medicine

Bates, Don, ed. *Knowledge and Scholarly Medical Traditions.* Cambridge: Cambridge University Press, 1995, esp. 277–343

Chattopadhyaya, Debiprasad. *Science and Society in Ancient India.* Amsterdam: B.R. Gruner B.V., 1978

Chowdhury Amiya Kumar Roy, and K. Ray Chawdhury. *Man, Malady, and Medicine: History of Indian Medicine.* Calcutta: Das Gupta, 1988

Filliozat, Jean. *La doctrine classique de la médecine indienne: Ses origines et ses parallèles grecs.* Paris: Ecole française d'extrême orient, 1975

Gupta, K.R.L. *Hindu Anatomy, Physiology, Therapeutics, History of Medicine, and Practice of Physic.* Indian Medical Science Series no. 2. Delhi: Sri Satguru Publications, 1986

– *Madhava Nidana: Ayurvedic System of Pathology.* Indian Medical Science Series no. 7. Delhi: Sri Satguru Publications, 1987

Lambert, Helen. 'The Cultural Logic of Indian Medicine: Prognosis and Etiology in Rajasthani Popular Therapeutics.' *Social Science and Medicine* 34 (1992), 1069–76

Meulenbeld, G. Jan, ed. *Medical Literature from India, Sri Lanka, and Tibet.* Proceedings of the 7th World Sanskrit Conference, Kern Institute, 1987. Leiden and New York: E.J. Brill, 1991

Savnur, H.V. *Ayurvedic Materia Medica: Principles of Pharmacology and Therapeutics.* Delhi: Sri Satguru Publications, 1984

(iii) North American Aboriginal Medicine and Its Interfaces

Coppermine: Consequence of Contact with the Outside. Videofilm, based on research by Walter J. Vanast. Montreal: National Film Board of Canada, 1992

Herrick, James William. 'Powerful Medicinal Plants in Traditional Iroquois Culture.' *New York State Journal of Medicine* 78 (1978), 979–87

Isaacs, Hope L. 'Comparative Perspective on American Indian Medicine Concepts.' *New York State Journal of Medicine* 78 (1978), 824–9

Kunitz, Stephen J. *Disease and Social Diversity: The European Impact on the Health of Non-Europeans.* New York: Oxford University Press, 1994

Macdonald, Elizabeth. 'Indian Medicine in New Brunswick.' *Canadian Medical Association Journal* 80 (1959), 220–4

'Plants and the Indigenous Peoples of North America: Proceedings of Botany 80 Symposium.' *Canadian Journal of Botany* 59 (1981), 2189–325

Vogel, Virgil J. *American Indian Medicine.* Norman: Oklahoma University Press, 1970

Waldram, James B., D. Ann Herring, and T. Kue Young. *Aboriginal Health in Canada: Historical, Cultural, and Epidemiological Perspectives.* Toronto: University of Toronto Press, 1995, esp. 97–121

(iv) African Medicine

Feierman, Steven, and John M. Jantzen, eds. *The Social Basis of Health and Healing in Africa.* Berkeley: University of California Press, 1992

Fontenot, Wonda L. *Secret Doctors: Ethnomedicine of African Americans.* Westport, Conn. : Bergin & Garvey, 1994

Makinde, M. Akin. *African Philosophy, Culture and Traditional Medicine.* Athens, Ohio: Ohio University Center for International Studies, monograph no. 53, 1988

Yoder, Stanely P., ed. *African Health and Healing Systems. Proceedings of a Symposium, 1980.* Los Angeles: University of California at Los Angeles African Studies Center, 1982

(v) Alternative or Complementary Medicine

Bynum, W.F., and Roy Porter, eds. *Medical Fringe and Medical Orthodoxy, 1750–1850.* London: Croom Helm, 1987

Cayleff, Susan E. *Wash and Be Healed: The Water-Cure Movement and Women's Health.* Philadelphia: Temple University Press, 1987

Connor, J.T.H. '"A Sort of Felo de Se": Eclecticism, Related Medical Sects, and Their Decline in Victorian Ontario.' *Bulletin of the History of Medicine* 65 (1991), 503–27

Cooter, Roger, ed. *Studies on Alternative Medicine.* Basingstoke and London: Macmillan, 1988

Fuller, Robert C. *Alternative Medicine and American Religious Life.* New York and Oxford: Oxford University Press, 1989

Gevitz, Norman. *The D.O.'s: Osteopathic Medicine in America.* Baltimore: Johns Hopkins University Press, 1982

– ed. *Other Healers: Unorthodox Medicine in America.* Baltimore and London: Johns Hopkins University Press, 1988

Inglis, Brian. *Fringe Medicine.* London: Faber, 1964

Kaufman, Martin. *Homeopathy in America: The Rise and Fall of a Medical Heresy.* Baltimore: Johns Hopkins University Press, 1971

Martin, Stephen C. '"The Only Truly Scientific Method of Healing": Chiropractic and American Science, 1895–1990.' *Isis* 85 (1994), 206–27

Micozzi, Marc S., ed. *Fundamentals of Complementary and Alternative Medicine.* New York: Churchill Livingstone, 1996

Risse, Guenter B., Ronald L. Numbers, and Judith Walzer Leavitt, eds. *Medicine without Doctors: Home Health Care in American History.* New York: Science History Publications, 1977

5 Some Online Resources for History of Medicine*

American Association for the History of Medicine
  http://www.histmed.org/
Bibliography of Recent Secondary Works in the History of American Medicine and Related Health Fields
  http://www.medlib.iupui.edu/hom/biblio.html
Bulletin of the History of Medicine
  http://calliope.jhu.edu/journals/bhm/
Canada Wide Health and Medical Archives Telephone Information Network
  http://www.fis.utoronto.ca/research/ams/chmain/

---

* Website addresses are subject to change, but good search engines should be able to locate the new site with the name.

Canadian Medical Hall of Fame
    http://collections.ic.gc.ca/medical/
Canadian Museum of Health and Medicine, Toronto
    http://www.cmhm.org/
Directory of the Medical Humanities
    http://endeavor.med.nyu.edu/lit-med/
Great Canadian Scientists
    http://www.science.ca/
Hanna Chair, History of Medicine, Queen's University, Kingston
    http://meds-ss10.meds.queensu.ca/medicine/histm/
Hannah Institute for History of Medicine, Toronto
    http://www.ams-inc.on.ca
HISTLINE (History of Medicine Online) National Library of Medicine
    http://www.nlm.nih.gov/pubs/factsheets/histline.html
History of Health and Medicine Unit, McMaster University, Hamilton
    http://www-fhs.mcmaster.ca/histmed/
History of Science, Technology and Medicine (WWW Virtual Library)
    http://www.asap.unimelb.edu.au/hstm/hstm_ove.html
History of Science Society
    http://depts.washington.edu/hssexec/
Links to Medical Images (New York Academy of Medicine)
    http://www.nyam.org/library/images.html
Literature, Arts, and Medicine Database
    http://endeavor.med.nyu.edu/lit-med/lit-med-db/topview.html
Museum of Health Care for Eastern Ontario
    http://139.15.161.15/newhosp/hosmus.html
National Archives of Canada, Ottawa
    http://www.archives.ca
National Library of Canada, Ottawa
    http://www.nlc-bnc.ca
National Library of Medicine-History of Medicine Division, Bethesda, MD
    http://www.nlm.nih.gov/hmd/hmd.html
Nobel Foundation – Electronic Nobel Museum Project
    http://www.nobel.se/
Online Images from the History of Medicine (National Library of Medicine)
    http://wwwihm.nlm.nih.gov/
Osler Library, McGill University, Montreal
    http://www.health.library.mcgill.ca/osler/welcome.htm
Social Studies of Medicine, McGill University, Montreal
    http://www.mcgill.ca/ssom/
Wellcome Institute Library, London UK
    http://www.ull.ac.uk/ull/his/welhis.html

Educational Objectives of This Book

1: Introduction: Heroes and Villains in the History of Medicine

The overall educational objectives of this book are:
1 to raise awareness of history (and the humanities as a whole) as a research discipline that can enrich our understanding of the medical present
2 to instill a sense of scepticism with regard to the 'dogma' of the rest of the medical curriculum

The objectives of each chapter are given below.

2: The Fabricated Body: History of Anatomy

To understand that

- anatomy has not always been important to medicine
- dissection has been viewed with ambivalence by many societies
- anatomical knowledge was applied first to physiology, then to medicine
- even today, not all diseases can be linked to a physical change

To recognize reasons for

- the relationship between art and anatomy
- the importance and impact of *De humani corporis fabrica* (1543) (The structure of the human body) by Andreas Vesalius

To know that

- to overcome sanctions against dissection medical students and professors resorted to grave-robbing and murder

3: Interrogating Life: History of Physiology

To understand

- that functional explanations of disease vary with culture and time
- the meaning of the terms 'vitalism,' 'mechanism,' 'empiricism,' and 'teleology'
- the reasons for and significance of William Harvey's discovery of the circulation of blood
- how positivism influences modern methods of experimental physiology

To recognize

- the role and limitations of chance in scientific discovery

4: Science of Suffering: History of Pathology

To understand

- how pathology links medicine to science
- the potential distinction between 'disease' as an idea and 'illness' as suffering
- two theories of disease relating to the perceived sufferer: organismic (individual) and non-organismic (population)
- two theories of disease relating to the perceived cause: physiological (disease from within the patient) versus ontological (disease as a separate entity from outside the patient)
- how eighteenth-century nosologists thought of diseases as constellations of symptoms
- that anatomy was not useful to pathology until diseases had been linked to organic change
- the nineteenth-century change in disease concepts: from subjective symptoms described by the patient to objective organic changes detected by the doctor
- the advent and impact of germ theory (Pasteur, Lister, Koch)
- the meaning of 'social construction' of disease
- criticisms of the medical model that react against its reductionism, its lack of subjectivity, and the apparent exclusion of the patient's feelings

5: First Do No harm: History of Pharmacology

To understand

- that most therapies have been discovered by empirical methods

- that the social factors play an important role in perceived need for remedies
- that most therapeutic 'discoveries' have non-scientific precursors
- the impact and problems of 'magic bullets' (vitamins, hormones, and antibiotics)

6: On Being a Doctor: History of Health-Care Delivery

To understand that

- the history of being a doctor is the story of a contract between doctor and patient
- power, authority, and self-governance are privileges given to doctors in exchange for satisfying society's expectations
- expectations have changed from hope for relief to demand for cure
- medical privileges are threatened by past abuses and by present-day scepticism of science and medicine
- an increase in information does not mean an increase in knowledge

7: Plagues and Peoples: Epidemic Diseases in History

To know that

- epidemics have had a major impact on populations and on economic, social, intellectual, and political aspects of life
- panic and breakdown of social order typify human reactions to epidemic disease
- smallpox was the first human disease to be eradicated by medical methods
- incidence of infectious disease can be related to changes in wealth, hygiene, and nutrition
- 'new' diseases are rarely as new as they first seem to be
- public health measures are the product and legacy of prior epidemics
- legislated controls are influenced by current notions of disease transmission and can incorporate social prejudice
- public health measures have not always been effective; in some instances, they have been detrimental
- knowledge of a microbial cause is not essential for the prevention of infectious disease

To understand

- the meaning of 'social construction' of disease (also discussed in chapter 4)

- the role of germ theory and antibiotics in control of epidemics
- the implications of the term 'innocent victim'

8: Why is Blood Special? Changing Concepts of a Vital Humour

To understand that

- blood has always been awarded special status in anthropological, social, mystical, and intellectual terms
- blood has always related to theories of disease (e.g., the Greek theory of humours; modern theories of immunity and tissue typing)
- transfusion was promoted in response to wartime needs
- red cells were linked to oxygen and to respiration through hemoglobin
- the hemophilia of the European royal families may have had an impact on the political history of the West
- the identification of clotting-factor deficiencies depended on simple mixing studies

To know that

- mismatch, clotting, and infection have been (and continue to be) the main dangers of transfusion
- work on hematological problems has been awarded a disproportionately large number of Nobel Prizes

9: Technology and Disease: The Stethoscope and Physical Diagnosis

To know that

- technological inventions, such as Laennec's invention of the stethoscope, depend on
  1 changing concepts (e.g., anatomical disease)
  2 prior technology (e.g., percussion)
  3 social factors (e.g., the French Revolution)
- Laennec's discovery also depended on his knowledge of anatomy, pathology, and clinical medicine, and on his personal skills as an observer and a musician
- Laennec identified most breath sounds recognized today, but his interpretation of the heart sounds was different
- the use of auscultation and X-Rays spread quickly
- technology has been intended to introduce diagnostic acumen and objectivity

- technology tends to distance the patient from the doctor

To understand how

- new technologies emerge from changes in disease concepts
- established technologies can alter disease concepts by creating new possibilities for the definition of disease

10: Work of the Hand: History of Surgery

To know that

- surgical practices in the care of trauma can be traced to prehistory
- some surgical techniques have been developed to deal with the trauma of war
- trephination and circumcision are elective procedures of great antiquity
- some ancient and folk recipes for wound dressing are beneficial
- early methods of healing conceived of a need for 'laudable' pus and burning oil, and Paré's accidental discovery altered that perception
- pain and infection were major obstacles to the development of surgical techniques
- anesthesia was promoted by dentists before it was adopted by surgeons
- anesthesia was adopted after a long prehistory in the late 1840s
- two decades after anesthesia, Lister contributed to the development of surgical antisepsis and related it to germ theory
- the advent of antisepsis and anesthesia brought a period of tremendous surgical innovation
- surgical practices are modified by economic and epidemiological factors

11: Women's Medicine and Medicine's Women: A History of Obstetrics and Gynecology

To understand

- that history is about the present as well as the past
- that the past may have a variety of interpretations
- the reasons for the introduction of midwifery in Canada

To know that

- for most of history, birthing was the domain of non-medical women

- birthing women can die of bleeding and infection
- obstetrical forceps may have been used in antiquity, but their use was kept secret by the Chamberlen family
- Ambroise Paré's description of podalic version was intended to save both mother and child
- eighteenth-century atlases contributed to an understanding of the normal anatomy and function of the pregnant uterus
- doctors could transmit childbed fever to birthing mothers via instruments, but acceptance of this notion was slow
- the use of anesthesia in birthing was controversial
- birth-control methods were (and in some situations still are) controversial
- modern reproductive technology raises many questions.
- women were initially allowed to enter the medical profession with the expectation that they would care for other women

12: Wrestling with Demons: History of Psychiatry

To know that

- ancient words for diseases of the psyche, such as melancholia, hysteria, and mania, still have currency in our time
- understanding mental disturbances often relies on a conceptual separation of mind and body
- lunatic asylums resembled prisons
- concepts of madness have incorporated prejudicial notions of race, gender, culture, morality, and class
- psychiatric patients have been blamed for their condition
- the introduction of humane measures to care for the insane was a conscious project of the late eighteenth and early nineteenth centuries
- Charcot's studies of hysteria are now considered to have been problematic
- many attempts have been made to link disorders in thought and behaviour to physical change
- physical treatments for mental disorders have been and are used with benefit (e.g., ECT, phenothiazines, lithium)
- some physical treatments for mental disorders are now considered to be ineffective and unethical (e.g., ECT, ovariotomy, insulin shock, lobotomy)
- 'decarceration' movements are the product of medical discoveries, financial concerns, and changes in social attitudes
- the classification of mental diseases is dependent on an analysis of symptoms felt by the patient or behaviours observed by others

To understand

- the pervasive impact of Freud's theories of the unconscious
- the origins and continued impetus of antipsychiatry movements

13: No Baby, No Nation: History of Pediatrics

To understand that

- the history of pediatric medicine is intimately related to social attitudes toward childhood and children
- the eighteenth-century awareness of child mortality fostered a rising interest in disease prevention and recognition of the social determinants of health
- medical pediatrics was shaped by specific definition of childhood diseases; surgical procedures for congenital abnormalities; and discoveries in hormones, vitamins, and genetics

To know

- the factors that have helped and hindered the decline in child mortality in the twentieth century in developed countries and elsewhere

14: A Many-Faceted Gem: Decline and Rebirth of Family Medicine

To understand

- the contexts of 'general practice' in the nineteenth century
- how family medicine can be seen as a new discipline and how to recognize forces that led to its development
- the challenge of research in academic family medicine
- the influence of family medicine on health-care delivery and on training, certification, and continuing education in other fields

15: Sleuthing and Science: How to Research a Question in Medical History

To understand

- some conceptual and methodological issues in medicohistorical research and writing
- some common pitfalls in medicohistorical research and writing and how to avoid them

Index